Follow The What ? -- An Introduction

By

Anab Whitehouse

Published 2023

Published by One Draft Publications in Conjunction with Bilquees Press

Although the practice of allopathic medicine is critically reflected upon throughout the following pages, such a perspective is not intended to serve as a blanket condemnation of all medical practitioners. Like any set of occupations, on the one hand, medicine is populated both with individuals who are competent, ethical, and caring practitioners who are willing to critically question the foundations of science and medicine, and, on the other hand, medicine is also populated with an array of people who are not competent, ethical or caring human beings, and, in addition, seem to exercise a willful blindness to any idea that runs contrary to their ideological biases concerning the nature of medicine. I have had experiences with each of the foregoing kinds of individuals, both while employed in several different hospital settings as well as when I was patient in an array of different medical facilities.

Furthermore, nothing which is said in this book is intended to serve as either medical or legal advice. Throughout this book, my focus is solely on: (a) Exploring some of the conceptual possibilities that seem to be entailed by what it might mean to "follow the science" as well as (b) trying to promote the sort of discussion concerning the nature of medicine and biology that might be constructive rather than ideological.

Whatever might be wrong with what follows is entirely my responsibility. Whatever might be correct with what follows is the result of a Mystery that is above my pay grade.

Table of Contents

Chapter 1: The Abyss Stares Back -- page 9

Chapter 2: Framing Analysis – page 29

Chapter 3: Technocracy as a Theocracy of Control – page 53

Chapter 4: Terrain Theory vs. Germ Theory – page 65

Chapter 5: Enderlein, Rife, and Naessens – page 87

Chapter 6: The Great Influenza – page 129

Chapter 7: Piecing Together the Alleged 1918 Virus - page 165

Chapter 8: Virology -- The Game Is Afoot – page 191

Chapter 9 : Seeking to Save Appearances – page 221

Chapter 10: Debunking Some Modern Research – page 235

Chapter 11: There Is No Immune System – page 251

Chapter 12: De-stabilizing Vectors of Toxicity – page 319

Chapter 13: Epigenetics, An Adaptive Learning System – page 363

Chapter 14: Frequency Following Behavior – page 397

Chapter 15: Energies of Life – page 433

Chapter 16: Fields, Quantum Dynamics, Transducers – page 461

Chapter 17: Interfering with Following the Science – page 531

Chapter 18: Rights, Medical Practice, and Public Health – page 583

Bibliography -- page 641

Chapter 1: The Abyss Stares Back

Frederick Nietzsche is reported to have said: "Whoever fights monsters should see to it that in the process he does not become a monster. And if you gaze long enough into an abyss, the abyss will gaze back at you."

Information, misinformation, disinformation, data, evidence, fact-checking, methodology, and science have all been cast into an abyss of hermeneutics – that is, an opaque, churning whirlpool of seemingly unending arrays of critical reflection on theories concerning the nature of interpretation, along with some of the forces that shape those kinds of inquiries. Now, as any given person struggles to separate truth from falsehood or vice versa, the aforementioned abyss appears to be gazing back at that individual, taunting her, his, or their efforts.

What does it even mean to 'follow the science'? Science understood as what, and by whom, and according to what criteria and what set of metrics, or with what sorts of justification?

The struggle to control the narrative concerning the nature of science has turned some people into monsters. Unfortunately, the general public, as well as even some so-called scientists, are not quite certain of the identity of the ones to whom the term "monster" should be applied since in many ways the notion of science has been turned into nothing more than a pissing contest through which different sides seek to mark their territories and assert their right – presumably through the authority of some kind of natural law -- to control whatever principalities, institutions, and people might fall within the range of their sprays of detoxification.

Moreover, as would be explorers get caught up in the potentially treacherous currents and riptides that are set in motion by competing streams of discharge, individuals who are being tossed about by the tumult of the swirling, unpredictable rapids of controversy that have ensued, many of those individuals are being induced to follow a dynamic of unknown provenance and, as a result, run the risk of becoming monsters themselves should they end up being swept along by a current that, initially seemed safe and civilized, only to become toxic within a very short period of time.

Some years ago, I used to watch a television program called "House". For those who are unfamiliar with the show, the general plot of the series concerned the exploits of an unorthodox medical doctor (more on this shortly) who put together a team of talented consultants who sought to diagnose, and, then, to treat certain difficult cases that came before them at the hospital which employed them. Almost invariably, the cases with which the diagnostic team dealt took a number of twists and turns over the course of the hour program (minus time for advertisements), and, consequently, the assembled team of physicians were required to make a series of diagnoses based on what they understood of the patient's condition at various points in time, only to have to change the character of their diagnosis, and accompanying treatment, to something else based on the outcomes of whatever tests were run subsequently or based on the patient's problematic response to whatever treatment, following a given diagnosis, was being administered.

Although the leader of the aforementioned medical team was scripted as a genius when it came to diagnosing medical problems, and, in addition, the other individuals on the team were portrayed as being more than competent in their own right, dramatic tension was built into the show because the main character – Dr. House – was something of a psychopathic or narcissistic, drug-abusing, Machiavellian individual who wasn't always right and who, at times, placed his patients, his colleagues, and the hospital at risk due to his self-absorbed ways of going about his job. Most of the time, Dr. House's method was vindicated, and the patient would be cured of whatever mysterious, rare malady might have descended upon the hapless individual, but there were times that patients were put through medical hell because of mistakes that were made by different members of the team, including Dr. House, and, on a few occasions, patients died, or the quality of their lives was ruined in some fashion, as a result of those mistakes.

There was an on-going source of dramatic tension embedded in the show due to the differences of medical opinion that would emerge between Dr. House, the leader of the team, and the other members of his consulting group. Sometimes, Dr. House listened to and accepted the advice offered by his colleagues, while on other occasions, no matter what his colleagues might have been concerned about in relation to the medical treatment for a given patient, Dr. House would simply overrule them and instruct his underlings to carry out his instructions irrespective of their feelings and worries, and the latter individuals would feel compelled to comply with the indicated course of treatment or be confronted with the risk of losing their jobs or positions. Most of the time, those doctors were not willing to run such risks and, consequently, they would cow tow to the edicts of the one with power over their lives as well as over the lives of the patients they treated.

From time to time, the foregoing sorts of problems were exacerbated further because of the perspective of people higher up in the hospital hierarchy who were concerned about matters such as liability and/or public image in conjunction with whatever mistakes might be being made – or could be made -- by the diagnostic team at issue. Consequently, another source of tension would be created within the television series when hospital administrators, some of whom were medical doctors themselves, took issue with Dr. House's maverick, medical inclinations and wanted to place constraints on some of those adventures, while, simultaneously, Dr. House would seek to do an end around such constraints in various duplicitous ways.

Oftentimes, Dr. House proved to be successful with his way of going about medicine – that is, after some trial and error on the part of the medical team, the patients either would become sufficiently improved that they would be discharged from the hospital or those patients would be pronounced to have been cured in some fashion despite whatever 'unethical' decisions might have had to be made along the way by the "good" doctor in order to achieve such an outcome. On some occasions, the consultants with whom Dr, House worked were able to prevail upon the good doctor and, eventually, able to convince him – frequently via a reluctant concession on his part – to move in some other direction of diagnosis or treatment than the one to which Dr. House initially had been committed. Alternatively, sometimes, the members of the hospital administration would step in and countermand whatever Dr. House had set in motion, and although the patient might have benefitted on some of those occasions, in other instances, the administrators proved to be wrong in their medical decision to intervene, and they had to be bailed out by Dr. House and/or the rest of his consulting team.

I've worked in several hospitals (as an orderly), and I have gone through a few medical procedures of my own (some of them quite serious), and, furthermore, I have a few friends who have served as doctors within different hospital settings. All three of the foregoing sources of experiential information provide data which indicate that egos often (but not always) tend to be on prominent display in such facilities among various facets of the medical staff (usually in the form of doctors).

The main character in the "House" television series might be a fictional invention, but the truth, unfortunately, seems to be that: (1) there are all too many House-like doctors who are caught up in their own little narcissistic bubble and, consequently, appear to believe they are entitled to go about their activities as if they were God, and (2) despite whatever favorable pronouncements medical doctors (whether House-like or not) might like to offer concerning the nature of their work, medicine is inherently experimental.

A diagnosis is experimental in nature because doctors who make such diagnoses, don't necessarily know whether he, she or they are correct, or not, with respect to such judgment calls, or whether an initial diagnosis will be able to stand the test of time or have to be changed because of what transpires over time with a given patient Furthermore, treatments are also highly experimental because different people react differently to the same sort of treatment, and doctors have no way of knowing whether a given course of treatment will have to be altered as a medical case unfolds over time because events take place which indicate that either a given diagnosis and/or course of treatment is problematic if not just plain wrong.

Based on different studies, various estimates have been given, that indicate how in the United States alone many people die at the hands of doctors using what are considered to be fully approved courses of diagnosis and treatment – known as a 'standard of care'. These estimates run anywhere from 250,000 people per year to more than 700,000 people per year.

Such fatalities are referred to as deaths due to iatrogenic causes – that is, these sorts of tragic outcomes are due to doctors practicing medicine in an officially approved fashion, and, yet, nonetheless, the patients who die are not dying from whatever malady with which they might have been afflicted. Instead, the patients died because of unintended or unexpected problems that arose involving either the form of the diagnosis and/or treatment protocols that were administered to the patient despite being in compliance with existing standards of care.

Over a ten year period, the foregoing statistics indicate that in the United States anywhere from 2.5 to 7 million people will have died as a result of the kind of care they received from the medical establishment. In short, they died, because they came out on the wrong end of the experimental activity of the medical establishment.

Stated in another way, notwithstanding the alleged best efforts of the medical industry, more Americans have died at the hands of the medical establishment than have died in any war in which Americans have ever been involved, including the Civil War (about 600,000 deaths). In fact, if one were to put aside the number of civilian fatalities that occurred in World Wars I and II, more American civilians have died at the hands of the medical establishment using standard methods of care during each and every decade for the past 100 years than have died in the same set of ten-year time periods in conjunction with wars that have taken place anywhere in the world.

In other words, if one accepts the generally stated figure of some nine million civilians who were exterminated in the concentration camps run by the Nazi government during World War II, then, for many decades now, American civilians have undergone a holocaust-like tragedy every ten years, and, yet, almost nothing is said or constructively done about the situation.

Instead, under the provisions of such legislation as the 2004-5 PREP Act, the medical industry has been freed from any liability for causing the death of civilians during times when the declarations of alleged pandemics have led to the implementation of emergency authorization protocols as was done in 2020 in America and which have continued to be extended into at least the early part of 2023 by the Biden administration. People have been locked up and tortured in Abu Ghraib, Guantanamo, and Bagram Air Force Base in Afghanistan -- not to mention a lot of CIA black sites -- for being caught up in a cloud of suspicion for, possibly, having done involved in something far less lethal, for far less a period of time.

Anyone who supposes that medicine is not an experimental enterprise does not understand medicine. Every diagnosis is done on the basis of available information which is always limited in nature, and, therefore, there is no way to avoid the uncertainties, unknowns, and therefore, opportunities for mistakes which surround such a diagnosis, and, as well, every proposed treatment is ensconced in a risk-benefit analysis that often is based on incomplete information concerning how any given patient will fit, or not, into the safety and effectiveness profile of a given form of treatment.

The chapters which follow the present chapter will explore different aspects of medical science, as well as some dimensions of the biological sciences that tend to underlie and inform medicine. Therefore, a pertinent question which could be asked at this point is the following one: What are my qualifications for undertaking such a daunting task?

Aside from, possibly, having slept at a Best Western Motel previously, and aside from having worked in several hospitals, as well as having had several friends who worked in the medical industry for decades and with whom I have had a number of extended discussions concerning that industry, and aside from having been processed by medical institutions on a number of occasions in several different countries, and aside from my exposure to such fictional creations as, among others:: House, Dr. Kildare, Ben Casey M.D., The Terminal Man, and Coma, there are some additional considerations which might be added to the foregoing résumé. For example, I had something of a front row seat with respect to the manner in which my mother was often treated by the medical system.

She had a bevy of medical issues, including a severe form of rheumatoid arthritis which afflicted her, in one way or another, for most of her adult life and, finally, forced her into a wheelchair during the latter part of her 83-odd years of Earthly existence. She went to a number of different specialists as well as interacted with various General Practitioners or Family Physicians, and while she was laudatory of a few of them, she also had running battles with a number of them – battles about which she wrote to me and in relation to which she would engage in discussions when we talked on the phone.

My mother was an intelligent, talented woman who was a feminist well ahead of that movement's sort of public inception during the late 1950s and early 1960s. She read, investigated, and reflected on all manner of topics, and she was often the bane of the existence of individuals who served as editorial page editors for this or that newspaper, or individuals who were involved with government, in some manner, whether on a local, state, or federal level.

She was the one who had done some reading somewhere which indicated that Harvard might be interested in an individual like me, and, as a result, suggested that I should fill out an application to the school. Sorry, Harvard, but I didn't even know of your existence until my mother mentioned you to me, but, nonetheless, I did as my mother suggested, and the rest is, as some say, history – in other words, much to my surprise, as well as the mystification of many others, I was accepted by Harvard for the Class of 1966.

But, I digress. The running battles that she had with some of her medical (dare I say it) "care-givers" tended to be about issues involving drug safety, drug cross-reactions, and informed consent. She often brought a copy of the *Physician's Desk Reference* concerning drugs with her to doctor appointments and sought to question her doctors about some of her concerns with respect to either the drugs that she was on or drugs which some of her doctors wished to put her on. Moreover, she would back up her questions not only with some of the contraindications that were listed for the aforementioned sorts of drugs, but with information she had gleaned from other medical references as well.

Some of her doctors took her queries in stride and actually would engage her in rational, give-and-take sorts of discussions concerning her questions. Some of her doctors tried to shut her down immediately and resented being questioned about anything that they said or proposed – apparently, feeling that they had the right to experiment on my mother in any manner that they wished -- and some of those doctors were quite brutal in their treatment of her.

My own experience with the medical system (both as an employee and as a patient) tends to lend support to the foregoing bi-polar nature of the medical system. In other words, I have found that while some doctors have been very open, willing to discuss issues and, if possible, allay concerns as well as being actively prepared to address, as best they could, whatever questions might be raised, nonetheless, there were other doctors who were fairly arrogant about such matters and tried to give the impression that they, and they alone, knew the answers to all questions, issues, and problems, and as far as they seemed to be concerned, the patient was there for the doctor's experimental purposes and not for the patient's purposes involving actual matters of well-being.

My extended discussions involving some of my medical friends provide additional evidence that tends to back up the experiences of both my mother and myself with respect to the medical industry. Those friends have tended to concur with the perspective that some dimensions of the medical industry are amenable to engagement with patients about what might be the best way to move forward with a given issue and, in the process, are committed to all the nuances entailed by the idea of informed consent, while other facets of the medical industry appear to believe that it is their right to engage in experimental activities in relation to patients and, as a result, feel they are entitled to impose whatever treatments that they, in their infinite wisdom, deem to be appropriate, and while, for legal purposes, they might permit the patient to say whatever they like, nonetheless, in the end they appear to be prepared to herd those patients toward whatever experimental cul-de-sac fits in with a given doctor's theory of medicine, as long as that theory can be reconciled with the prevailing standard of care concerning such issues so, that the doctor will be able to keep her, his, or their jobs and/or not be sued, or be able to defend themselves in court, for the way in which they have conducted their experimental approach to medicine.

However, as noted previously, irrespective of whether patients are fortunate enough to interact with aspects of the medical system that are genuinely interested in listening to, and working with, the concerns of their patients, or such patients are unfortunate enough to have to deal with members of the medical industry who are not all that interested in the concerns of their patients, the medical system is inherently experimental in nature. Diagnoses are given which might, or might not be correct, and even if correct, might have to be modified as new information arises during the course of treatment, and, as well, there is no such thing as a form of treatment which has a 100% safety and effectiveness profile, and, moreover, because people respond to treatments differently, those treatment protocols often have to be modified, adjusted, or discontinued in favor of other approaches that might have a better chance of addressing whatever health issues are present For all of the foregoing reasons, the art and science of medicine are always experimental in character.

Given the unavoidably experimental nature of the practice of medicine, any member of the medical industry who believes that it is somehow impertinent of the individuals who are to be experimented on to presume that they (i.e., patients or prospective patients) don't have sufficient standing to engage in critical reflections concerning the activities of the medical industry is someone who, perhaps, does not have the right moral or intellectual orientation to engage in such experimentation. Consequently, one of the qualifications that I – or any human being – has for having the right to engage in a rigorous critical exploration concerning the experimental world of medicine is precisely because they either are, or could become, the objects upon whom such experimentation takes place.

Let's take a brief look at some other facets of the qualification issue which might surround my writing the present book. Aside from having an inalienable right to raise questions concerning the medical industry's inherently experimental nature, someone might ask what is there about my experiential background that might qualify me, at least to some degree, to engage in a critically reflective study of various parts of medicine, medical science, and some of the biological sciences that help form the foundations of those medical endeavors?

People who become medical doctors have read textbooks and articles on molecular biology, biochemistry, biophysics, cell physiology, membrane functioning, immunology, virology, mathematics, genetics, evolution, and so on. I've done that as well, and, actually, have done so, on and off, for over five, or more, decades.

People who become medical doctors have watched lectures or talks by experts or engaged in lengthy discussions with various medical personnel that delve into an array of medical and scientific fields. I have done that as well.

People who have become medical doctors have often won National Science Scholarships – or some other kind of award -- to study this or that topic, or they have participated in special science and math programs that have been supported by their local and state governments. I also have been awarded similar sorts of scholarships (mine was to study the theory of semi-conductors) as well as participated, during high school, in advanced programs focusing on science and mathematics.

People who have become medical doctors have done research concerning different facets of science or medicine and have published their results. I also have done that, and, in fact, I have managed to write, in addition to some 33 other kinds of works, ten, or so, books on various aspects of science and medicine, most of which (that is, most of the 45 books that I have written) have been accepted into the collection of books known as Widener Library at Harvard University.

People who have become medical doctors have engaged in clinical settings involving life and death issues. I have done that as well.

My participation in the latter sorts of activities might have been limited to taking and recording: Pulse, temperature, and respiration, along with making beds, talking with patients, changing their bed pans, giving massages, engaging in shift work, interacting with doctors and nurses, along with sterilizing instruments in an autoclave, but I also was involved, peripherally, in situations that entailed emergency as well as life and death events that were taking place in my presence, and I did it for $25 to $30 dollars take-home-pay a week.

Am I a doctor? No, I am not – despite, as indicated previously, my claim of having slept in a Best Western Motel (a claim which might not be true but may have been offered for attempted comic relief).

Nevertheless, I have been exposed to many of the same or similar sorts of textbooks, articles, lectures, ideas, and experiences to which doctors have been exposed. The foregoing activities were not undertaken because I was in a degree program or seeking a career in medicine but because I had an interest in medical and scientific issues and, as a result, I pursued those sorts of matters, along with other issues, in a somewhat methodically chaotic manner.

Were my aforementioned experiences and exposures as intensive or as expansive or as rich as those of individuals who would go on to become doctors? Probably not, but, nonetheless, I feel that based on my education, experience, and research, I have earned a certain standing, amateurish or semi-pro though it might be, which entitles me to critically explore a variety of issues that involve medicine and medical science.

Notwithstanding the aforementioned considerations, based on more than half a century of varied experiences, I also have garnered some degree of insight into the way academic institutions, government institutions, corporations, and media institutions often tend to operate. Those experiences and insights provide the sort of background that helps to shed light on how medicine, among other industries (e.g., academia, media, corporations), often tends to operate as an institutionalized system that is more interested in controlling situations than being controlled, and, in addition, oftentimes, are not always fussy about the nature of the justifications that are used to assert such control or to avoid being regulated in some objective fashion.

Perhaps, a few illustrative examples might provide some context concerning the foregoing indications. For instance, when I was doing doctoral work at the University of Toronto, I was the chairperson for a student group that brought forward considerable evidence indicating that a professor in the university's Department of Middle East and Islamic Studies was guilty of plagiarism with respect to several articles that he had written for a book of which he was the primary editor – a book that was promoted as being able to serve as source material for students and professors alike with respect to not only the Islamic religious tradition, but, as well, in relation to various economic, political, legal, historical, and social considerations associated with that religious tradition.

Part of the evidence which was published by the aforementioned student group – that is, in addition to the actual line-by-line comparative account of the material that had been copied largely verbatim involving several other published works – was the release of information by the student group to which I belonged. This information indicated that we had shared our findings with various professors at different universities in North America.

A number of the professors that we contacted wrote back to us and indicated how they agreed that the evidence provided in conjunction with the University of Toronto professor definitely demonstrated plagiarism. In fact, a professor from a university in New York directed our attention to, yet, another instance of plagiarism that had been committed by the same professor who was featured in our exposé.

Initially, based on the package of material that the student group to which I belonged had put together, several prominent national newspapers in Canada declared that they were very interested in covering the plagiarism issue. One of the papers even indicated that they were interested in gaining exclusive coverage rights to the story.

Unfortunately, at this point, politics and religious bigotry seemed to take over. University of Toronto authorities apparently got in touch with the newspapers and, presumably, informed those companies that the student group in question – The Sufi Study Circle of the University of Toronto -- was a Muslim group and, apparently, the recommendation was pointedly given that the group should be engaged with some degree of circumspection, and, as a result, the papers began to distance themselves from the story. This process of distancing by the media did not take place because of a lack of evidence – as the letters of support we got back from a variety of professors clearly demonstrated and as the initial interest of the newspapers initially indicated -- but, rather, the obstacles to some sort of objective media coverage took place because of other considerations that had nothing to do with the primary issue of plagiarism.

Indeed, the newspaper that had been so keen on covering the story based on the package of information which had been given to the paper initially (a package that provided a considerable number of examples of such plagiarism), and, as a result, expressed interest in having some sort of exclusive coverage, that newspaper disengaged from any further contact with the student group to which I belonged.

The other media outlets which we had contacted concerning the story also ghosted us.

To make a longer story much shorter, the individual who had committed the plagiarism was not held accountable by the University of Toronto. To add insult to injury, the University decided to promote that person and made him – wait for it – the faculty liaison for the administrative body that had oversight over student honor violations at the University involving, among other things, cases of plagiarism.

A number of months later, I read about one of the activities of that University of Toronto administrative body which had been mentioned in the previous paragraph. The body decided to reject, or withdraw acceptance of, the doctoral thesis of a candidate who had been accused of plagiarism, proving, apparently, that what is good for the goose is not necessarily good for the gander.

The Ontario Provincial government took exception to the foregoing sorts of activities involving the student group to which I belonged, and, as well, did not appreciate the activities of another extra-curriculum group to which I belonged, namely, the Canadian Society of Muslims which had written and published a report that was critical of some of the books that were being used in the provincial education system and which contained misinformation and unfounded, derogatory content about Islam and/or the Prophet Muhammad (peace be upon him). One of the avenues of retaliation that was directed against the Sufi Study Circle of the University of Toronto and the Canadian Society of Muslims was go try to get me expelled from the graduate program in which I was enrolled as well as to try to create difficulties for the President of the Canadian Society of Muslims who was tenured professor at the Department of Middle East and Islamic Studies at the University of Toronto.

I knew about the attempt to have me thrown out of the University because the individual who was my thesis advisor at that time confronted me one day concerning the matter. He asked me what in the heck was up with me because he had just been contacted by the Director of the Institute in which I was enrolled as a doctoral candidate and that also was part of the University of Toronto , and the Director had informed my advisor that the Minister of Education for the Province of Ontario had been making inquiries with him as to why

I was still a student at the University of Toronto, apparently suggesting that, maybe, something should be done about the situation.

It seems that the 'something that was to be done' about the situation was to place obstacles in the way of my getting a doctoral degree. For example, my thesis advisor kept jerking me around for years by, among other things, agreeing to meet at a certain time on a particular day, only to cancel out of the meeting at the last minute, and, this tactic was used on a multiplicity of occasions.

In addition, my, then, thesis advisor took exception with my critical reflections concerning certain scholars to whom he was partial. He wanted to know whom I thought I was that I should have the audacity to be critical of certain books that such esteemed individuals had written, and, here I was, foolishly thinking that critical reflection played a crucial role in the process of education, and, as such, education, -- at least, theoretically – presumably involved (to a degree) a process of engaging those ideas by means of a dynamic focused on a critical examination of those sorts of perspectives.

Finally, although I went ahead and wrote a dissertation on the subject that had been agreed upon when my advisor initially assented to be my advisor, he refused to read what I had written. As a result, I ran out of official time and became what is known as a "lapsed status Ph.D. candidate" – that is, someone who is in academic limbo, and, as such, has no right to access any of the facilities or personnel of the university regarding a thesis but who, if the appropriate university authorities were amenable, could apply at some future date in order to seek reinstatement for purposes of having an orals examination of said dissertation.

It took me approximately 17 years to obtain my doctoral degree, but, as Leonard Cohen's line indicates in his song: "Democracy" (comes to the U of T): "... I'm as stubborn as those garbage bags that time cannot decay." Consequently, by the Grace of Allah, the ordeal came to an end. That ordeal was the way that the provincial government and the University of Toronto apparently had selected to use as retaliation for my participation in a student group and an extra-university group which pursued activities that were inimical to the vested interests of a provincial government, an academic institution, and the media.

Consequently, in light of the foregoing 17 years of experience, I do have some degree of experience and insight concerning how institutions such as universities, the media, and the government often collude together to protect their respective interests. This constitutes experiences and insights that I believe are eminently transferable to some of the dynamics that take place in conjunction with medicine and medical science.

By way of an addendum of sorts, I might note that my orals committee consisted of two physicists, two professors with expertise in the philosophy of science, a linguist, a historian, and a professor of adult education. The latter individual remarked during the oral defense that he "... had never encountered a thesis like mine and hoped to never do so again" but, he, along with the six other members of the orals committee, all voted in favor of accepting the dissertation.

I might also add that the dissertation ran some 700 or 800 pages. I was later informed that not all that long following the occasion when my oral defense took place, the University of Toronto passed an edict concerning the maximum length of a dissertation. Conceivably, my thesis might have played a role in helping to inspire or contribute to the University of Toronto's decision to introduce such a rule.

My dissertation – the one that actually got read and accepted -- sought to explore the idea of a field theory concerning the nature of understanding. In order to develop the foregoing possibility, the thesis delved into, among other things, topics such as: Maxwell's theory of electromagnetic energy, special relativity, chaos, quantum mechanics, chronobiology, holographic dynamics, gauge theory, morphogenesis, various facets of mathematics, and hermeneutics. The foregoing list of topics helps to explain, perhaps, why there were several physicists who were members of the oral defense committee, as well as several individuals who had a background in philosophy of science, along with an individual with some expertise in linguistics.

If I were to try to reduce my critically reflective orientation concerning medical science down to a somewhat manageable statement – but one that would need to be fleshed out in a variety of ways (say, in a book like the present one) – I might proceed in the following manner. More specifically, all too many facets of the sorts of medicine that hold sway in the United States (as well as in many other countries) and which, to a large extent, are rooted in what is known as the allopathic approach to health, tend to commit the same sort of error – namely: They are nothing more than narratives held together by assumptions that cannot be justified.

The overlords of the medical industry have the power or capacity to induce a large number of aspiring medical professionals to operate in accordance with such a narrative (through an array of techniques involving indoctrination, propaganda, compulsion, bribery, and/or threats to career). As a result, such "professionals" never seem to rise to the occasion and question – at least, in any official manner – the often fraudulent theories and practices that are imposed on unsuspecting patients, and this state of affairs would seem to reveal more about the abuse of power and cult-like behavior within the medical industry than it discloses anything of probative value with respect to the actual nature of health and disease.

Perhaps, before proceeding further, one might lend a certain amount of concreteness to the allusions which are being made in conjunction with the idea that many aspects of the medical industry are little more than narratives that are held together by assumptions which cannot be justified. For example, the evolutionary narrative tends to be ubiquitous in modern-society and shapes many facets of the understanding, discourse, and practice that frame hermeneutical orientations, governing the institutions which populate that milieu, including medicine.

However, in many, if not most ways, evolutionary theory is little more than a narrative (replete with technical terms) that is tied together by assumptions that cannot necessarily be justified. More specifically, one might claim, with some justification, that DNA/RNA play fundamental, essential roles in evolutionary theory with respect to the process through which life forms are believed to evolve through a series of random mutations to the ribonucleic acids that help make up the aforementioned DNA and RNA molecules such that over millions and billions of years, the cumulative effect of those mutations leads to the emergence of biological systems that are capable of generating the sorts of proteins that, when organized into certain sequences or pathways of dynamics, give expression to anabolic (building up) and catabolic (breaking down) actions that appear to have proven themselves to be able to offer effective ways of adapting to prevailing environmental circumstances, and, thereby, provide some advantage to the possibility of a given species that has developed such pathways to be in a position to leave behind progeny that are capable of continuing on with the evolutionary journey with something of a competitive advantage.

Two of the assumptions that are present in the foregoing description of the evolutionary process are, on the one hand, that there is such a thing as random mutations, and, on the other hand, that when considered collectively or cumulatively then, eventually if given enough time, such mutations will be capable of generating functional metabolic pathways. To begin with, one can never actually prove that any sequence of events is random, but, rather all one can demonstrate is that one has not, yet, discovered any algorithm or set of algorithms (that is, any set of sequentially ordered instructions that is capable of producing various evolutionary events to which one might be alluding).

In addition, one faces an explanatory challenge when trying to account for how so-called random mutations are capable, when considered cumulatively over large spans of time, to be able to produce functional metabolic pathways capable of explaining how life might have made the transition from, say, Chemotrophs (obtain energy by the oxidation of organic or inorganic electron donors in the environment) to phototrophs (obtain energy through the harvesting of photons via, for example, photosynthesis), or might be capable of explaining the advent of Archaea organisms (whether considered as having arisen independently of bacteria or as species that, somehow, have branched off from bacteria) which are different from bacteria in significant ways (e.g., their ability to thrive in extreme environments involving radiation, cold, heat, acid or alkaline conditions that are fatal to most other forms of life).

Or, one could point to the differences between prokaryotic forms of life marked by, among other things, the absence of a nucleus, and eukaryotic forms of life that do have a nucleus and go about the business of life in a way that is markedly different from prokaryotes and wonder what the step-by-step dynamics were that could account for how eukaryotic life forms might have developed from prokaryotic organisms. The endosymbiotic theory of Lynn Margulis which proposes that more complex forms of life – for example, eukaryotes – might have arisen through the symbiotic interaction of different, lesser forms of life – for example prokaryotes – is often mentioned as a way of bridging the differences between prokaryotic and eukaryotic forms of life, but, all of the details are missing in such theories with respect to not only how different prokaryotic forms of life originated in the first place but how those different forms of life came together in a symbiotic manner to establish functional metabolic systems of a eukaryotic nature.

Moreover, there are a whole bevy of unstated, but implicit assumptions in the evolutionary narrative entailed by the challenge of having to account for how five ribonucleic acids (thymine, adenine, guanine and cytosine in DNA and uracil in RNA which replaces the thymine in DNA) have come to stand for, mean, or signify some 20-plus varieties of amino acids which are totally different modalities of molecules (made from peptides and not ribonucleic acids) when the aforementioned ribonucleic acids are put together in sets of three (either in the form of DNA or RNA) and read by an appropriate cellular mechanism ... such as a ribosome. Why should a set of three DNA molecules or a set of three RNA molecules – both of which are different from one another in relation to thymine in DNA and uracil in RNA – be able to stand for one, or another, of some 20-plus amino acids which are quite different from DNA and RNA molecules?

How did this language or code which enables DNA and RNA molecules to be translated into amino acid molecules come about? What was the step-by-step dynamic that established such a translation process?

One might put forth an analogy of sorts that helps indicate how extraordinary the relationship is between sets of three DNA or RNA molecules and one of some 20-plus possible amino acids. More specifically, in a sense that relationship is like saying that if one placed three different kinds of dogs together in a given sequence, they would be capable of being translated into one, or another, species of cat.

I've been reading books and articles on evolutionary theory for more than 40 years. In addition, I have written several books on evolutionary theory.

Nonetheless, I have, yet, to come across anything in the so-called scientific literature that is capable of being able to account, in a plausible manner, for the emergence of such a coding or translation dynamic. One could claim, of course, that the foregoing process is a function of a series of random mutations, but by proceeding in that fashion, not only would one be unable, as indicated previously, to show that such a series is, in fact, random in nature, but making claims that are dependent on a plethora of assumptions, concerning allegedly random events doesn't actually provide any sort of detailed explanation that is not dependent on thousands, millions, if not billions and trillions – if not a googleplex – of assumptions in order to make such an account seem to work,

All one ends up with is a narrative. Moreover, despite the presence of a great deal of technical detail, there really is no science involved … it is just a narrative tied together by assumptions which cannot be justified.

As different chapters in the present book will seek to demonstrate, there are many facets of so-called medical science that are really very like the foregoing example drawn from evolutionary theory. In other words, as the current work will endeavor to show, there are any number of examples that can be introduced which indicate or suggest that some of the fundamental facets of allopathic medicine appear to be little more than narratives which are glued together by and array of assumptions that cannot necessarily be justified, and, as a result, such a reality carries numerous, far-reaching implications for the issue of well being and heath care.

Chapter 2: Framing Analysis

Although I am not a sociologist by trade, nonetheless, I have some degree of familiarity with, and appreciation for, the work of Erving Goffman, a Canadian researcher who was born in 1922 and died in 1982. I especially have been attracted to his notion of "framing analysis" that -- in somewhat altered and piecemeal forms -- appeared in many of his earlier writings such as: *Presentation of Self in Everyday Life* (published in 1959), *Asylums* (released in 1961), *Stigma* (published in 1963), and *Interaction Ritual* (released in 1967), but which did not become more fully delineated until *Framing Analysis* was published in 1974.

While, hopefully, the idea of framing analysis will shortly become a little more concrete and visible, one should note that even though that idea can be applied to the dynamics of social interaction – for example, as a way in which a psychiatrist might evaluate (or frame) the behavior of patients in mental asylums -- nonetheless, Goffman clearly indicates that framing analysis ultimately has to do with a broader process of organizing experience in general. Therefore, framing analysis should not be limited to just the phenomena of social dynamics.

As such, one might describe 'framing analysis' as the process of reflecting on the ways in which we – both individually and collectively – attempt to understand, interpret, create, and critique the dynamic perceptual/conceptual/linguistic/emotional/intentional structures that are used to bring organization to, and confer meaning upon, our experiences as we seek to figure out the nature of our relationship with reality at any given juncture of our experiences – whether considered individually or collectively.

Ideas, concepts, perceptions, assumptions, beliefs, values, emotions, motivations, theories, hypotheses, principles, paradigms, world views, interpretations, and methodologies all give expression to frames of organizing experience that can be used to analyze and critically reflect on the nature of experience. The question that haunts all of the foregoing possibilities is the following: What do such ways of framing experience have to do with coming to grips with, or understanding, what is taking place at any given instance of on-going experience?

Frames of experience can be given to us by others, such as during formal modalities of schooling or through articles that are published via one media outlet or another (e.g., television, the internet, magazines, radio, newspapers). Frames of experience also can be created by us as, for example, when we generate interpretations concerning what we believe might be happening during an on-going experience.

The framing process can be active or passive. In other words, on the one hand, we might passively – that is, do so without objection and, perhaps, not even with conscious consent – accept frames of experience that are imposed on us (such as might be done through various modes of education, indoctrination and propaganda), or which we are induced to adopt through the dynamics of undue influence when power relationships, of one kind or another, are used in unethical ways by individuals for purposes of manipulating someone's behavior ... individuals who might be in the form of parents, neighbors, peers, teachers, doctors, scientists, religious figures, corporations, employers, and/or government agents. On the other hand, frames of experience also can be actively constructed by us – whether done individually or done in co-operation with others during formal and informal inter-subjective projects such as science, education, religion, medicine, commerce, sports, and politics.

There is no guarantee that any frame of experience, or the analysis of such a frame of experience, will be correct. Goffman, sometimes, uses the term: "fabrication," in order to refer to framing processes during which we – whether considered individually or collectively – generate false beliefs or mis-framings concerning the actual nature of what is transpiring at any given moment (or series of moments).

Such 'fabrications' need not be intentional – although they might be. However, 'fabrications' also might be forthcoming via the most sincere of intentions (despite being incorrect).

Seen from the foregoing perspective, the sorts of iatrogenic fatalities which were discussed somewhat in the Introduction – that is, deaths caused by the medical industry despite following protocols involving established standards of care – could be construed as "fabrications" in Goffman's foregoing sense. In other words, whatever the theories, ideas, understandings, or standards of care that might have been playing an essential role while governing or shaping the manner in which patients were being treated prior to their deaths, those fatalities were due to the fact that the doctors and medical establishment had no idea that their protocols would be the very thing that led to the deaths of such individuals, and, consequently, what can one call such false or mistaken ideas, if not delusional thinking, concerning their way of medically treating such soon-to-be-dead patients except as a form of 'fabrication'. In short, the reason such patients died is because the individuals treating the former were operating on the basis of one, or more, fabrications that the medical personnel had accepted and which they were treating as truths, but were not, in fact, actually true, and, as a result, led to tragic results.

Frames of experience sometimes have the capacity to conceal the truth in certain ways via, for example, the previously noted process of 'fabrication'. Alternatively, when done appropriately, frames of experience can, in a sense, unmask the character of what is taking place and, in the process, reveal (within certain degrees of freedom and constraints) different facets of the truth.

Frames of experience are the focus of our exchanges with ourselves as we reflect about on-going phenomenology. In other words, these frames of experience are forms of conscious awareness that gives expression to modalities off existential streaming that are taking place in the present or which involves memories – frames – concerning the past that are playing out or being recalled in the present.

Frames of experience also give expression to the character of our communications with other human beings. We use such frames of experience to convey something of ourselves to others or to ourselves – for example, as a function of the role or roles that we play in different social contexts -- and, in addition, we use such frames of experience to convey something about our understanding of the nature of the relationship between human beings and the Ocean of Being within which such framing processes take place.

Framing analysis is also a means of trying to distinguish – to whatever degree this is possible – between, on the one hand, one's essential self that might be at the heart of one's capacity for personhood, and, on the other hand, one's social self as given expression through the roles, rules, rituals, and so on that are learned in order to be able to navigate one's way through the highways and byways of the social milieu that tends to vary from one society to the next – although there might be some degree of commonality or overlap with respect to the nature of such social highways and byways that exist within various societies. Framing analysis is also the attempt to distinguish between, on the one hand: (a) the sorts of frames that are being imposed upon experience – and experience is, by default, one's point of contact with reality or Being – and which, in the process, obscure or obfuscate the nature of that reality, and, on the other hand: (b) the sorts of frames of experience that seem to unmask or reveal or reflect or resonate with some 'real' dimension of that which makes such experiences possible.

Framing analysis is the process of critical reflection that seeks to engage, consider, understand, question, evaluate, and organize all of the foregoing considerations. The purpose of such a dynamic process is to work toward being able to grasp – to whatever extent this is possible – the degree to which such forms of framing analysis are capable of uncovering or reflecting the nature of our relationship with both social as well as, possibly, even more fundamental physical and metaphysical dimensions of experience, Being, or reality.

Thus, every instance of medical diagnosis and/or treatment protocol is an exercise in framing analysis in the foregoing sense. Every medical practitioner is engaging their experience – including patients – through the manner in which their process of framing analysis induces the practitioner to pay attention to some aspects of experience to the exclusion of other facets of experience – a framing analysis that when considered in its entirety defines how any given individual – medical practitioner or otherwise – is oriented toward what they consider the truth to be with respect to the nature of their experiential relationship with the universe, Being, or Reality.

A simple example of framing analysis might involve a painting. More specifically, paintings are framed by different materials in ways that are intended to orient a viewer with respect to the qualities of a painting as well as to separate that particular painting from other properties of the surrounding environment – such as the wall on which the painting hangs, as well as other, near-by paintings.

However, such a framing process can involve more than the molding materials that are used to mark the visible boundaries of a painting. For example, the lighting that is used to illuminate a given painting could be considered to be part of the framing process, and depending on the character of the light which is shining on a painting, different facets of the painting might be given emphasis over other aspects of that same painting.

Furthermore, molding materials that "frame" a painting could be hiding defects along the edges of that artwork. If so, the painting would have to be de-framed in order for those defects to be discovered, and without such a process of de-framing to unmask the true nature of the painting, the molding material serves as a form of fabrication because it conceals various hidden facets of the painting that might lead an observer to have a different impression of the painting than if such defects were also visible to the observer.

Similarly, lighting also can both reveal and hide different aspects of a given painting. Change the nature of the lighting that illuminates a painting, then the features of a painting to which a viewer's attention is being drawn might also change, and, in fact, artists have long indicated that the time of day in which something is painted will affect how and what a painter sees, and, therefore, even the act of creating an artwork is a process of framing what is experienced at the times that an artwork is being rendered.

Whistleblowers in the medical industry are, to use the term provided previously, de-framers. In other words, medical whistleblowers are individuals who talk about the defects which are present in the medical industry despite the best efforts of the medical industry to frame over and, thereby, hide those defects from the public.

For example, Dr. William Thompson is such a whistleblower or de-framer. He revealed that the CDC had been hiding data for more than a decade indicating that the thimerosal -- a mercury based preservative -- which was present in certain vaccines was, despite the denials of the CDC, indeed, responsible for the emergence of autism in certain demographics (e.g., young black males).

Or, consider the perspective of Dr. Marcia Angell who has served as another de-framer – that is, a person who discloses defects that lie hidden beneath the forms of framing analysis that are used by the medical industry to, among other things, cover up its faults and short-comings. She was the first woman ever to be appointed to serve as the editor-in-chief of one of the most prestigious medical journals in the world – namely, the *New England Journal of Medicine*.

In her 2004 book: *The Truth About the* Drug Companies, she documented how the corporate world has financially corrupted the processes of both medical research and education, not only in the United States but all over the world. She also once stated that: "It is simply no longer possible to believe much of the clinical research that is published, or to rely on the judgment of trusted physicians or authoritative medical guidelines. I take no pleasure in this conclusion, which I reached slowly and reluctantly over my two decades as editor of the *New England Journal of Medicine*" – which is as about as severe a form of de-framing as one might offer.

One might also consider the 2018 book *Dopesick* by Beth Macy as an exercise in the dynamics of de-framing – that is, an exposé concerning the ways in which different aspects of the medical industry (including an array of hospitals and doctors, as well as the FDA and a pharmaceutical company,) colluded together for several decades to ignore, if not actively resist and hide, information concerning the destructive impact which OxyContin was having on Americans. Thus, for instance, while tens of thousands of Americans were dying as a result of problems surrounding the use of OxyContin -- deaths about which the FDA had been apprised of on many occasions -- certain FDA officials were, nonetheless, busy with generating an official labeling profile for the drug that hid the actual truth concerning the drug's addictive, debilitating, and lethal potential ... not to mention the impact the drug was playing in pushing crime statistics higher and higher as users who became hooked on the drug looked for ways to subsidize their addiction. Furthermore, when the FDA subsequently was provided with a second opportunity to properly re-label the drug with respect to the drug's actual dangers, the federal organization once again just continued on with its enabling activities and provided a form of labeling that, apparently, helped the drug to achieve increased sales.

Many more examples of the foregoing sorts of de-framing activities could be provided here, but, perhaps, enough has been said to indicate that the sorts of problematic framing processes which have been actively pursued through different facets of the medical industry within the United States are not a matter of isolated cases that don't accurately describe the "normal" manner in which the medical industry operates, but, instead, tend to paint a picture of a corrupt, systemic dynamic in which many doctors, hospitals, pharmaceutical companies, universities, media outlets (both technical as well as general), and government agencies such as the CDC, the FDA, and the NIH have become entangled within a set of conflicts of interests, and other kinds of unethical practices which have had, and continue to have, devastating effects on the well-being of American citizens.

A further complication concerning the foregoing considerations concerns how the process of framing analysis might spill over into the notion of a 'palimpsest'. Although normally speaking the term "palimpsest" refers to contexts in which what previously had been written on a piece of parchment has been completely or partially scraped off from that piece of parchment in order to free-up space for some new form of text to be placed on the parchment, nevertheless, one could apply the palimpsest notion to artists when they take an old canvas on which something previously had been painted and, then, proceeded to paint over the earlier creation.

Sometimes the foregoing process is done in order to free-up space on a canvas in order to be able to have an opportunity to give expression to, or unmask, some new artistic creation. Sometimes, however, something of value is concealed – whether intentionally or unintentionally – by painting over some artwork, and the earlier artwork will only be discovered – if at all – by a painstaking process of removing the paints that have been used to cover up the earlier artwork.

As such, intentions are capable of becoming part of a framing process. For instance, if, for whatever reason, someone deliberately decided to cover up some earlier artwork that had been recorded on a given canvas, then such intentions become part of a framing process and such processes were undertaken in order to hide something from view.

Without wishing to try to argue that all forms of alternative medicine are necessarily reliable and, in addition, keeping in mind that there are unprincipled individuals who populate virtually every strata of society who seek opportunities that are amendable to the exploitation of unsuspecting people who are seeking medical assistance of some kind, nevertheless, a very strong case can be made (and constructing such a case will be attempted in some of the subsequent chapters of the present work) that following the Carnegie Foundation-supported, but Rockefeller serving, *Flexner Report* published by Abraham Flexner in 1910, a power-struggle ensued in which an allopathic approach to medicine sought to erase from competition, if not existence, any form of medical practice that was inconsistent with what the *Flexner Report* indicated medicine should be and the manner in which doctors ought to be trained.

The sort of allopathic medicine which was being promoted in the *Flexner Report* constituted – allegedly -- a science-based system of medicine. However, what was actually being promoted was the establishment of a power system for controlling what could and couldn't be considered to be acceptable forms of medical education and practice, and, therefore, what was meant by the idea of a science-based system of medicine was left to be worked out by the individuals who either were in, or who soon would be in, positions of power within government, corporations, hospitals, the media, as well as educational institutions, and, as such, allopathic medicine was not necessarily so much science-based as it was to become power-based and the ones in power got to determine what the notion of being "science-based" did and did not mean.

In other words, allopathic medicine sought to create a palimpsest in which all forms of previously existing medical ideas were to be painted over because those idea or practices were deemed to not comply with what the new overlords of medicines insisted was to constitute how everyone needed to understand the nature of medicine and, therefore, outlined how new medical images, ideas, and textual accounts should be laid down. Moreover, the foregoing new way forward for medicine was to be established irrespective of whatever constructive elements earlier medical ideas and practices might have entailed, as well as irrespective of whatever problematic, if not unsuccessful, elements might be introduced through allopathic medicine.

Although, initially, what follows might seem to have nothing to do with the issues at hand, I would like to offer a more complicated and personal example concerning the issue of framing analysis that is drawn from the life of my spiritual guide. More specifically, when he was doing doctoral work in England back in the 1950's and 1960s – and prior to when I met him for the first time in the early 1970s -- the occasion had arrived for him to give an oral defense of his doctoral thesis. His dissertation was on, among other things, the life and teachings of Shaykh Ahmed Sirhindi (may Allah be pleased with him) a Sufi saint who lived in India during the 16th and 17th centuries.

One of my future spiritual guide's examiners was Professor A.J. Arberry, who was considered, by a general consensus of experts at that time to be one of the leading academic authorities on, among other things, the Sufi mystical tradition. During the process of translating the Qur'an into English, Professor Arberry had converted to Islam, and for a time, that conversion was hidden from his fellow academics through a process of social framing due to the existence of stigmatizing prejudices concerning Muslims and Islam that existed at the time – and, unfortunately, continue to exist -- in the institution of higher education where Professor Arbitrary taught.

Following the aforementioned oral examination of my future spiritual guide's dissertation, Professor Arberry indicated that the thesis which he, along with others, had been examining was the best work on the Sufi tradition that Professor Arberry had seen in the English language up to that point in time. For a number of years after receiving his doctorate, my future teacher had sought to publish his doctoral thesis, but, due to various biased machinations – jealously being one of those dynamics -- that were taking place within the academic department to which my future spiritual guide belonged, the thesis was not published even though, at one point, a prominent English publisher of such textual materials had indicated its interest in publishing the work but that interest was undermined subsequently by the activities of some of the individuals who belonged to the same academic department as my future spiritual guide.

When my future spiritual teacher was informed by his own Sufi teacher in the late 1960s that my soon-to-be teacher had been given the responsibilities of being a shaykh or spiritual guide, he began to observe some of the more rigorous forms of practice entailed by the Sufi path, including the discipline of spiritual seclusion. During this form of observance, the individual goes by himself or herself into a room from which all the distractions of modern society have been removed while wearing the two sheets of cloth known as Ihram (worn during the Hajj) and, then, spends one's time engaged in constant remembrance of God, prayer, and other acts of worship.

In addition, the individual fasts from two hours, or so, prior to sunrise until sunset, and, as well, the person keeps the night vigil. Adhering to such a discipline also requires that an individual refrain from interacting with other human beings.

The structure of seclusion is such that an individual eats less, drinks less, sleeps less, and spends less time with people. As a result, a person's time is freed up to concentrate on God more, and one does so through the processes of fasting, ritual prayers, remembrance or zikr, night vigils, reading the Qur'an, as well as through meditation and contemplation.

The foregoing set of observances may last for a day, three days, five days, seven days, eleven days, nineteen days, twenty-one days, and forty days. Almost invariably the length of the seclusions observed by my spiritual guide lasted 40 days, although, occasionally, the foregoing 40-day seclusion --which was usually done during the summer months when the university's regular programs were not in session – would be augmented by a shorter period of seclusion lasting 19 or 21 days on other occasions during the year (for example, during Christmas break).

Spiritual experiences of one kind or another sometimes are undergone during such periods of seclusion. Furthermore, quite irrespective of whether those experiences take place, the time spent in seclusion tends to be an intense time of learning about oneself and the nature of one's relationship with Reality or Being.

Every time that my spiritual guide came out of seclusion, he would, at some point or other in the following weeks and months, begin to think about revising his doctoral thesis in the light of what had been learned during his period of seclusion. The problem with such an idea was that following the next round of seclusion, he would have had, by the Grace of Allah, further spiritual experiences and/or additional intense forms of learning, and, as a result, he, once again, would be faced with the prospect of having to revise whatever he might have previously revised in his thesis based on experiences and learning that had taken place in conjunction with earlier periods of spiritual seclusion.

Eventually, after a number of periods of spiritual retreat, my shaykh gave up, altogether, on the idea of revising his doctoral thesis. He understood that no matter how many times the dissertation might be revised, those revisions would not be able to keep up with what was being learned during various subsequent periods of seclusion.

During the time that I knew him, he observed some 15 or 16 periods of 40 day seclusions as well a number of lesser 19 and 21 day periods of seclusion, and, in addition, prior to the time when I first met him, he already had observed a number of 40-day periods of spiritual retreat. So, by the grace of Allah, a great deal of learning is likely to have taken place during those many instances of seclusion.

In a sense, despite the dissertation of my future shaykh having been described by Professor A.J. Arberry as being the best text on the subject of the Sufi mystical tradition in the English language that the professor had encountered, nonetheless, my spiritual guide's original doctoral thesis was, to a considerable extent -- a conceptual process of framing analysis involving the life and teachings of Shaykh Ahmed Sirhindi (may Allah be pleased with him). However since each period of spiritual seclusion through which my guide went gave rise to newer mystical forms of framing analysis, then, as his conceptual understanding was opened up to an expanded set of experiential modalities of learning, then, so too, did the way in which he understood the nature of his relationship with Being also undergo transitions.

With each instance of seclusion, the process of framing analysis which was taking place within my guide was turned back on itself in a critically reflective manner. Consequently, as a result, whatever that process of framing analysis might have indicated previously changed as a result of subsequent experiences and learning that took place during ensuing periods of seclusion.

The foregoing process went on until my spiritual guide was informed, in a vision that took place in India, that his work on Earth had been completed. He had been on sabbatical when the foregoing event occurred and was not expected to return to Toronto for a number of months, but he returned to Toronto unexpectedly, spent the month of Ramadan with his initiates (of which I was one), and, then, passed away nineteen days after the month of fasting had concluded.

The term "fitra" is the Islamic/Sufi term that refers to the inherent, essential potential of a human being. In a sense, whether one approaches the idea of fitra from the perspective of framing analysis or through the notion of 'palimpsest', the purpose of the Sufi path is to assist an individual's journey back to one's original nature and its concomitant potential in order -- through a complex dynamic of interacting experiences – to discover the essential character of one's relationship with Being or reality.

Therefore, the practice, observance or discipline of seclusion can be understood as a rigorous form of a reflexively reiterative process in which one seeks -- over time and God willing -- to remove (through fasting, prayer, keeping the night vigil, remembrance, reading the Qur'an, mediation, contemplation, and so on) all of the different kinds of framing analysis or modalities of palimpsest that have been superimposed on fitra, or one's essential nature, due to the beliefs, values, ideas, motivations, understandings, feelings, roles, rituals, rules, methods, theories, systems, and interpretations that arise as a result of maturation, schooling, acculturation, peers, parenting, as well as imagination, and in the process have come to obscure, or generate, an array of 'fabrications' – or false beliefs -- concerning, the nature of what or who one, in essence, is.

Every time that my shaykh went into seclusion, he was engaged in an exercise of seeking to remove – or have removed -- more and more of the fabrications or false systems of understanding that tend to build up in us over time due to the way we engage experience as a function of different kinds of theories, theologies, presuppositions, likes, dislikes, and so on. As such, he was seeking to remove – or have removed, God willing -- forms of framing analysis and palimpsest that led away from truths entailed by one's fitra or essential nature because such fabrications induced one to wander away from fundamental truths or to become distracted away from such truths despite – when properly unmasked or unveiled -- their very palpable presence.

I can attest to some of the foregoing considerations, because in my own very limited way, I have gone into spiritual seclusion for – compared to my spiritual guide – only relatively short periods of time. Nevertheless, I have observed the discipline of seclusion and the intense manner in which it helps a person, if God wishes, to begin to learn how to differentiate, at least within certain parameters, between various fabrications and truths concerning one's way of having engaged experience prior to such observances or practices.

Notwithstanding the foregoing considerations, I also can truthfully say that I am far from being a realized human being. In other words, I am a work in some sort of, God willing, progress through which I continue to try to critically reflect -- via an array of different spiritual practices -- on the different forms of framing analysis and palimpsests that have been, and are being, imposed on (sometimes by others and quite often by me) my own essential nature or fitra that emerged due to various experiential forms of socialization, acculturation, schooling, propaganda, parenting, as well as individual choices that, each in their own way, have helped – in part or completely – to conceal, obfuscate, distort, and mis-frame one's essential nature, and, therefore, have gotten in the way of trying to understand the nature of my relationship with Being or Reality.

Socialism, communism, feudalism, mercantilism, capitalism, democracy, fascism, corporatism, anarchy, monarchy, oligarchy, plutocracy, legalism, constitutionalism, trans-humanism, methodology, scientism, schooling, artificial intelligence, militarism, spiritualism, philosophy, journalism, mythology, science, banking, medicine, economics, politics, rationalism, empiricism, materialism, evolution, education, and religion are all ways of framing experience. Furthermore, seeking to induce people to engage reality – or advocating that people should pursue such forms of engaging reality -- through the foregoing sorts of framing processes or dynamics has the potential for obfuscation that is rooted in the understandings, ideas, emotions, hermeneutical renderings, and perspectives to which the aforementioned systems of framing and palimpsest formation give expression.

The current portion of the present presentation is also an exercise in framing, as is the topic on which this part of the current presentation is about to critically reflect – namely, technocracy. Framing is not necessarily inherently evil or immoral – although it can be -- but, instead, framing analysis seeks to draw attention to the manner in which almost every – if not every -- way that we engage reality imposes various kinds of conceptual, hermeneutical, emotional, and epistemological obfuscations onto reality (that is, so many layers of fabricated conceptual palimpsests), and, in the process, even when such understandings accurately convey certain aspects of the truth, nonetheless, we are required to realize that various facets concerning the nature of reality are simultaneously being concealed, if not distorted, as a result of the different forms of the conceptual, emotional, epistemological, and experiential frames or palimpsests through which we engage, perceive, and analyze Being, or Reality, or experience.

The process of trying to understand ourselves is like – to state a mouthful that requires unpacking -- a multi-leveled reverse palimpsest dynamic. The French philosopher Paul-Michel Foucault would likely refer to such a dynamic as an expression of the "archaeology of knowledge", whereas the German existential phenomenologist Edmund Husserl might employ the notion of a series of phenomenological and cognitive bracketing processes that were intended to enable a person – or, so, the hope went -- to work his, her, or their way down, or back, to some semblance of experiential apodicticity, or necessary certainty, concerning the nature of experience and what the result of such a bracketing process might have to say, if anything, about the character of one's relationship with Being or reality.

In other words from the perspective of the Sufi path, human beings begin life with an original manuscript page – namely, our fitra or essential nature. However, as we go through life, we begin to paint over, re-text, or re-frame our original nature, or fitra, so that the manuscript of original potential can be repurposed, instead, to give expression to the imprint of some other set of individual and/or social modalities of – metaphorically speaking – existential expressions of texting over, painting over, or re-framing the character of our essential nature ... the source of our personhood ... our true selves.

Instead of removing what has been imposed on -- and, therefore, does not belong with -- the original manuscript page (in other words, our essential relationship with Being), we become busy with developing or acquiring new conceptual and emotional texts, images, and imaginings to the existential parchment that covers up or obfuscates fitra or original nature. Such texts, images, and creative efforts may allow some facets of the potential of the original manuscript to shine through, but, on the whole, such frames and palimpsests tend only to add new forms of conceptual and emotional texts, images, and imaginings that are inclined to obscure – rather than reveal -- the nature of the original manuscript page ... that is, the true nature of our experiential relationships with Being or reality.

The foregoing overview of several aspects of mystical science has to do with the Sufi spiritual tradition. However, one can find counterparts to all of the foregoing methodological features in a variety of spiritual traditions such as: The Vedanta, Yoga, Taoism, Buddhism, Judaism, Christianity, Janism, and any number of other kinds of indigenous spiritual traditions that can be found in North America, South America, Australia, New Zealand, and so on.

All of the foregoing spiritual traditions have at least one commonality. The discipline and methods entailed by those systems of understanding are all geared toward helping the individual to undergo a series of de-framing exercises through which one seeks to undergo an archaeological exploration concerning the palimpsest layers of understanding (many of which are self-imposed or other-imposed "fabrications" in Goffman's sense) that have been laid down previously and, in the process, covered over or covered up one's essential potential and, thereby, have served to obstruct one's search for the truth concerning the nature of one's relationship with Being, Reality, or the Universe.

Many people today believe that science and religion stand at opposite ends of any process of inquiry. For example, many individuals might claim, among other things, that science is rooted in methodology whereas religion is a function of theology. Or, alternatively, many people maintain that science seeks to provide hard evidence and work out rigorous proofs in support of various claims, whereas religion bases its assertions on professions of blind faith and speculation.

While I am quite willing to concede that there often is a great deal of truth in the foregoing ways of characterizing and comparing science and religion, I don't feel that such a perspective necessarily does justice to the discipline of authentic mysticism. Although the impression of some people concerning the nature of mysticism is that it tends to be entangled in notions of flights of fancy of one kind or another, the essential nature of authentic mysticism is, I believe, quite different from those sorts of considerations.

For instance, the previous discussion concerning the nature and rigors of the spiritual practice of seclusion – which is just one of many practices that might be mentioned – indicates that such a methodology is far more advanced and demanding than anything which medical school or medicine has to offer as a way of cleansing, calibrating, activating, and learning how to use different facets of the instrument that is primary to any sort of endeavor – medical or non-medical -- and this has to do with the instrument of the self. While medical school and the practice of medicine might involve, in some minimal fashion, engaging the occasional course, seminar and/or text concerning the idea of medical ethics, none of those courses, seminars, or texts actually require a person to go through a demanding, methodological discipline, such as spiritual seclusion, in which a fundamental emphasis of the exercise, is to not just to induce one to think about ethics but to actively engaged in purifying the instrument – namely, the self – through which an ethical or moral perspective is to be expressed and applied to everyday situations.

I am wondering how many medical doctors and medical practitioners there would be if they had to go through just one extended exercise of seclusion in order to be able to obtain a medical license, and, as well, were required to participate every year, or so, in additional exercises of a like nature in order to be able to keep their medical license. Any doctor who claims objectivity with respect to the practice of medicine and who alludes to various principles of ethics which, supposedly, govern medical practice, but who is unwilling to undertake a rigorous set of methods, like spiritual seclusion, to help purify the primary instrument – namely, the self – that is to be engaging in allegedly objective and ethical activities, is really doing little more than whistling past the cemetery and, while doing so, engaging in an elaborate form of fabrication.

If one were to characterize scientific methodology, one might indicate that it consists of the following sorts of procedures or protocols: (1) empirical observation; (2) the use of instrumentation; (3) recursive methodology; (4) objectivity; (5) a community of expertise; (6) experimental replication, and (7) reliable prediction. Surprisingly, to some extent at least, such a methodology is not the exclusive preserve of so-called material sciences, but actually represents the essence of authentic mystical methodology of whatever traditional form of spirituality one might wish to mention.

However, unlike material sciences, the thrust of authentic mystical sciences of whatever species (and, yes, to complicate matters there are some counterfeit forms of such spiritual sciences) is that the entire methodology is directed toward cleansing, calibrating, and learning how to use the only instrument which matters, and that instrument is the self and its associated faculties. In the absence of a purified and calibrated self, then, in many ways, science begins at no beginning and works toward no end, and, instead, for the most part, becomes little more than an exercise in self-posturing irrespective of how dazzling, in some respects, that posturing might appear to the uninitiated.

My spiritual guide not only engaged in steps 1-6 of the foregoing procedures for scientific methodology in every single spiritual seclusion which he entered in order to be in a position to become open to spiritual possibility if, God willing, something in that regard might be offered. However, he engaged in the discipline of spiritual seclusion as a rigorous way to continue to hammer away at whatever fabrications that might be lurking in his understanding of the nature of his relationship with Being or Reality.

To be objective, one needs to eliminate as many sources of bias, prejudice, distortion and error as is possible. The search for truth must be freed from all forces which would compromise the integrity of that search.

Thus, through an exacting process of empirical observation, my spiritual guide sought to purify and calibrate the instrument of the self by means of the process of spiritual seclusion again and again (i.e., recursively), in order to whittle away at whatever biases might be present. Such attempts at achieving objectivity would, then, be measured against the standards that have been evinced by the community of those (for example, authentic spiritual guides) who have, by the Grace of Allah, been able to achieve various levels of knowledge, and, in the process would (via steps 1-5) work toward replicating the experiment that constitutes the dynamics of spiritual seclusion and which every member of the community of those who have real knowledge also have replicated again and again.

Just as the goal of a mystic is to de-frame experience and understanding so that one might gain access to one's essential potential and, thereby, discover the nature of the truth concerning one's relationship with Reality or Being, so too, the goal of a medical practitioner is to de-frame experience and understanding in order to try to discover the actual nature of health and disease with respect to the essential potentials of the body. As different chapters in the present book will attempt to indicate, allopathic medicine appears to fail miserably with respect to such a quest, and, as a result, its understanding of health and disease is, quite frequently, a function of fabrications rather than being a function of a rigorous de-framing process that seeks to bring one closer to more essential truths concerning the nature of health and disease.

Before delving into a few considerations concerning the nature of technocracy (see Chapter 3) in which much of allopathic medicine seems to be deeply ensconced, perhaps being able to take a look at some of the meanings to which religion supposedly gives etymological expression might be instructive. The reason why this might be instructive is because I believe that when the notion of technocracy is properly understood it can be seen as a form of theocracy, and since much of allopathic medicine plays a fundamental role in that theocracy, one needs to have some appreciation for the way in which allopathic medicine has many of the qualities of a religious, evangelical activity.

Words are ways of linguistically and conceptually parsing reality or the universe. Therefore, trying to understand the structural character of the logic that is inherent in different ways of engaging and parsing experience might prove to have heuristic value.

To begin with, various individuals claim that the etymology of religion rests with the Latin word **re**-li-gare. The central sense of the foregoing Latin word refers to a process of tying or binding oneself to something.

The obvious questions are: What is being tied, and what is the nature of the tying process? The foregoing questions might be best engaged through another Latin word: "re-li-gi-o-nem" that conveys a sense of reverence for that which is considered sacred.

When combined together, the foregoing two etymological possibilities give expression to the idea of becoming bound or tied to that for which one has reverence or that which one considers to be sacred because one believes that that to which one is binding oneself is true in some sense. At the heart of this condition of being tied or bound is a state of belief, understanding, commitment, knowledge, and/or faith concerning one's relationship with that which is considered to be sacred or worthy of reverence.

Another etymological possibility involves the term "religion" that comes from the Old French and refers to a process of devotion or piety, as well as refers to communities in which that devotion and piety plays a central role. Devotion and piety both give expression to a sense of being bound or tied to that which is sacred or worthy of reverence, but, as well, piety alludes to a set of behaviors, some of which are moral in nature, that are intended to manifest conscientiousness concerning the presence, and requirements that emerge in relation to the realm of the sacred.

When discussing the meaning of religion, some individuals make reference to Cicero's use of the word *"re-le-gere"*. This term refers to a process of going through a text or a textual reading more than once.

Perhaps, the idea of reading something again is intended to make reference to a process of taking care with, and critically reflecting on, the possible meanings inherent in a text. In other words, one goes through a reading again and again in order to make sure that one understands what is being said ... and, perhaps, in order to try to be certain that one has arrived at the truth of a given text.

The foregoing sense of things might be relevant in contexts in which the texts being studied have to do with issues considered to be sacred in nature. One wants to bind oneself or tie oneself to the truths – assuming there are some -- that are being given expression through various sacred themes contained in a given text or practice, and one does not want to become bound or tied to some distorted or false understanding concerning those matters.

Consequently, there is a need to exercise care in how one reads a given text or parses a given experience. One engages the material again and again to work toward a correct understanding of, on the one hand, what is being said, and, on the other hand, the possible nature of the relationship between what is being said and the nature of Being or Reality.

The *Oxford English Dictionary* indicates there are some question marks surrounding the etymology of the word: "religion". Nonetheless, one should keep in mind that etymological factors have to do with how certain root ideas associated with this or that word were used in the past and, in the process, shaped the way in which language was used to parse experience.

Nonetheless, while etymology can help create a sense of some of the possible meanings that might be woven into the semantic and syntactic fabric of a word, one might note that words tend to evolve or change over time. As this occurs, words become used in a variety of ways that often juxtapose, if not blend, older senses of a word with newer nuances, leading to different understandings and ways of describing experience.

Today, there are a growing number of people who are of the opinion that the general idea of "religion" has acquired what they consider to be a deserved aura of negative connotations ... if not problematic denotations. Those individuals seem to believe there is something inherently defective in the process of binding or tying oneself to a sense of the sacred in a manner that establishes parameters of piety and moral behavior for purposes of engaging the sacred in an appropriately reverential manner.

An obvious question that arises in conjunction with the foregoing considerations is what -- if anything -- is the relationship between "the sacred" and "the nature of reality"? Does that which is considered to be sacred necessarily give expression to some dimension of the real or is the notion of sacredness merely a human construction that, ultimately, tends to obfuscate the nature of the truth concerning what one's relationship with Reality, Being, or the Universe?

If there are dimensions of reality that are worthy of reverence and, thereby, give expression to the sacred, then, identifying the actual nature of those dimensions becomes a very important process. If one reads or parses reality in the wrong way, then, one's sense of the sacred will be skewed or tarnished.

Consequently, one must be careful to distinguish between, on the one hand, what, if anything, reality actually requires of us, and, on the other hand, what, if anything, we are imposing on reality through inappropriate hermeneutical dynamics. If there is a sacred dimension to reality, then binding or tying oneself to that dimension in a manner that distorts the nature of that sort of a reality, is likely, sooner or later, to lead to problems of one kind or another, both for oneself as well as for others.

Perhaps Cicero was on to something when he mentioned the idea of going through the reading of a written text or reality (which is a text of another kind) more than once. Becoming bound to the sacred should be done in accordance with the nature of the sacredness to which reality actually gives expression – to the extent that it does this -- rather than in accordance with some human construction that is arbitrarily imposed on reality.

In many ways, the general idea of religion might carry a lot of negative connotations for so many people precisely because all too many individuals have done such a poor job of: Reading reality, understanding its dimensions of sacredness, and determining what, if anything, the idea of sacredness requires from us. In and of itself, the idea of binding oneself to the sacred and developing a sense of reverence in that regard is not necessarily the problem.

After all, everyone binds himself or herself to a hermeneutical orientation or set of beliefs that they consider to be sacred and deserving of reverence, and, therefore, commitment. Consequently, the essential issue is: What, if anything, does one's sense of the sacred have to do with the actual nature of reality?

The foregoing question can be translated into the manner through which framing analysis might address that query. More specifically, framing analysis is the attempt to distinguish between: (a) the sorts of frames that are being imposed upon experience by oneself or others (experience, as the default point of reference, is one's point of contact with reality or Being), and which, as a result, obscure or obfuscate one's understanding of such experiences, and (b) the sorts of frames of experience that seem to de-frame, unmask, reveal, reflect or resonate with some dimension of that which makes such experiences possible, and which some might refer to as "Reality"..

In other words, framing analysis is the process of critical reflection that seeks to engage, consider, understand, question, evaluate, and organize all of the foregoing considerations. The purpose of such a dynamic process is to work toward being able to grasp – to whatever extent this is possible – the degree to which such forms of framing analysis are capable of uncovering the nature of our relationship with both social as well as, possibly, even more fundamental physical and metaphysical dimensions of experience, Being, or Reality.

Consequently, someone's conception of medicine or medical practice gives expression to that person's beliefs about how one ought to bind or connect to what is considered to be an appropriate framing of reality (that is, without what is believed to be any obfuscations) and, as such, is worth binding to and, therefore, being treated as something which is sacred (that is, something which should be treated with deference and reverence), and because it is sacred (that is, worthy of being bound to conceptually, emotionally, socially, and so on), then, that form of framing analysis constitutes a way of orienting and informing oneself when it comes to one's sense of duty and obligation that should govern one's actions medically and in other ways as well.

Medicine – as is true for any kind of science, philosophy, political theory, theology, spirituality, or conceptual system – is an attempt by an individual or group of individuals to seek that which is considered to be the truth in relation to the nature of an individual and/or a collective relationship with the Universe, Reality, or Being ... however one wishes to state the matter. As heretical and distasteful as the foregoing sort of claim might appear to some – perhaps many -- that medicine is a species of religion, nonetheless, such an observation is not without its merits. In other words, I don't believe one is unnecessarily distorting the nature of medicine to indicate that -- just as is the case with any sort of understanding concerning reality -- medicine is a species of parsing dynamic which frames the way one understands how, or believes that, one is bound to the nature of reality, and, in the process, not only establishes one's sense of the sacred, obligation, duty, and the like, but, as well, might come to motivate one to become quite evangelical concerning one's willingness to spread that perspective to, if not impose it on, others.

In addition, one might suppose that -- and this would be in line with the ideas of Cicero mentioned earlier -- medicine as theology becomes something that one reads over and over again. This process is not only a means of trying to make sure that one understands what is being said, but it also induces the one who is going through the review process is seeking to inculcate and reflect on the theological fabrications that are being taught concerning one's alleged relationship with Reality as understood by or through the framework of medicine.

Just as religious theologies exist, so too, do medical theologies tend to exist. Medical theology is the body of beliefs that tend to shape and orient many facets of medical understanding and practice, and while the notion of "objectivity" tends to serve as a watchword which supposedly protects medicine from descending into a system of blind beliefs concerning official medical doctrine, how can one honestly speak of "objectivity" or morality when so much of medicine is – as previous examples have pointed out – caught up in a systemic process of corruption, conflicts of interest, bribery, indoctrination, desire for power, influence-peddling, propaganda, palimpsest activity, and "fabrication?"

Chapter 3: Technocracy as a Theocracy of Control

According to Patrick Wood in his work: *Technocracy: The Hard Road To World Order*, (and Patrick Wood has written a number of other works on the issue of technocracy prior to the aforementioned book), one of the primary shaping forces that operates in conjunction with various manifestations of technocracy that have been taking place, and are continuing to take place, in the world can be traced to the creation of the Trilateral Commission by David Rockefeller and Zbigniew Brzezinski in 1973. The essential purpose of the Trilateral Commission is to create a new, globalized economic system that will replace the sovereignty of nations, states, and individuals with the economic system that is being given expression through the Trilateral Commission.

Prior to the formation of the Trilateral Commission, Brzezinski had written a book that was published in 1970 which was entitled: *Between Two Ages: America's Role in the Technetronic Era*. The term "Technetronic" refers to the manner in which societies are shaped politically, legally, economically, financially, psychologically, and culturally by the impact of technology, especially electronic technology. However, instead of having the foregoing sorts of impact occur in unpredictable and uncontrolled ways, the Trilateral Commission was created in order to bring order to the process of change that was to take place through the use of technology.

Brzezinski believed that systems such as socialism and communism were merely stop-gap measures that arose on the way to the sort of economic system that needed to emerge in conjunction with the impact of technology. Some people – for example, Klaus Schwab, the founder and Executive Chairman of the World Economic Forum – refer to the aforementioned economic system as the "Fourth Industrial Revolution"

The first industrial revolution concerned the emergence of the steam engine and the impact which that discovery and its various applications had upon society. The second industrial revolution arose with the advent of the electrification of businesses, societies, and individuals. Finally, the third industrial revolution became established through the digitalization of many aspects of life that occurred in conjunction with the introduction of computers and other related forms of electronic technology.

The fourth industrial revolution seeks to fuse quantum computing, artificial intelligence, robotics, genetic engineering, nanotechnology, medicine, and other kinds of physical and biological technology into a unified, ordered framework of economic, social , legal, and political connectivity within which human beings will be induced to move and exist. Moreover, this fourth industrial revolution will operate in accordance with an array of partnerships involving private entities (i.e., corporations) and public agencies (i.e., various forms and levels of governance).

In the book, *Technocracy:: The Hard Road To World Order*, Patrick Wood indicates that the notion of technocracy predates, on the one hand, Brzezinski's aforementioned work which, as indicated previously, introduces the term: "Technetronic Era" and, on the other hand, the idea of technocracy also predates the advent of the Trilateral Commission. Thus, Patrick Wood notes that in 1932 Nicholas Butler, who at the time was President of Columbia University, released a public statement announcing the intention of the university to lend its full support to a new economic system that was being, and would continue to be, designed as well as implemented by an array of engineers and scientists and that the forthcoming system would replace all previous systems of economics, including socialism, communism, and capitalism.

The system would be known as "technocracy". Brzezinski's notion of the "Technetronic Era", Klaus Schwab's Fourth Industrial Revolution, and the Trilateral Commission's notion of economic globalism were just variations and elaborations of that original concept of technocracy. Irrespective of the term or terms that have been used, the operating system that is held in common by each of the foregoing treatments of technocracy is the idea that scientists and engineers would, supposedly, solve the political, legal, economic, and social problems of the world within a framework of unified government that was to be directed by the dynamics of technocratic understanding and organization.

In effect, technocracy was a system of social engineering. According to technocracy, one of the ways in which society could be engineered would be through the manner in which goods and services would be generated by, and distributed among, the people of the world, and, therefore, seen from that perspective, technocracy was an economic theory that would use the methods and discoveries of scientists and engineers to determine not only how goods and services would be produced and distributed, but, as well, the purposes to which such goods and services should be directed.

Although what Patrick Wood says in his aforementioned book is in line with some of the historical sources that he cites in his work, nonetheless, Patrick Wood tends to restrict, if not reduce, the idea of technocracy to being merely a system of economics, and doing so seems to distort and obfuscate the extent of the social engineering which modern proponents of technocracy appear to have in mind. In other words, however technocracy might have been conceived of originally, nonetheless, currently, technocracy gives expression to a system of dynamic organization that seeks to fuse corporations and legal/constitutional agencies into a network of fascist rule that seeks to take the ideas, beliefs, values, theories, methods, and creations of scientists as well as of engineers and impose those conceptual products onto the members of society without the informed consent of the latter and, in the process, technocrats seek to re-shape, in fundamental ways, the understanding, existential orientation, and activities of people concerning what they believe to be the nature of their relationship with Being and Reality.

As such, technocracy seeks to control what and how people think, feel, and act. Indeed, the extent of the social engineering that is entailed by technocracy transcends the production and distribution of goods and extends into issues of purpose, belief, values, aspirations, motivations, psychology, philosophy, religion, law, governance, culture, and society.

Technocrats wish to re-fashion human beings in accordance with the way in which such technocrats wish to fuse an array of digital, physical, and biological considerations. For example, the transhumanist dimension of technocracy maintains that the present state of the human species is not an end point but, instead, is merely a way station along an evolutionary path through which human beings can be transformed into a novel species that is augmented in different ways through applying to the human condition various techniques of genetic engineering, nanotechnology, pharmaceuticals, artificial intelligence, and other forms of technology to human beings.

The foregoing possibilities give expression to what might be technically possible, either now, or in the future. However, neither technocracy, nor its transhumanist dimension, nor any of the other facets of technology which various technocratically-inclined individuals are advocating, actually rigorously address whether any of the foregoing technocratic aspirations should be pursued, or whether such would-be social engineers have a viable way of justifying (that is, by means of something that is other than through methods which are tautologically self-serving) their desire to impose their philosophical, religious, political, economic, financial, medical, pharmacological, psychological, and legal system onto others through a fascist system of control that undermines the sovereignty ability of people – both individually and collectively – to place limits on what is being done to the general population.

Even more importantly, technocrats are inherently incapable of resolving the problem of how to deal with the unforeseen consequences of their actions – which there always are – because the very nature of such consequences is that they are unforeseen, and, therefore, cannot be planned for ahead of time. The foregoing sorts of unforeseen consequences tend to give expression to Black Swan events that evade, in catastrophic ways, one's ability to predict and control, and the collateral damage that ensues from such events is just one of the forms of pollution that are generated by technocracy ... forms of environmental damage (including damage to human beings) for which technocracy has an extremely poor record of handling in ways that do not just add to environmental problems rather than resolve those issues in a constructive fashion that is to everyone's benefit.

According to Patrick Wood, ideas such as "sustainable development," "Technetronic Era," "global warning," "one world government," "globalization," "Transhumanism," "Agendas 21 and 30," as well as the "Fourth Industrial Revolution" are all different manifestations of the notion of "technocracy". The foregoing ideas have been, and are being, pushed by a variety of organizations such as: The League of Nations (introduced in 1920), the United Nations (first instituted in 1942), The Bilderberg Group (established in 1954), The World Economic Forum (founded in 1971), the Trilateral Commission (formed in 1973), The William J. Clinton Presidential Foundation (originally formed in 1997 but in 2013 was renamed the Bill, Hillary, and Chelsea Clinton Foundation), The Open Society Foundation (established by George Soros in 1998), The Bill and Melinda Gates Foundation (launched in 2000), as well as a number of corporations involving Big Tech (e.g., Google), Big Finance (e.g., BlackRock, Vanguard, or State Street Bank), Big Pharma (e.g., Pfizer, Moderna, Johnson and Johnson, AstraZeneca, etc.), as well as a variety of organizations/corporations that are involved in different aspects of security – including biosecurity – along with an array of activities involving intelligence gathering, data crunching, and surveilling human beings (e.g., via social media, facial recognition, digital passports, and so on).

The methodologies of technocracy are intended to measure – in arbitrary and, therefore questionable ways (for example, as a function of the notion of 'efficiency') everything which human beings: Produce, buy, consume, use, desire, observe, communicate, learn, feel, think, and do. Such information will be used by technocrats to induce human beings (through a combination of rewards and punishments) to comply with all aspects of technocracy, and, thereby, cede their agency to a system that wishes to dictate to human beings what the nature of our relationship with Being or Reality is or can be. The foregoing agenda will be generated through the Internet of Things as well as codified within so-called Smart Cities that are intended to be made tractable and capable of being processed by algorithmically-driven technologies like 5G and beyond.

From technocrats arises the web of permissible degrees of freedom and constraints that will define the sort of existence that human beings will be permitted to have. From technocrats emerge -- in best tradition of Orwellian forms of Newspeak -- the arbitrary definitions, characterizations, and meanings that words and thoughts can assume for human beings. One's understanding of existence, reality, Being, life, identity, purpose, justice, morality, duties of care, law, and potential will be assigned to those who manage to survive the transition period through which technocracy becomes established, and as far as the issue of managing to survive is concerned, a number of proponents of technocracy are calling for the elimination of nearly 7 billion human beings.

Given the foregoing considerations, technocracy and its web of technological pathways will become the only sort of reality with which human beings will be permitted to develop a relationship. The Reality that makes life and human potential possible, as well as makes possible the lives and potential of all other beings, phenomena, and dimensions of existence will become only what technocracy and technocrats say it is or can be.

During the course of Patrick Wood's book -- *Technocracy: The Hard Road To World Order* – he details many of the twists and turns that the unfolding of technocracy has taken since the 1930's when the term first came into currency – details that are far too extensive in number to be able to encompass within the present, relatively abbreviated work -- and to that end, the aforementioned book is well worth reading. However, there is one further idea that Patrick Wood touches on during the course of his foregoing work which is important and actually ties the idea of technocracy back to the discussion with which the current conceptual journey began, and this concerns the ideas of framing analysis and palimpsest.

About half way through his book, Patrick Wood mentions the term "infrastructure" in conjunction with the issue of Supply Chain Management. According to him, infrastructure has two important functions to perform: namely: (a) it must be able to efficiently move resources and necessary materials to places that manufacture and assemble such resources and materials into finished products of one kind or another, and (b) the infrastructure must be able to deliver such goods in a timely and efficient manner to consumers.

Patrick Wood points out that when governments communicate to their citizens about the issue of infrastructure, this is done in a context where people are induced to believe that those types of projects have to do with building highways and bridges, or fixing potholes, or improving sewage systems, or providing enhancements to the delivery of clean water. However, Patrick Wood goes on to say that when globalists and technocrats refer to infrastructure they tend to mean something that is very different from the way in which citizens have been led to understand the notion of infrastructure.

More specifically, technocrats and globalists see infrastructure as the system that ties the world together in a functionally efficient way that is capable of serving the needs of chain supply management with respect to the resources and materials that need to be gathered and delivered to places of manufacture and assemblage so that finished goods can be delivered to consumers in a timely fashion. In order to be able to accomplish the foregoing infrastructure functions, resources, corporations, financing, workers, manufacturing, transportation, consumer outlets, communication, legal issues, and different levels of governance must all be controllable.

As such, infrastructure is not just about manufacturing, transportation, and consumption. Rather, infrastructure functioning has to do with the entire network of social institutions (both private and public) that make the foregoing sorts of functions possible. Allowing nations and/or individuals to have sovereignty tends to interfere with the efficiency with which such an infrastructural system works, and this is why technocracy and technocrats seek to undermine and eliminate any potential for sovereignty among nations and/or individuals because the presence of such sovereignty is perceived by technocrats as having the potential to interfere with the efficient functioning of infrastructure as a global system of control which takes resources from raw materials to finished, manufactured products that can be made available to consumers in a timely fashion.

In light of the foregoing considerations, infrastructure is not just about highways and potholes, but it is also about the form of the global system that the technocrats consider necessary for society to be able to function effectively and efficiently. Moreover, in order to engage the notion of infrastructure in terms of its more global system for managing the supply chain of resources, manufactured products, and modes of distribution to consumers as outlined previously, one begins to realize that, for the technocrat, the notion of infrastructure encompasses all manner of: Scientific, educational, financial, political, philosophical, legal, methodological, environmental, social, cultural, militaristic, religious, medical, and media forms of activities.

In order for technocrats to be able to do what they want to do, everything must become an efficient, working, compliant cog within infrastructure operations so that the supply chain of goods and services can be properly – that is efficiently – run. Anything which undermines or interferes with such infrastructure operations will adversely affect efficiency.

By necessity, technocrats must impose their understanding of infrastructure on everyone and everything if their system is to operate in the way that they envision. This means that the infrastructure which the technocrats wish to impose on people must become a Leviathan-like palimpsest that covers over, obliterates, and obfuscates every trace of the original existential manuscript with which human beings came into this world.

Technocrats need to set the degrees of freedom and constraints that are available for the sorts of framing analysis that can be used by any individual or group of individuals, for if they do not set such limits, their system cannot function in the way they wish the system to function. Under technocracy, framing analysis can never be permitted to be pursued to a sufficiently rigorous extent that would enable a person to work toward discovering the possible character of one's essential nature independently of the infrastructure palimpsest and systems of framing that technocrats insist be imposed on every human being and through which their experiences are to be forcibly filtered.

Technocracy – and, therefore, technocrats -- will not permit human beings to explore any modality of framing analysis that would enable individuals to come to understand the differences between possible fabrication and possible truth. As noted earlier, fabrication has to do with the generation of mis-framed instances of experience that lead to false beliefs about the character of one's relationship with reality, whereas truth is what the actual nature of reality gives expression to and which we try to engage, to varying degrees, through our conceptual, emotional, behavioral, psychological, social, and spiritual activities.

Unfortunately, technocrats cannot see, or do not tend to have insight into, anything which lies beyond the boundaries that are set by what technocracy requires for its system to be able to effectively continue in order to be able to control what people think, feel, say, and do. All that technocrats can perceive is in accordance with the quality of the light that is given off by technocracy's notion of economic efficiency, along with its quantitative, arbitrarily construed, utilitarian notion of whatever is considered to constitute the greater good.

As such, to say that arbitrary conceptions of economic efficiency or the alleged greater good should become the only permissible modalities for engaging – whether individually or collectively -- the nature of our relationship with reality is like saying that the only form of music that should be permitted as a metric for evaluating the quality and worth of the melodies and instrumentation entailed by classical, jazz, rock and roll, pop, rap, hip hop, blues, religious, spiritual, or musical offerings from different cultures must be some sort of elevator Muzak. Reality is calling to us to explore its complex potential as well as is calling us to explore our complex relationship with it, but all technocracy has to offer is an existential and epistemological cul-de-sac enclosed within a dazzling – but toxic -- array of technological sweet nothings whose only purpose is to control, oppress, and destroy whatever comes into its spheres of influence.

Day after day, technocracy is busily going about its mundane business of generating newer and newer modes of oppressive and controlling technological palimpsests that are being imposed on human beings in the attempt to erase the message of our original, essential nature or fitra and replace it with a counterfeit message that serves the interests of the technocratic overlords. To preserve one's humanity in the face of such a destabilizing assault upon our souls – both individually and collectively -- one has no choice but to become equally busy in the search for whatever tools of 'framing analysis' that one can find (whether scientific, methodological, philosophical, medical, psychological, political and/or spiritual in nature) which might offer one some kind of constructive assistance with respect to developing a capacity for acquiring the quality of discernment or de-framing that is necessary to be able to constructive meet the challenge of learning how to tell the difference between frames of understanding that are fabricated (by ourselves and/or others) and frames of understanding that resonate in essential ways with the properties of reality, and as such, are important way stations in the human journey toward realizing, in part or more completely, the nature of one's relationship with reality.

Contrary to the claims of Patrick Wood, technocracy is not just an economic system. Rather, technocracy is a system of total control in which economics of a certain kind has a role to play as part of that system's dystopian sense of order. Within that system of oppression, human beings (at least those who are not in control) are nothing more than deposable resources, of a sort, whose sole function is to maintain, protect, promote, repair, and serve such a system in order to ensure that it continues on in the prescribed manner.

Technocrats often seem to believe they are deriving order from chaos. In reality, however, technocracy is merely an elaborate, technologically based and algorithmically driven form of coping mechanism that, among other things, seeks to limit the unknown nature of future experiences as well as to limit where the latter might lead if those experiences were engaged by minds, hearts, and souls that aspired to seeking the truth concerning the nature of their relationship with reality rather than being forced to comply with an oppressive system of technocratic delimitation that exists only to serve the existential insecurities, impoverished set of interests, and psychological deficits of the overlords who have assigned to themselves the task of ensuring that everyone operates in accordance with the notion of order with which the technocratic overlords -- in a completely self-serving manner -- feel most comfortable.

Allopathic medicine has come to play a fundamental role in the technocrats desire to establish a theocracy in which all that is considered to be sacred, deserving of reverence, worthy of being bound to -- and the ultimate, absolute source of one's sense of duty, obligation, and morality -- is a function of a technology that is to be imposed on individuals quite independently of any considerations of informed consent. The proof of the foregoing claim can be found in the details of the alleged COVID-19 pandemic in which medical technocrats sought to claim that everyone should treat unjustifiable proclamations of the alleged medical "experts" concerning PCR tests, the wearing of masks, social distancing, lockdowns, as well as their forced mandates involving treatments (whether through mRNA jabs or the use of remdesivir and respirators in hospitals) that were shown, again and again, to be agents of unsafe, ineffective, and averse, if not fatal, outcomes [for further details in support of the foregoing claims, please see my book: *Observations Concerning My Encounter With COVID-19 (?)* In addition, in order to provide a somewhat broader perspective concerning allopathic medicine and a few related issues, one might take a look at: *Explorations in Medicine, Evolution, and Mind*].

During the course of the so-called COVID-19 pandemic, fundamentalist proponents of, and evangelical shills for, allopathic medicine have managed to turn the two-weeks that were said to be needed to flatten the curve into a three-plus year adventure in which such intellectually and emotionally challenged individuals sought to exploit every: Institutionally rooted, media-based, governmental-related, corporate-oriented, educationally biased, and arbitrary form of medical science to engage in a process of fabrication that has unnecessarily destroyed the lives, finances, and sovereign rights of millions of human beings in order to protect society from an alleged "virus" which – even if one granted them their fairy tales concerning so-called infectious diseases – constituted a potential (but not necessarily an actual) threat to a miniscule part of less than one percent of the people.

The following chapters of the present book are an attempt to engage in a series of de-framing exercises concerning some of the claims of many fundamentalist-inclined proponents of allopathic medicine who are seeking to impose onto everyone in society a technocratic view concerning the alleged nature of a human being's relationship with Reality or Being (i.e., a technocratic form of religion) by means of a medical theocracy that is intended to control how that theocracy believes everyone should become bound to, as well as to treat as sacred (and, therefore, have a sense of duty to, and obligation toward), various technocratic-allopathic ideas concerning health, disease, biological functioning, and human nature. So, let us "not go gentle into that good night" … and let us "rage, rage against the dying of the light."

Chapter 4: Terrain Theory vs. Germ Theory

In order to try to put the problem in perspective through which allopathic medicine has entangled and endangered society, consider the following list of diseases that are claimed to be caused by viruses – a claim that, as will be demonstrated in a subsequent chapter, has **never** been vindicated – and I emphasize NEVER. The reason why the following list is so essential to understanding the magnitude of the problem that allopathic medicine has so egregiously imposed upon society, is because **if** none of the following diseases can be shown to be caused by a virus, then, much of the diagnostic and treatment infrastructure that surrounds those diseases is rooted in total ignorance, and, therefore, given the foregoing premise concerning the issue of ignorance, then, when medical doctors diagnose such conditions as being caused by a virus, then, apparently, they don't actually know what they are talking about, and, furthermore, if they propose treatments for those sorts of disorder that are rooted in antiviral strategies, then, they are literally experimenting on people in unconstructive ways because the diseases that are being diagnosed are caused by something other than a virus.

The list of alleged viral diseases being alluded to in the foregoing paragraph include: Mumps; Hepatitis A, B, and C; HIV/AIDS; colds (some of which, supposedly, are due to various forms of coronaviruses); influenza (e.g., swine flu, bird flu); small pox; measles; polio; chicken pox; HPV (human papillomavirus); rabies; certain forms of meningitis; viral pneumonia; SARS 1 and 2; Epstein-Barr; mononucleosis; RSV (respiratory syncytial virus); an array of hemorrhagic fevers including Ebola, Lassa Fever, and Marsburg; hantavirus; yellow fever; dengue fever; some researchers believe that 15% of cancers are due to viruses of one kind or another; West Nile Virus; Zika; Western Equine Encephalitis; Herpes Simplex Virus I and II; shingles; roseola, as well as monkeypox, Many other viral candidates could have been added to the foregoing list, but enough diseases have been identified that supposedly link to alleged viral disorders to be able to indicate that if viruses do not exist, then, the medical establishment really has no clue as to what the nature of the illnesses are to which the foregoing names are alluding nor do they have any idea about what might cause those illnesses.

Furthermore, if such illnesses are not actually caused by a virus, then, to whatever extent treatments for the foregoing diseases are based on antiviral strategies, then, those treatments are contraindicated because patients are being treated for something that they do not have – namely, a viral infection. Moreover, while treatment protocols (which are successful, to varying degrees, some of the time, but not always so) often arise in clinical settings that are based less on what is causing an illness than on what seems to help alleviate some of its symptoms, one still needs to clearly note that such treatments have little to do with any medical understanding of what is causing a given set of symptoms, and, in a very fundamental sense, those treatments give expression to the experimental side of medical practice in which patients are the subjects of such trial-and-error treatment procedures.

In the light of the foregoing considerations, let's take a look at some of the early history that led to the rise of germ theory. Doing so, might begin to establish some of the groundwork that will help to work toward the development of a critically reflective orientation toward the notions of health and disease.

More particularly, let's explore some of the differences of perspective between two individuals. One of these individuals (namely, Louis Pasteur) is an icon within the hagiography of modern, medical orthodoxy, while the other individual (Antoine Béchamp) is hardly mentioned, if at all, in conjunction with the origins of modern medicine, and, examining some of the possibilities as to why there is a lack of awareness concerning the latter individual within the halls of medicine might be fairly instructive.

According to various biographies of Pasteur, a number of foundational discoveries concerning biology and medicine are attributed to him. For example, he is credited with being among the first to provide a scientific account for the process of fermentation, and, as well, he is described as having developed successful treatments for silk worm disease, chicken cholera, anthrax, and rabies.

Furthermore, Pasteur's investigations into the foregoing topics were believed to be instrumental in helping him to develop a germ theory of disease. This theory entailed the notion that many diseases are caused by the capacity of certain microorganisms in the environment to be able to invade and infect human beings, as well as to infect other forms of animal and plant life. In addition, his germ theory of disease indicated that for each modality of infectious malady there was a single kind of microorganism that was responsible for any given manifestation of such an infectious disorder.

Apparently, Pasteur's way of understanding both germ theory and the development of countermeasures in relation to the presence of germs was aided by a chance observation in 1879. More specifically, Pasteur, reportedly, was trying to establish methods of inoculation for chicken cholera that might be safer – and more effective -- than the form of inoculation that he initially had used in conjunction with that disease.

During his search for a safer/more effective process of inoculation, he had instructed an assistant to inject a certain group of chickens with a fresh culture of the bacteria that was thought to be responsible for chicken cholera. For whatever reason, the assistant forgot to do as instructed and, instead, left for a holiday.

When the assistant returned from his vacation a month later, he did get around to injecting the chickens with the culture that previously had been prepared. Surprisingly, the chickens did not become seriously ill following the injection of the culture. Seemingly, the bacterial culture had lost some, if not much, of its virulence during the period during which the vacation had taken place, and, as a result, the chickens only displayed mild symptoms in conjunction with what was considered to be a fairly lethal disease.

Over the course of a month, the original bacterial culture somehow seemed to have become weakened. Pasteur theorized that exposure to oxygen had rendered the bacterial culture less virulent.

When the foregoing chickens were subsequently injected with a fresh batch of chicken cholera bacterial culture, the birds did not get sick. The unexpected consequences of the assistant's mistake served to give new life to the fledgling study of immunological issues which had begun – at least to a degree – with the experimental work of Edward Jenner in conjunction with cowpox some one hundred and twenty years earlier and, consequently, Pasteur's work was considered by many to constitute something of a turning point in medicine.

Pasteur continued to explore the foregoing process in which an attenuated live bacterial culture would be used to help an animal to adapt to the presence of such a culture in order to be able to resist more virulent exposures of the same kind of bacteria later on. For example, in 1881 he played a role in developing an anthrax culture that was used to help cows, goats and sheep to – allegedly -- resist the presence of virulent strains of anthrax bacteria.

Furthermore, while doing research on rabies in 1885, Pasteur developed a treatment that could be applied to humans (his first such treatment) using the principles that had emerged through his work with chicken cholera. However, unlike both chicken cholera and anthrax which were believed caused by the presence of a certain kind of bacteria that could be identified with the use of a microscope, Pasteur was never able to identify the presence of any particular microorganism to which a cause of disease might be attributed in the case of rabies.

Nevertheless, Pasteur proceeded with a similar set of protocols that he had followed in the case of chicken cholera and anthrax. He removed fluids from the spinal column of rabbits that were believed to have been infected by whatever sort of microorganism might have caused the condition from which the rabbits were believed to be suffering (in other words, the animals were diagnosed as being rabid on the basis of unknown considerations.)

The fluids removed from the rabbits were put through an attenuation process. Those fluids were, then, injected into another animal.

As circumstances would have it, close to the time of the aforementioned research, a nine-year old youth had been attacked by feral dogs which, apparently, were suffering from rabies – or, so, the diagnosis went. Many people believed that if the boy were not helped in some way, he would surely die an agonizing death from hydrophobia, as the illness of rabies was sometimes called in the case of humans.

Since Pasteur claimed to have successfully treated a number of dogs using his rabies protocol – a series of injections that had increasing degrees of virulence and were administered over a number of days – Pasteur agreed to use the protocol with the young boy given that the only alternative to doing so was, supposedly, the boy's death due to the pathological ramifications which emerged followed being infected with rabies. Fortunately, he young boy did not develop any symptoms of hydrophobia following treatment, and, as a result, Pasteur became a medical hero.

Initially, the rabies protocol was referred to as "Pasteur's Treatment." However, as a gesture of homage to Edward Jenner's 1796 work that used the milder, less virulent cowpox material -- which Jenner referred to as Variolae vaccinae -- as a way of allegedly helping human beings to develop resistance to the more virulent and deadly small pox microorganism, Pasteur decided that the generic term for the set of protocols that were intended to help human beings resist the onslaught of virulent pathogens in the environment should be known as "vaccines."

Of course, there are a number of questions that might be asked in conjunction with the foregoing account of Pasteur's discovery of a treatment for rabies. To begin with and as already indicated, Pasteur never was able to identify the microorganism that supposedly was responsible for the diseased condition that, allegedly, was induced by the presence of rabies, and, consequently, we don't really know the causal identity of whatever symptoms might have been present in the rabbits.

One possible reason why Pasteur was not able to identify the microorganism that might cause rabies is because at the time of his investigation into that disease the purported causal entity was too small to be detected. For example, in 1898, M.W. Beijerinck coined the term "virus" to refer to the extract from an ill tobacco plant that could not be filtered out and was able to survive the filtration process and go on, apparently, to induce illness in healthy tobacco plants.

Life forms that could be filtered out from a fluid were referred to as filterable organisms. Entities that could not be filtered out from such cultures and, as a result, seemed to be able to continue to exhibit varying degrees of toxicity (as, for example, in the case of Beijerinck's toxin that affected tobacco plants) were referred to as toxins or viruses

Later, in the mid-1930's the electron microscope began to be used to probe entities that existed on the nano-scale (i.e., beginning at one billionth of a meter), and various images of "objects" that were produced during the photographic process which were used in conjunction with those kinds of microscopes suggested to some individuals that viral particles were being depicted. However, such images might have been artifacts of the imaging process since, among other things, heavy metal dyes and some enzymes were used in the image-fixing process, and there was evidence to indicate that some of the objects being observed in the electron microscope images actually captured features that were due to the dynamics of, and conditions created by, the heavy metal dyes, enzymes, vacuum, and temperatures that were involved in the photographic fixing process rather than giving expression to the actual structural properties of whatever aspect of biological nature that researchers supposedly were trying to photograph.

Moreover, even if the objects being depicted via the electron microscope photographs actually constituted some facet of biological life, the objects being depicted in those photographs were never properly assayed—that is, a rigorous analysis of the inner properties of the objects being depicted in those images was never pursued. Consequently, no one knew, for sure, what the objects being depicted actually were, nor did researchers know anything about the internal nature or properties of those objects in the electron micrographs.

Of course, starting with the work of John Enders in the mid 1950s, viral entities supposedly were being isolated in culture studies. Nonetheless, as a few subsequent chapters in this book will demonstrate, Ender's claims – along with the claims of all other virologists -- concerning the isolation and purification of viruses is highly suspect.

Notwithstanding the foregoing considerations concerning the possibility that the rabies-causing microorganism which Pasteur sought – unsuccessfully -- to find might, or might not, have been a virus of some kind, we still don't know what was, or was not, in the fluids and materials that were taken from the spinal columns of the sick rabbits. Furthermore, given that Pasteur had not been able to identify the microorganism which was believed to be responsible for rabies, we don't know whether the dogs treated with such attenuated materials were actually suffering from rabies. In addition, if we cannot assume that the feral dogs that attacked the nine-year old boy actually had rabies, then, we cannot assume that rabies was necessarily transmitted to the boy through the bites and cuts received from the feral dogs.

Finally, we cannot be sure that whatever was being injected into the boy from the materials that were extracted from the rabbits contained the unidentified microorganism that was believed to be responsible for rabies or hydrophobia. As a result, we really don't know whether the boy was being protected against the presence of rabies-causing microorganisms that allegedly had been transmitted to him via the supposedly rabid dogs.

Irrespective of whether, or not, the claim is true that Pasteur successfully treated a human being who otherwise would have died from rabies – or, so, the legend goes – that historical incident sparked the interest of researchers all over the world. As a result, scientists began to search for not only microorganisms that might be the cause of this or that disease, but, as well, they tried to discover treatments for those diseases in the form of this or that mode of vaccine.

Aside from the questions that have been raised above concerning the "Pasteur Treatment" for rabies, there are actually many other questions that might be raised in connection with the hagiography of Pasteur, for the overview of Pasteur's life that has been presented so far turns out to not be even remotely like his actual research activities … activities that have been largely hidden by those who have assigned to themselves the role of serving as gate-keepers for historical data. We will begin with the issue of fermentation and journey on from there.

Briefly stated, contrary to various "historical" accounts, Pasteur did not discover the cause of fermentation. Instead, what he did do is try to take credit for – if not plagiarize -- some earlier research of a contemporary French scientist, namely: Antoine Béchamp.

In addition, Pasteur did not even properly understand the research that he had pilfered from another researcher. As a result, he modified that research in problematic ways.

Béchamp first began exploring the issue of fermentation in 1854. The prevalent theory of the day was that when, for example, cane sugar is dissolved into water, then – after a suitable period of time had elapsed – the solution would spontaneously (as in "magically" or inexplicably) transmute into an evenly divided mixture of fructose and glucose sugars. However, on the basis of observations that had been made in conjunction with starches, Béchamp became skeptical about the idea that the dynamic through which cane sugar was transformed into two other sugars (known as "invert sugar") was spontaneous or inexplicable in nature.

Accordingly, he set up something which is referred to as the "Beacon Experiment" that began in May of 1854 and carried over into February of 1855. During this investigation, he established both experimental and counter controls for his studies.

In the experimental aspect of that research, he dissolved cane sugar in a bottle of water which was closed (i.e., stoppered) with respect to the environment outside the container but which, nonetheless, had a small pocket of air above the water within the bottle. In the control setting, he had the same arrangement as the experimental focus of his study, but the control bottles also contained a chemical (e.g., salts such as potassium carbonate).

After approximately a month's time had passed, the experimental bottle contained elements of mould. However, the control bottles with the added chemical did not show any signs of mould formation.

Béchamp wanted to know why mould formed in one set of bottles – the experimental group – but did not form in the bottles with the added chemical. Consequently, he carried out an additional series of experiments beginning in 1856, as well as a further set of experiments that began in 1857 and, along with the experiments started in 1856, carried over into 1858.

In the foregoing trials, the experimental bottles, as was the case in the earlier trials, contained nothing more than water, cane sugar, and a little air in a stoppered bottle. In the stoppered control bottles there was no air pocket above the water that contained dissolved cane sugar.

Once again, after a period of time, mould began to form in the experimental bottles, but no mould emerged in the containers without any air pocket above the water in the stoppered bottles. Apparently, the presence of air seemed to have something to do with whether, or not, mould would form in a bottle containing dissolved cane sugar, and, furthermore, his experimental results seemed to indicate that whatever was happening was not spontaneous because if this were the case, then, mould would have emerged in both experimental and control containers, and this did not occur.

Up until the time of Béchamp's foregoing experiments, Pasteur and other researchers had included albuminoids (globular albumin proteins that are soluble in water and salt solutions) in their fermentation experiments. On the bases of those experiments, many researchers had come to the conclusion that fermentation could not occur unless such albuminoids were present.

However, given the possibility that the presence of such albuminoids might have entailed some sort of fermenting potential, Béchamp did not add those kinds of protein to his experimental and control bottles. Yet, notwithstanding the absence of such albuminoids, the containers that held dissolved cane sugar (and nothing more except a pocket of air above the water) went on to give rise to mould, whereas the bottles of dissolved cane sugar that contained no air pocket above the water did not generate mould.

At one point, Pasteur referred to fermentation as being a process involving life without oxygen. Béchamp, on the other hand, had shown through his various experiments that fermentation actually seemed to have something to do with the presence of oxygen – that is, fermentation was, in some way, connected to the air that was present in the experimental bottles.

Despite the research of Béchamp, Pasteur proclaimed in a memoir which he penned in 1857 – the same year as Béchamp's foregoing experimental findings were released -- that the formation of mould, as well as the process of fermentation, took place spontaneously. Clearly, given the nature of Béchamp's research indicating that the presence of air was necessary both to the emergence of mould in the sugar solutions as well as to the inducement of the process of fermentation, Pasteur did not understand what was transpiring during either kind of process – that is, the formation of mould or the dynamics of fermentation.

Béchamp documented the findings of his various experiments in a paper that was submitted to the French Academy of Science in December, 1857. During the course of describing his foregoing set of experiments, Béchamp provided an account of how the presence of microorganisms in the stoppered bottles which contained nothing more than a small amount of air above some water with dissolved cane sugar was responsible for the formation of mould and the inducement of fermentation. In fact, he described those processes as being due to the way such microorganisms went about their life cycle within the bottle and, among other things, absorbed certain contents of the bottled water and, then, subsequently, released certain kinds of waste products into the stoppered bottle.

. Twenty years earlier in 1837, a German physician by the name of Theodor Schwann had hypothesized that microorganisms in the air might be inducing fermentation. However, unlike Béchamp's experience twenty years later, Schwann had not been able to experimentally prove his conjecture.

Three years later (1860), Pasteur ran some experiments that were variations on a theme of what already had been accomplished, starting five years earlier, by Béchamp. It was at this point that Pasteur began to retreat from his 1857 claims that fermentation was a spontaneous process and, instead, moved toward the position that fermentation was a function of the presence of microorganisms in the air, but Pasteur did not completely relinquish his belief that spontaneous generation was, somehow, still involved with the process of fermentation until 1864.

Notwithstanding the foregoing considerations, Pasteur perjured himself and, in process, committed scientific fraud when he announced during a November 22, 1861 meeting at the Sorbonne that it was he – and not Béchamp – who had discovered that the process of fermentation could occur in a stoppered bottle that was devoid of albuminoids and contained nothing more than a pocket of air above water containing dissolved sugar cane. When -- during the aforementioned meeting -- Béchamp tried to remind Pasteur concerning the experiments that Béchamp had conducted in 1857 (and earlier) which established precisely what Pasteur was claiming credit for in 1861, Pasteur merely offered a dissembling sort of response that sought to throw shade on Béchamp's way of conducting research.

Pasteur also maintained – without proof – that each kind of fermentation was a function of a different species of microorganism. Béchamp, on the other hand and on the basis of actual evidence, argued that whatever differences emerged during the process of fermentation were due to the nature of the medium in which fermentation took place rather than being due to the idea that one needed to posit a singular sort of microorganism for each kind of fermentation. Moreover, on the basis of his own observations via microscopy, Béchamp indicated that a microorganism could change its shape and form in response to the character of the medium or biological terrain in which it existed.

In effect, Pasteur -- on the basis of conjecture – was putting forth a monomorphic theory of microorganisms in which every different manner of fermentation and alleged infection was due to the presence of a singular kind of microorganism that did not, and could not, alter its morphological structure and was, alone, responsible for each specific kind of fermentation and infection process. In contrast, Béchamp was putting forth a pleomorphic perspective – based on considerable empirical work -- in which any given microorganism was capable of changing its shape and structure in response to different environmental circumstances involving the biological terrain in which such an organism might exist at a given time.

Pasteur continued his plagiaristic, if not fraudulent ways when he published a paper in 1872 which had the title: "*Experiments to Demonstrate that the Yeast Germ that Makes Wine comes from the Exterior of Grapes.*" However, Béchamp already had conducted a series of experiments involving grape diseases more than eight years earlier (and which were published in 1864) that firmly established how the process of fermentation could be affected by the presence of microorganisms on the skins of grapes.

Of course, one might hypothesize that Pasteur knew nothing of the research of his fellow countryman in this regard but merely had arrived at the same conclusion in a manner that was completely independent of Béchamp's previous research. On the other hand, given that Pasteur's countryman was the very individual with whom Pasteur had publically clashed in the 1861 Sorbonne meeting concerning the issue of priority with respect to the discovery of fermentation's causal underpinnings, a certain amount of incredulity tends to seep into the foregoing hypothetical possibility.

During Béchamp's earliest experiments (dating back to 1854) that eventually led to his discovery concerning the process of fermentation, he had placed various salts – such as potassium carbonate – in some of his control bottles. He noted that neither the emergence of moulds nor process of fermentation took place in those containers.

In 1866, he repeated his 1854-55 experiments by replacing potassium carbonate with calcium carbonate (chalk), and he observed the phenomenon of fermentation taking place in bottles filled with a solution of cane sugar plus calcium carbonate but which had no air pocket above the water in the container. This dynamic occurred even when Béchamp added creosote (a growth inhibitor) to the contents of those bottles.

If, in his experiments, Béchamp replaced calcium carbonate that came from the Earth with pure calcium carbonate, he noted that fermentation did not take place. Yet, when he used calcium carbonate which was taken from the Earth, and even if such a specimen had not been exposed to air while in the Earth, fermentation took place, indicating that something appeared to be present in the natural chalk that was not present in the purified chalk.

In another set of experiments, Béchamp heated the natural chalk. He, then, observed that when natural chalk is heated sufficiently, it lost its capacity to induce the process of fermentation in a solution of cane sugar.

When Béchamp examined unheated samples of natural chalk (calcium carbonate) with a microscope, he discovered tiny bodies that had the power of movement but which were considerably smaller than the microorganisms that were present during the process of fermentation. He published his findings in a paper called "*On the Role of Chalk in Butyric and lactic Fermentations*" and during the course of that paper, he referred to the little bodies that he had discovered as "microzymas" – that is, 'small ferment'.

Béchamp began to examine a wide variety of living and dead samples of biological materials. He found the aforementioned microzymas to be ubiquitous in those samples, and often they were found in conjunction with different forms of bacteria.

On the basis of the foregoing research, Béchamp developed a theory of microzymas. More specifically, he believed that the microzymas were the basic unit of life rather than the cell, and, in fact, he not only believed that cell tissue was generated through the activities of the microzymas, but, as well, he maintained that bacteria – indeed all of life – arose as a function of the activities of the microzymas.

Furthermore, Béchamp through a variety of experiments was able to show that bacteria came into being after microzymas passed through several stages of development. Other researchers considered such stages of development to be giving expression to different species of microorganism, but Béchamp and his research associate (Professor Estor) maintained that all of the different entities being observed (from microzymas, to several intermediate states, to bacteria) were transformations of one, and the same, microorganism, and, therefore, those entities (collectively considered) were indications that microorganisms were governed by principles of pleomorphism rather than monomorphism, and the latter perspective – i.e., monomorphism -- governed the conceptual framework of those researchers (such as Pasteur) who considered all of the different entities as being separate, independent species of microorganism.

Béchamp believed that the microorganisms that were present in the air pocket above the dissolved sugar cane in the stoppered bottles that were used in the fermentation experiments and the microorganisms which also were present in natural (unpurified) samples of calcium carbonate or chalk were possible because of the microzymas that seemed to exist everywhere in both living and dead tissue> Furthermore, he hypothesized that such entities were released into the air (and elsewhere) when tissues decomposed.

On the basis of further experiments that were conducted over a period of seven years – from June 1875 to August 1882 – Béchamp noted that while cells disintegrated when tissues die, the microzymas that were present do not die or disappear and, for this reason, he considered the microzymas to be more fundamental than cells. Furthermore, on the basis of experiments that were run during the aforementioned seven year period, he felt that he had successfully demonstrated how bacteria actually arose as a function of the activities of microzymas because he had gone to considerable lengths in various experiments to ensure that there were no bacteria present in the materials being studied and noted that bacteria only were observed to arise in his experiments subsequent to the active presence of microzymas.

Finally, Béchamp maintained that the bacteria which emerged as a result of the activity of microzymas were not vanguards of an invading army of infectious microorganisms but were actually present for the same reason that those entities arose within nature generally. In other words, bacteria emerged – whether within human beings or within nature -- in order to play various roles with respect to either the anabolic or catabolic processing of dying tissue, or in conjunction with the dissolution and removal of, dead tissue.

Béchamp believed that bacteria never attack healthy tissue (that is, a healthy form of biological terrain). Instead, he maintained that changes in the condition or viability of the medium or terrain in which bacteria existed were responsible for inducing microorganisms to operate constructively or problematically.

To fill in a few more details concerning the competence and character – or lack thereof – of Pasteur, let's take a look at several, additional historical incidents. For example, beginning in 1855 and continuing on for a decade, the silkworm industry in France had been adversely affected by some sort of disease that was interfering with the production of silk.

In 1865 Béchamp began his own self-financed investigation into the foregoing matter. Based on his previous, extensive research into microorganisms as well as his understanding that creosote was capable of inhibiting the growth of certain microorganisms, he suspected that he might know both the nature of the cause and solution to the silkworm disease problem, and, as a result, during a 1865 session of the Agriculture Society of Herault he announced that silkworm disease was due to the presence of a parasite and that if one were to expose the silkworms to a thin vapor of creosote, the disease would disappear.

Pasteur, who had leveraged his fraudulently-gained reputation as the discoverer of the cause of fermentation into helping him to become a darling of the French government, and, especially, its emperor, was appointed and financed by the government in June of 1865 to look into the silk worm problem. Despite having had no experience with, and knowing absolutely nothing about, silk worms, Pasteur claimed that the cause of the disease was akin to some sort of cancerous-like phenomenon which had nothing to do with ferment-like dynamics.

At this point, Pasteur had to withdraw from the issue for a period of six, or so, months because two of his daughters, as well as his father, had passed away. However, in February of 1866, he, along with some fellow researchers, once again began to study the silkworm problem.

Initially, they made very little progress with their research. Eventually, however, Pasteur published a paper entitled: *"New Studies on the Disease of Silkworms"* and sent it off to the French Academy of Science, and in the paper he indicated that there was no microorganism-based cause of silkworm disease.

Béchamp countered with a paper of his own. This latter work – *"Researches of the Nature of the Actual Disease of Silkworms"* – provided additional evidence to indicate that a parasite was the cause of silkworm disease.

Following the release of, yet, another paper by Béchamp which lent further support to his assertion that the microorganism involved in silkworm disease was capable of fermenting sugar, Pasteur seemed to see the light. Pasteur demonstrated his new-found understanding of the silkworm disease through the contents of a early 1867 letter that he wrote to the French Minister of Public Instruction which provided an overview of the general nature of the perspective which Béchamp had been championing for the better part of a year and, then, Pasteur proceeded to take credit for that very same idea.

In April 1867, the French Academy of Science published, yet, another paper penned by Béchamp that provided an even more detailed account concerning the cause of the silkworm problem. Notwithstanding Pasteur's previous claim of having discovered the cause of silkworm disease in his aforementioned early-1867 letter to the French Minister of Public Instruction, nevertheless, the very same publication of the French Academy of Science that contained Béchamp's newest research on the silkworm issue also contained a note from Pasteur which apologized for some of his own earlier errors concerning the silkworm problem and that, in the near future, he would be providing a complete account of the silkworm affair.

Béchamp followed up his earlier papers on the silkworm issue with two further works. One of those papers – namely, *"New Facts to Help the History of the Actual Disease of Silkworms and the Nature of the Vibrant Corpuscles"* not only put forth evidence that the microorganism involved in silkworm disease came from the mulberry leaves with which silkworms are often associated, but, as well, Béchamp indicated that there was a second disease capable of affecting silkworms.

During a subsequent paper, Béchamp provided a more detailed account of the second kind of silkworm disease. This work was published on June 8, 1868.

On June 24th, 1868, Pasteur wrote a letter to a government official indicating that he – Pasteur – should be considered the discoverer of the cause of the silkworm disease. In addition, the letter insisted that a note he alleged to have sent to the Agricultural Society of Alais on June 1st, 1868 be printed – a note for which there was no actual evidence that it had ever been written – in order to lend "credence" to Pasteur's alleged priority concerning the silkworm issue.

Béchamp responded to the foregoing exercise in chutzpah by publishing another paper – *"On the Microzymian Disease of Silkworms, in Regard to a Recent Communication of M. Pasteur."* In this paper, Béchamp referred to his silkworm publications of April 11, 1867, July 13, 1867 (revised March 28, 1868), as well as his papers of May 13 and June 10, 1867, all of which preceded any of Pasteur's published work.

As is often the case today and as was also often the rule in the time of Pasteur, politics rather than actual science ruled the day. Because Pasteur was a close friend of Napoleon, government officials and various researchers (not wishing to offend government officials who often funded research) sided with Pasteur's claims concerning priority with respect to the cause of silkworm disease. When Pasteur published a monograph on the silkworm issue he not only sought to reassert his claim of priority concerning the discovery of the cause of silkworm disease, but, at well, he couldn't resist belittling Béchamp's much earlier assertion that creosote was capable of resolving the silkworm problem and, thereby, indicated, once again, that he had no understanding of how creosote served as a growth inhibitor when the microorganisms responsible for silkworm disease were exposed to the vapors of creosote.

Due to Pasteur's supposedly groundbreaking research into the silkworm problem, the government put him in charge of resolving the crisis. Since Pasteur allegedly "knew" – based on pronouncements that he had made in his monograph on silkworms that creosote would not serve as an appropriate countermeasure to silkworm disease -- Pasteur went in search of other methods that might be used to attack the disease (and did so unsuccessfully), and, as a result, the production of silk plummeted precipitously.

In 1850 – prior to the onset of silkworm disease – French industry had produced 30,000 million kilograms of silkworm cocoons per year. However, by 1866-1867 that production had been cut in half as a result of the disease that plagued the silkworms in those cocoons.

After Pasteur was placed in charge of "saving" the French producers from silkworm disease and proceeded to experiment with various ways of dealing with the problem, the production of cocoons plummeted still further to, first, 8 million kilograms in 1873, and, then, down to 2 million kilograms in subsequent years -- 1/15th of the original production amounts of 1850 prior to the onset of silkworm disease. Yet, many alleged "narratives" concerning this period in French history describe Pasteur as not only having been the one who discovered the cause of silkworm disease but, as well, according to such "histories," he supposedly was the one who had "saved" the silkworm industry by, ironically, pushing it into near-extinction because he didn't know what he was doing and because he had elected to ignore the solution that had been put forth many years earlier by Béchamp – and which Béchamp already had shown to be effective and commercially viable.

One could add to Pasteur's continuing legacy of incompetence and failure by referencing his studies concerning, and recommended solution for, the disease of anthrax. In 1838, Henri-Mamert-Onésime Delafond discovered some rod-like structures in the blood of animals that were said to be suffering from charbon or splenic fever which is now referred to as anthrax.

A subsequent researcher – Devaine – conjectured that the rod-like structures might be parasites and could be responsible for splenic fever/charbon/anthrax. He referred to these entities as "bacterida," but he could not establish a causal link between the bacterida and the disease.

In 1878, Robert Koch noted that he had observed some spores amidst the bacterida which were present in the blood of animals that had been diagnosed with splenic fever/charbon. Pasteur responded to the Koch report by advancing his own idea of monomorphism that each disease was caused by a different microorganism, and, consequently, anthrax was a function of the presence of bacterida, just as trichinosis was due to the presence of trichina and itch was caused by the presence of its own special acarus or mite.

Pasteur went on to argue that if one were to put together a conglomeration of aerobic microorganisms (i.e., the aforementioned bacterida) as well as certain anaerobic microorganisms) and inject this material into animals sick with anthrax, then, the contents of that injection would not only neutralize the virulence of the disease but would, as well, protect the animals against further pathological encounters with anthrax. Pasteur's perspective concerning anthrax was challenged by another researcher (Dr. Colin) who indicated that he (Dr. Colin) was aware of cases in which anthrax was quite virulent but this took place in the absence of the bacterida which Pasteur was claiming to be the cause of anthrax.

In May of 1878 Dr. Colin further claimed that Pasteur had falsified or induced someone to falsify the public record in relation to what had been said by Dr. Colin during a previous, public meeting of scientists. In essence, Dr. Colin indicated that Pasteur had suppressed a number of criticisms which Dr. Colin had voice in conjunction with Pasteur's perspective concerning anthrax.

Approximately a month and a half later -- April 30, 1878 – Pasteur made a presentation to the Academy of Science entitled: "*A Theory of Germs and their Application to Medicine and Surgery.*" In the paper he formalized his position with respect to diseases such as anthrax – a position which had been alluded to when Pasteur responded to Koch's previously noted discovery of spores amidst the bacterida that were found in the blood of animals which had been diagnosed as suffering from anthrax and which were believed to be the cause of anthrax.

Once again, Pasteur failed to give any credit to the prior work of Béchamp. Instead, he merely referred to his own alleged discoveries concerning the cause of the fermentation dynamic, and failed to offer any actual evidence that was capable of substantiating his monomorphic notions concerning the causal mechanism of disease.

In 1882 Pasteur presented a talk in Geneva with the title: "*How to guard living creatures from virulent maladies by injecting them with weakened microbes.*" Not too long after the delivery of the foregoing speech, Robert Koch released a document asserting that not only were the vast majority of Pasteur's claims concerning the latter's anthrax vaccine not demonstrable, but, even worse, Koch charged Pasteur with having suppressed data showing that the results from using the vaccine were not anywhere nearly as successful as Pasteur had been claiming was the case.

During March of 1892, a number of faculty members at the University of Turin in Italy put Pasteur's anti-anthrax vaccine to the test. They found that all of the test animals – both vaccinated and unvaccinated died – and, therefore, their results indicated that Pasteur's vaccine was a useless, if not fraudulent, "remedy".

The foregoing researchers published a report in June 1883 covering their work involving the anti-anthrax vaccine. It was entitled: "*Of the Scientific Dogmatism of the Illustrious Professor Pasteur,*" and, among other things, it not only cited many of the contradictory statements which Pasteur had made at different times over the years concerning the issue of anthrax, but, as well, put forth a set of arguments that completely countermanded Pasteur latest theory concerning anthrax.

The University of Turin paper was translated into French. However, Pasteur managed to survive the problems raised by the translated paper and continued on recommending and distributing his anti-anthrax vaccine to desperate farmers.

In 1888 some of Pasteur's anti-anthrax vaccine was sent to a locale in southern Russia by an institute based in Odessa. 4,564 sheep were vaccinated in southern Russia with the Pasteur treatment, and fairly quickly 3, 696 of those animals were dead.

The farmers in southern Russia were probably never properly compensated for the lost of their animal livestock, Apparently however, Pasteur was required to properly compensate many French farmers whose animals died as a result of using his anti-vaccine concoction.

Pasteur lied about his work involving fermentation and sought to take credit for something which he did not do and, which, apparently, he did not even understand. Pasteur also lied about his work involving silkworm disease and proceeded to push the silkworm industry into near extinction with his ill-considered "solutions" and stubborn, self-serving insistence on ignoring what Béchamp had shown, already, to be a successful, affordable treatment for silkworm disease via the use of creosote.

Moreover, evidence emerged in Italy, at the University of Turin, as well as in southern Russia which demonstrated that not only did Pasteur not understand the pathology of anthrax, but, as well, the anti-anthrax vaccine that was concocted on the basis of his lack of understanding with respect to the dynamics of anthrax was an abject failure. Furthermore, as discussed earlier in this chapter, Pasteur never actually proved that he understood rabies or that he could cure it.

There are other historical data that could be added to all of the foregoing material which add further evidence that Pasteur was better at plagiarism, self-promotion, suppressing evidence, defrauding people, and currying government favor than he was at actual science. In addition, Pasteur never brought forth a case that was capable of establishing his monomorphic theory of germs in a persuasive manner which was able to demonstrate, irrefutably, how every form of disease was due to the infectious character of a specific microorganism.

Conversely and, scientifically speaking, Pasteur had done absolutely nothing to demonstrate that microorganisms were incapable of altering their morphology into different shapes with different properties as Béchamp had been arguing for a number of decades. Alternatively, Béchamp, unlike Pasteur, had put forth considerable evidence, research, and studies in support of the pleomorphic perspective which held that microorganisms, under the right conditions of an organism's biological terrain, were able to alter their morphology and modality of functioning.

Consequently, based on nothing of a substantive nature, Pasteur on the one hand, was leading many subsequent scientists and researchers into a scientific and medical cul-de-sac. However, on the other hand, he, simultaneously, was providing future investigators with the worst kind of role model but a role model which, unfortunately, all too many individuals from the future worlds of academia, medicine, research institutes, government officials, and the media would take to heart as Dr. Marcia Angell -- long-time, senior editor for the *New England of Medicine* -- sadly confirmed in a quote cited in Chapter 1 of the present book concerning the utter absence of integrity and overwhelming presence of corruption which exists in relation to the vast majority of modern, medical research.

Chapter 5: Enderlein, Rife, and Naessens

Antoine Béchamp passed away on April 15th, 1908. However, research into the pleomorphic perspective did not stop with his death, and one might even argue that there is evidence to indicate that the notion of the germ theory of diseases was being questioned even before its formal inception by Pasteur. For instance, in 1860, nearly two decades before Pasteur proclaimed his monomorphic notion of germ theory, Florence Nightingale has been quoted as stating: "Is it not ... a continual mistake to look upon diseases, as we now do, as separate entities, which must exist, like cats and dogs, instead of looking at them as conditions, like a dirty or clean condition ...?" (Page 18, *The Persecution and Trial of Gaston Naessens* by Christopher Bird) – or stated in an alternative fashion, 'as conditions like an unhealthy or healthy condition of terrain'.

Notwithstanding the foregoing sort of prescient insight, there were a variety of individuals who continued on with developing Béchamp's pleomorphic approach to microorganisms by generating concrete, empirical data in support of that position, and perhaps the most notable of those sorts of individuals – at least during the ensuing century following Béchamp -- were: Günther Enderlein, Royal Rife and Gaston Naessens. Royal Rife and Gaston Naessens are especially noteworthy in this regard because they each, independently of one another, developed advanced forms of microscopy which were not only capable of engaging events on the nano-scale but which, unlike electron microscopes that study objects on such small scales as well, the microscopes of Ride and Naessens also were capable of enabling scientists to observe microorganisms while the latter were alive, whereas the process of electron microscopy kills whatever living organisms it seeks to observe due to the use of various kinds of enzymes, heavy metal dyes, as well as conditions of vacuum, directed energy bombardment, and heat that are necessary to generate micrographs or images of whatever is being engaged via an electron microscope.

Not only, for previously stated reasons, are electron microscopes incapable of observing living dynamics as they take place, but, in addition, there are problems of interpretation which emerge in conjunction with that kind of technology. More specifically, as was pointed out previously in this book, one is not always able to determine whether, on the one hand,, what is being depicted in an electron micrograph (i.e., image) is a distorting or arbitrary artifact that has been created by an image-fixing process used in relation with such technology or whether, on the other hand, such images accurately reflect the structural properties of whatever is being engaged through such a microscope.

Notwithstanding the foregoing considerations concerning the issue of microscopy, Günther Enderlein did use a form of darkfield microscopy that while not nearly as powerful (in terms of nano-scale potential) as the technology employed by Royal Rife and Gaston Naessens, nonetheless, such darkfield microscopy enabled Enderlein to observe the dynamics – and especially the transformations – that took place with respect to the pleomorphic nature of microorganisms. Normal light microscopes are unable to pick up on the foregoing sorts of transformative dynamics because, among other things, the lenses used in normal run-of-the-mill light microscopes are not quartz in nature, and, therefore, were unable to "see" objects that only become visible in the ultraviolet light range of frequency that is present with the use of special lenses made of quartz.

For nearly 60 years, Enderlein – who had expertise in microbiology, entomology, zoology, and medicine – conducted research and pursued practical, successful forms of therapy in accordance with the principles of pleomorphism. In other words, through microscopy, he empirically observed microorganisms transforming into different shapes, with different functional properties, and, then, on the basis of such studies he developed therapies that were actually capable of resolving or healing various forms of clinical pathology that were due to such transformations in microorganisms.

While Enderlein was born in 1872, he did not begin serious research into the topics that would occupy his time for nearly 60 years until the year 1914 which was 6 years after Béchamp had passed away. Although Enderlein had volunteered to serve as a bacteriologist at the start of World War I, he, instead, was given a laboratory by the German government to pursue various medical issues, and, in addition, Enderlein put together a laboratory in his own place of residence, and, as a result, Enderlein would often commute each day between the two labs in order to research different topics.

According to Pasteur, the blood of a healthy person is pristine or sterile. In other words, Pasteur maintained that there were no microorganisms in the blood of a healthy individual, but this was more of a conjecture based on what he could see with a normal, light microscope rather what could be seen through the more revealing process of darkfield microscopy.

As a result, Pasteur, along with many of his colleagues and later researchers, were allowing their physical and intellectual vision to be framed by a form of technology which was very limited in what it could show. Pasteur and others were looking but they couldn't really see what was taking place in the slides beneath their microscopes because their vision and understanding were being warped – that is, framed – by the properties of the lenses that they used in microscopy.

On the basis of actual evidence using darkfield microscopy, Enderlein discovered the presence of tiny living entities in healthy blood samples that were capable of interacting with larger bacterial forms. However, when the foregoing sorts of dynamics took place, the resulting entity disappeared.

Using darkfield microscopy, Enderlein discovered that the foregoing interaction resulted in the formation of much smaller entities which disappeared from sight when using regular light microscopes. He referred to the new forms as "spermits", and these small life forms possessed flagella which enabled them to move about.

Along side of the foregoing discoveries, Enderlein observed, as well, several microorganisms of plant origin that also could be seen in the blood of healthy individuals. These were: Mucor racemosus Fresen and Aspergillus niger van Tieghem, and both were fungal in nature.

Enderlein referred to the two microorganisms, and a few others, as "endobionts" and noted that they were capable of exhibiting a variety of forms. However, apparently, he considered the Mucor entity to be somewhat more fundamental or primordial than the Aspergillus fungal microorganism.

He went on to develop a symbiotic notion of life forms – predating the work of Lynn Margolis and her theory of "endosymbiosis"

| Follow the What ? |

concerning the origin of, among things, mitochondria -- in which organisms were not in competition with one another and were not necessarily always trying to destroy or consume one another, but, instead, were seeking to create a ecological terrain in which different organisms could have existential balance with each other. He introduced and developed these ideas concerning the symbiotic nature of life in one of his major works that was released around 1925 – namely, *Bacteria Cyclogeny.*

The term "cyclogeny" refers to the way in which microorganisms go through life cycles which start out in forms that cannot be seen with a light microscope – but can be seen through darkfield microscopy – and which, according to the health of the conditions of the terrain in which such entities exist – develop into various apathogenic or pathogenic forms of microorganisms. The pleomorphic stages of development of a microorganism are known as valences, and as a microorganism assumes forms and structures that tend to be more visible, the direction of pleomorphic development is said to be in the direction of higher valences.

According to Enderlein, the normal state of organisms is to exist in a state of balance both within and in relation to other such organisms. However, when through, for example, the introduction of various kinds of poisons or toxins into a given ecology, the foregoing sort of symbiotic balance is disturbed, then, disease or pathology of some kind will occur, and this comes about through the pleomorphic development of a microorganism into higher and higher valences. The higher the valence of a developmental state of a given microorganism is, then, after reaching a certain threshold which demarcates apathogenic and pathogenic conditions, the more pathological is that condition of development. Moreover, as each higher, pathogenic form emerges, such forms are capable of releasing their own modalities of toxins and poisons which are capable of further destabilizing a given ecology or biological terrain and, thereby, exacerbate whatever toxins or poisons initially led to the departure from symbiotic balance and harmony in a given biological terrain.

Apathogenic forms of endobionts – such as spermits, chrondits, and fibrin (and the last entry has the highest form of, or valence for, apathogenic microorganism) – are considered by Enderlein to be essential for healthy forms of metabolism as well as various processes of biological defense and detoxification. These endobionts are assigned lower valence numbers relative to pathogenic forms of such microorganisms.

When conditions in an individual's biological terrain begin to change in an unhealthy direction (due, say, to the presence of toxins of some kind), then, pathogenic forms of bacteria and fungi (of higher valences) tend to emerge. Furthermore, if these conditions are left untreated or are treated inappropriately, then, more complicated illnesses, if not death, often result.

Beginning in 1955, Enderlein published a series of written works known as AKMON I – III. In that research he put forth his understanding concerning the nature of disease and how to treat it on the basis of his research into pleomorphic dynamics, starting with spermits or, as they also are called, "protits".

Like Béchamp before him, Enderlein maintained that the smallest unit of biological life was not the cell. Nonetheless, whereas Béchamp referred to the smallest units of life as microzymas, Enderlein argued that what he referred to as a colloid, which are of the order of .2 nanometers, were the fundamental unit of life.

A colloid is a mixture of microscopically small, insoluble entities that are suspended in some other kind of substance. According to Enderlein, the small entities that are suspended in another substance are the previously mentioned spermits or protits. Whether the spermits/protits of Enderlein are the same as the microzymas of Béchamp is uncertain.

At one point during his research, Enderlein asserted that "Medicine knows a lot about disease but nothing about life." The reason that he made such a claim is because he felt that medical practitioners were largely ignorant of endobionts and there modes of pleomorphic development, and, therefore, had little, or no, understanding concerning the value of endobionts with lower valences or the dynamics concerning the rise of pleomorphic forms of endobionts that had higher valences and, therefore, gave expression to, pathogenic properties.

According to Enderlein – and in opposition to modern microbiology – he believed that all bacteria have either a nucleus or a nucleic equivalent. On the other hand, modern microbiology maintains that bacteria have neither a well-define nucleus nor do any of the organelles that are contained with a given form of bacteria have well-defined membrane walls.

He claimed that bacteria are capable of reproducing either sexually or asexually. In 1946, Joshua Lederberg and Edward Tatum demonstrated – and subsequently won a Nobel Prize for their efforts -- that in addition to asexual forms of reproduction, bacteria also could reproduce through a process that is very similar to sexual reproduction, and, thereby, confirmed Enderlein's earlier claim in this regard.

Summing up, Enderlein empirically confirmed Béchamp's contention that, contrary to Pasteur's position – the blood of healthy people was not sterile but contained microorganisms. In addition, Enderlein brought forth considerable additional evidence to indicate that pleomorphism (i.e., the idea that microorganisms can change their morphological forms as well as exhibit different functional properties depending on the condition of the surrounding biological terrain), rather than monomorphism (Pasteur's theory that microorganisms were not capable of changing their morphological forms) governed the life cycles of microorganisms.

Together with Béchamp, Enderlein believed that the cell was not the smallest unit of life. Enderlein used the term colloids to refer to the suspension of spermits in different substances as giving expression to the most primitive form of life, whereas Béchamp talked in terms of microzymas as being the most primitive form of life, and, as noted previously, whether the two terms (spermits and microzymas) are equivalent to one another is not known. Furthermore, with Béchamp, Enderlein argued that disease of any kind was due to disturbances within the terrain that led to the formation of pathological forms of microorganisms and, therefore, was not due to the invasion of a given biological terrain by some form of externally attacking infectious microorganism.

Both Béchamp and Enderlein held that lower valence microorganisms do not attack healthy biological terrain or tissue.

Instead, they believed that when the condition of a given instance of biological terrain deteriorates (due, say, to a poor diet, or the presence of synthetic drugs and medicines, or the impact of continued stress, or as a result of the effect of various kinds of environmental toxins), microorganisms are induced by such a deteriorating terrain to enter into higher valence forms of their cycle which are non-symbiotic and, therefore, pathogenic in nature. Consequently, both Béchamp and Enderlein agreed with the earlier pronouncement of the French physiologist, Claude Bernard, which stipulated that the milieu or terrain is everything and the microorganism is nothing – something which, although this might be an apocryphal anecdote, Pasteur, supposedly, admitted on his death bed – namely, that 'Claude (Bernard) was right. The terrain is everything and the germ is nothing.'

One might note in closing this section of the present chapter, that Günther Enderlein is credited with curing many people during the course of his medical practice. His approach to medicine is referred to as Sanum Therapy, and it is predicated on: (1) Knowing the nature of the pleomorphic life cycle of the primordial unit of life that, under the "right" circumstances, can be induced to develop in different problematic directions according to the pathological condition of a given individual's biological terrain; (b) knowing what treatments are indicated at each stage of pathogenic development in a given microorganism which takes place during the cyclogeny or cycle of the primordial form of life so that a human being can be returned to a state of symbiotic balance or harmony in which only apathogenic endobionts are active and which constitutes nothing other than a condition of health or well-being.

There are many facets of the Royal Rife story which could be told, ranging from his deep desire to identify the cause of cancer as well as his dedication to establishing a form of treatments that would cure cancer once its cause was identified (efforts which began in the late 1920's and early 1930's and which he successfully demonstrated in 1934 – more on this shortly). Or, one could explore the way in which the head of the American Medical Association (Morris Fishbein) sought to acquire a financial interest in Rife's discoveries and when that proposal from the head of the AMA was turned down, the latter individual directed the full power of the AMA toward ruining Rife as well as completely suppress all knowledge about Rife's inventions, and, as part of this multifaceted attack, an engineer, who worked for Rife, was induced to betray the inventor and claim that the revolutionary optical device that was being used to make fundamental discoveries, as well the frequency treatment technology that had been developed by Rife for the purpose of curing cancer and which was complementary to the aforementioned breakthrough in microscopy were the result of the engineer's own work and not that of Rife. Alternatively, one might examinee the way in which Rife introduced improvement after improvement to both what came to be known as a 'Universal' microscope as well as the frequency mechanism that he used to cure cancer during the aforementioned period of decade-long attacks by the AMA. Finally, one might investigate the way in which, little by little, Rife's nerves began to become frayed as a result of the vicious legal and institutional attacks that were being leveled against him by the American Medical Association, and, eventually, he broke psychologically under the constant strain. Unfortunately, the only coping mechanism that Rife could find which was capable of quieting his nerves -- at least in the beginning) was through the consumption of alcohol and, in time, this led to years of substance abuse and some degree of institutionalization.

In the end the judge who was trying the Rife case indicated that the engineer who had betrayed Rife had not adequately demonstrated that the invention of the 'Universal microscope' or the frequency treatment device were the result of the engineer's work. However, the damage already had been done, and, notwithstanding a legal verdict in his favor, Rife's professional reputation had been torn to shreds and, as a result of the concerted efforts of the American Medical Association, the scientific and medical world had been induced – without actually objectively engaging the issues -- to ignore, reject, or distrust Rife's inventions and his work.

Let's begin with a simple overview of the essential issue. In 1934, a group of prominent bacteriologists and medical doctors conducted a cancer clinic at the University of Southern California. The work at the clinic demonstrated three things.

First, cancer was the result of the presence of a microorganism that could be observed using Rife's microscope. Rife labeled the different forms of the microorganism as BX or BY depending on whether a given instance of cancer involved a melanoma or a sarcoma.

Secondly, Rife had developed a form of frequency treatment which was capable of eradicating such microorganisms in a manner that was painless to human beings. The eradication process took just a short period of time.

Thirdly, the 1934 cancer clinic showed that the effects of cancer could be reversed. People who, previously, had been considered to be terminally ill with some form of cancer (and other serious forms of illness as well) were able to be restored to complete health.

For reasons that, shortly, will be indicated, the American Medical Association soon began to suppress the attempts of anyone who tried to inform people – professionals and potential patients alike -- about the discoveries and treatments entailed by the 1934 University of Southern California cancer clinic results. In addition -- and rather inexplicably unless one were to presume that the motivations for doing so had nothing to do with science, truth, or the well being of ill patients -- the American Medical Association along with like-minded confederates not only refused to put Rife's discoveries, instruments, and treatments to any sort of objective study, but, as well, they brought different kinds of pressure on doctors to discontinue pursuing the Rife approach to certain kinds of ill-health.

Millions of people die every year from cancer. Billions of dollars have been spent searching for variations on the cut (surgery), burn (radiation), and poison (chemotherapy) approach to cancer treatment that has become the so-called standard of care in medicine.

Yet, the American Medical Association in its infinite wisdom decided that it had the right – nay, the duty – to make sure that no one should be able to teach about, engage in research on, or publish material concerning the Rife microscope, his frequency-based treatment device, or the successful results that had been achieved through the Rife approach to cancer. The deaths which give expression to the colossal, tragic collateral damage which have ensued as a result of such hubris, jealousy, greed, ignorance, and a desire to have complete control all of medicine and science cannot really be considered to constitute an example of iatrogenic death but would appear to better represent a clear cut case of murder, theft of taxpayer money, and defrauding of the public by many members of the medical establishment.

Royal Rife was not the only individual who became a victim of the arbitrary wrath and Machiavellian tactics of the head of the American Medical Association. For a little more than 25 years (from 1925 to the 1949 when he was ousted at a convention in Atlantic City), Morris Fishbein ruled the AMA with an iron, inflexible, dictatorial vice-like grasp that forced everyone within his medical sphere of influence to bow down and worship his interests, beliefs, values, as well as his way of doing things or suffer some rather nasty consequences including: (a) The loss of their medical license; (b) the loss of research funds since, at the time, whether directly or indirectly, a lot of that funding came via the AMA., (c) the loss of access to being able to have research published in the pages of the Journal of the AMA; as well as (d) the loss of the opportunity to be hired to explore and reflect on such issues with aspiring medical students. Furthermore, whenever medical practitioners were able to develop successful treatments, Fishbein had established a sort of tithing system in which medical practitioners were forced to pay tribute to the AMA in the form of advertising revenues, and if a medical practitioner was unwilling to submit to such an arrangement, then no one would be permitted to find out about whatever form of successful treatment had been developed.

One might hope that after Fishbein had been removed from his position as the head of the American Medical Association, the course of medicine might have changed direction in the United States. Unfortunately, this was not the case, but, rather, the process of medical research, the teaching of medicine, the publication of medical papers, and the practice of medicine merely took on new overlords – including the 1930 transformation of the Hygienic Laboratory into the government run National Institutes of Health that took a few years to become organized, but, eventually, began to determine who would get research funding, and, as a result, came to control what got taught, and what got published, and who got hired, and who got to keep their careers, and what role pharmaceutical companies would have in the world of medicine.

The foregoing was especially true in relation to the manner in which the National Institute of Allergy and Infectious Diseases, a sub-division of the National Institute of Health, was run from 1984 to 2022 under the self-serving leadership of Anthony Fauci. In effect, although there were certain differences, Fauci conducted business at the NIAID with much the same kind of dictatorial ambience as Morris Fishbein had run the American Medical Association, and as was true with respect to the legacy of Morris Fishbein, so too, the fruits of that form of iron-handed control affected – in many negative, extremely destructive ways the development of medicine in America (the HIV causes AIDS fiasco being just one such tragedy and the COVID-19 travesty being another) – since researchers, practitioners, and teachers had to abide by the tenets of a medical form of theology which determined what ideas would be funded, and what ideas would be published, and what ideas would be taught at medical schools, and what forms of medicine would be suppressed.

However, before Fauci came along, there were other individuals such as Cornelius P. Rhoads who, for the decade lasting through the 1930s, acquired a perspective that was shaped substantially by the sort of petroleum-based pharmaceutical medicine that was being instituted at, and evangelically spread by, the Rockefeller Institute. Beginning in 1940, and continuing on through 1959, Rhodes took the razzle-dazzle of his petroleum-based pharmaceutical show on the road when he became the head of the Sloan-Kettering Cancer Center in New York.

From 1943 to 1945 he also served as the director of the chemical warfare service. This served to provide him with deeper insight into the capacity of chemistry to modulate, damage, and kill living systems.

After the war, he championed the process of using chemotherapy as a primary form of cancer treatment. As a result under Rhodes guidance – if such a description is actually warranted – Sloan-Kettering became the premiere center in the United States for testing cancer drugs.

As noted previously, Cornelius Rhodes not only had been inculcated or indoctrinated with the Rockefeller theory of medicine prior to becoming head of the Sloan-Kettering Cancer Center, but after he assumed control of the Center, he established deep connections with the American Cancer Society which had been established in 1913 by John D. Rockefeller as a means of promoting, and pushing for the development of petroleum-based pharmaceuticals in the treatment of, among other things, cancer.

Rhodes often attacked – verbally and in other ways as well -- anyone who had different ideas concerning the cause or treatment of cancer than he did. For instance, in 1950, he suppressed the research of Dr. Irene Diller when the Sloan-Kettering director made arrangements to stop her from addressing the New York Academy of Science concerning the discovery of a cancer-related microorganism – a discovery that resonated with the findings of Rife nearly 20 years previously.

The approach of Dr. Diller went contrary to Rhodes fundamental belief that cancer was in some way a cellular problem that was set in motion by mutational damage to some aspect of an individual's genome. As such, he maintained that cancerous cells needed to be destroyed through the use of chemotherapy – an idea that is inherently resistant to a perspective such as the one being put forth by Dr. Diller which indicated that a microorganism of some kind might be responsible for the emergence of cancerous tissue and, therefore, one had to address the issue of cancer through the specific activity of that microorganism instead of, indiscriminately – as Dr. Rhodes wished to do -- on the general cellular level.

The head of the Sloan-Kettering Cancer Center was up to the same sort of Machiavellian tricks in 1953 when he sought to undermine the work of Dr. Caspe who made a presentation in Rome involving the discovery of the same microorganism as Dr. Diller had sought to speak about three years earlier – a discovery that, once again, supported the work of Royal Rife several decades earlier. In retaliation, Rhodes arranged for the funding of Dr. Caspe's laboratory in New Jersey to be pulled, and, eventually forced the laboratory to shut down.

According to Barry Lynes who wrote the book: *The Cancer Cure That Worked!*, the Sloan-Kettering Cancer Center actually had run a series of tests in 1975 indicating that there was pleomorphic activity present in all of the blood samples of the cancer patients who were being tested. However, because the official position of the Sloan-Kettering Cancer Center had always been that the notion of pleomorphism was a myth and that the principle of monomorphism accurately reflected the nature of microbiological organisms,, officials at the Center buried the evidence of pleomorphism to which such tests had given expression.

Consequently, if one wished to become a non-entity within American medicine during the twenty's thirties, forties, fifties, sixties, and seventies all one had to do was disagree with people like Rhodes and Fishbein. Such ego-driven individuals had established an oppressive scientific and medical atmosphere that would continue on for another sixty years through people like Anthony Fauci at NIAID, and like-minded medical theocrats at the Center for Disease Control (CDC) as well as the Food and Drug Agency (FDA).

Initially, allusions to Royal Rife showed up – somewhat indirectly -- in Fishbein's medical crosshairs when the director of the AMA came to find out about an extraordinary cancer cure in relation to an elderly, 82year old man from Chicago where the headquarters for the AMA were located. The man had various cancerous growths on his face when he left to seek out the Rife frequency treatment via the facility that had been set up by Dr. R.T. Hamer in southern California based on Rife's work.

The elderly man wanted to take one last lunge of hope concerning the possibility of grabbing some extra time from the brass ring of life. When the man returned home from his encounter with the Rife frequency treatment at the Hamer facility in California, all of the cancerous growths were gone and there was nothing more than a small black mark on his face. The man's appearance had gone from grotesque to normal within a fairly short period of time.

The old man was so overjoyed with the result of the Rife treatment that he couldn't stop talking about his cure when he returned home. Fishbein, who lived in the same city, came to find out about the case and set up a dinner engagement with the gentleman in order to wine and dine the elderly man with the hope of finding out what that individual could reveal about the Rife treatment procedure,

Following the aforementioned dinner engagement, Fishbein, eventually, sent an operative from Los Angeles to meet with practitioners from the aforementioned Hamer facility who were successfully using the Rife frequency treatment. The operative had been instructed to put forth a proposal concerning Fishbein's desire to acquire a financial interest in their business – a proposal that was refused.

Up to that point in time, the Rife frequency treatment had not been advertised. In fact, the practitioners were being so overrun with a steady stream of new cases involving individuals who had heard about the effectiveness of the treatment through word of mouth that Dr. Hamer had to hire and train several new technicians to deal with the increasing patient load.

On average, forty patients a day were being treated at his facility. Although many of those patients previously had been diagnosed as being terminally ill or had not been helped in any appreciable manner by so-called mainstream or orthodox modes of cancer treatment, the Hamer facility was actually curing individuals who were being told that, among other things, they should begin to put their affairs in order.

However, under extreme forms of professional, legal and financial pressure applied by the American Medical Association at the direction of Dr. Morris Fishbein, Dr. Hamer was forced to discontinue his practice. This process of termination took place despite the fact that Dr. Hamer had a wealth of documented, successful outcomes in cancer cases, as well as in relation to various other kinds of pathologies thanks to the technologies that Rife had invented and which Dr. Hamer had been using.

The forms of dissuasion employed by the American Medical Association and those who came under its influence were not restricted to professional, legal, and financial dynamics. For example, one of the annual reports of the Smithsonian Institute contained some positive coverage concerning Rife's inventions, discoveries, and treatments, but shortly thereafter, the author of the article was shot at through the front windshield of his car, and, as a result, he never wrote about Rife again.

Against the backdrop of the foregoing sorts of machinations, one might note that during the late 1800s and moving forward for another 40 years, or so, pathogens were divided into two classes. On the one hand, there were micro objects that were capable of being filtered from, or out of, a biological sample (such as blood or some other fluid from an individual), and, on the other hand, there were micro objects present in such samples that were not capable of being filtered from the latter fluids.

The former objects consisted of various kinds of bacteria, parasites, and the like. The latter class of smaller objects constituted something of an unknown nature, but they were referred to as filterable viruses (that is, poisons).

Eventually, using the term "filterable" before the word "virus" was discontinued. However, the understanding being alluded to here by use of the term "virus" without the term "filterable" appearing in front of it does not necessarily have anything to do with the modern theory of a virus.

The original sense of the term "virus" had to do with some unknown kind of poison or toxin that was capable of by-passing the filtering process. The modern sense of the term "virus" refers to a nano-sized entity containing a sequence of DNA or RNA which is encapsulated within a protein sheath that, somehow, is capable of penetrating or gaining entry to the interior of cells and, supposedly, is capable of holding those cells hostage while such entities co-opt certain aspects of some of the biological mechanisms within the cells in order to be able to unleash whatever capabilities are supposedly present in the aforementioned DNA or RNA sequence that is believed to exist in the interior portion of the micro object that, theoretically, is surrounded by an outer protein sheath.

Rife referred to the microorganism that he had discovered and considered to be the cause of cancer as being a virus. However, he was not using that word in the modern sense of the term, but, rather, he was using the word in its original etymological sense of being a toxin or poison of some kind that was capable of passing through filters that were capable of separating out larger microorganisms from a biological specimen, but those filters were not capable of filtering out such smaller entities.

Bacteria that can be separated out of a biological specimen through the use of a filter are in the order of 1 micron, or so, in size. "Filterable viruses", understood in the original sense of that phrase, tend to have a size that is a thousand times smaller than the typical bacteria -- a size that falls somewhere between 10 nanometers and several hundred nanometers, or two tenths, or so, of a micron.

There are good reasons for resisting the idea that Rife's use of the term "virus" is equivalent to the modern notion of virus. For example, although, supposedly, viruses in the modern sense of the term require a cell to be able to propagate, Rife discovered that the small microorganism that he was observing and which could pass through filters that separated out larger bacteria, were capable of surviving, if not thriving, on something known as K-medium (the K standing for the inventor of the medium, Dr. Arthur Kendall, who collaborated with Royal Rife beginning in 1928), and K-medium was a non-cellular form of nutrient that the nano-sized microorganisms being studied by Rife could use to sustain themselves, but which would have been useless to viruses in the modern sense of the term.

In addition, the smaller-sized entities that were passing through the filters that separated out larger, bacterial forms of microorganisms seemed to be exhibiting many bacterial-like properties. Indeed, based on his own observations, Rife maintained that the microorganisms that were passing through the filters were actually transformed versions of the bacteria that previously had been observed on a larger scale and – when not undergoing transformation to a smaller, different morphology from its original status as a large bacterial form – could be filtered from a biological sample.

In other words, Rife's observations of the life cycles of microorganisms indicated that the latter were pleomorphic in character. They could change their morphology, as well as function, and in the process could, among other things, transform from, on the one hand, a bacteria whose size was such that it was capable of being filtered from a biological sample, to, on the other hand, a bacterial-like microorganism that was capable of passing through the very same filter that, previously, had been able to be separated out in the form of the larger version of the much smaller edition of that same microorganism.

Due to the influence of Pasteur's notion of monomorphism – a notion for which Pasteur put forth conjecture in place of evidence – modern microbiological orthodoxy held – again on the basis of no actual proof – that bacteria were incapable of changing their morphology and/or function. On the others hand, Béchamp had put forth considerable evidence to indicate that microorganisms were pleomorphic in nature, and as pointed previously in this chapter, Enderlein also had released a great deal more evidence to demonstrate that microorganisms were pleomorphic.

In addition, Rife was now providing live-action, microscopic proof concerning the existence of such bacterial transformations. These transformations were pleomorphic in nature rather than being monomorphic in character as Pasteur, without evidence, had misled subsequent generations of scientists and researchers to presume was the case and which, as a result, framed their understanding of microbiology in problematic ways.

The journal *Science* actually published (December 11, 1931) an account of the research of Dr. Kendall (a colleague of Royal Rife) concerning this issue. The research documented the transformation of larger bacteria into smaller editions of the same bacteria which -- following such a transformation -- could pass through a filter that previously separated out the larger form of that bacteria.

Dr. Kendall had been invited to attend the May, 1932 session of the Association of American Physicians at Johns Hopkins University in Baltimore, Maryland in order to speak about his research. Upon hearing about the foregoing presentation, Dr. Thomas Rivers of the Rockefeller Institute tried to have that scheduled address cancelled. When this attempt to derail things failed, Dr. Rivers subsequently insisted that both he and Harvard's Dr, Hans (a physician, bacteriologist, and author of many papers and books) should be allowed to speak to the members of the Association of American Physicians in response to whatever Dr. Kendall might say.

In December of 1926 – six years prior to the aforementioned May 1932 gathering of the Association of American Physicians -- Dr. Rivers had put forth a proposal to the Society of American Bacteriologists that supposedly established a set of criteria that would permit people to distinguish between bacteria and virus-sized entities. At the heart of his perspective were several beliefs. For example, at the December 1926 meeting, Dr. Rivers proclaimed – on the basis of what evidence is rather unclear -- that: (a) viral entities were functionally dependent on the presence of living cells in order to be able to reproduce; (b) entities known as viruses could not possibly be bacterial in nature because bacteria are inherently incapable of assuming viral-sized forms.

The problem, of course, with the foregoing perspective is that, as was discussed previously, the research of Royal Rife and Dr. Arthur Kendall indicated that bacteria were not only capable of assuming the size of virus-like entities (in the original sense of the term) and, therefore, were able to pass through filters that had been able to separate out typical forms of bacteria of a much larger size. In addition, according to Dr. Kendall, the smaller sized bacterial-like entities were capable of reproducing without the need for other cells to be present to help make such reproduction possible.

Obviously, the worldview of Dr. Rivers was being threatened by the research of Dr. Kendall. Consequently, he intended to vigorously defend the position that he had announced to the world during the aforementioned December-1926 meeting before the Society of American Bacteriologists concerning the alleged differences between bacteria and viruses because, in effect, research was now being released by Rife and Kendall indicating that Dr. Rivers didn't really know what he was talking about.

Upon request – or demand – Dr. Rivers and Dr. Zinsser were provided with the directions and information needed to replicate the methods used to generate the research results of Dr. Kendall's work in 1931. However, following the presentation of Dr. Kendall at the May 1932 meeting of the Association of American Physicians at Johns Hopkins University, Dr. Rivers and Dr. Hans Zinsser both sought to dismantle the perspective of Dr. Kendall by, among things, charging the latter individual with having perpetrated scientific fraud because neither Dr. Rivers nor Dr. Hans Zinsser had been able to replicate the results that were reported in 1931 by Dr. Kendall.

Dr. Edward C. Rosenow, Jr. – son of Edward Rosenow Senior, who had been a supporter of, and who collaborated with, both Dr. Arthur Kendall and Royal Rife – notes that he once had been a student of Dr. Hans Zinsser while attending Harvard. The younger Rosenow indicates that during this period of time, Dr. Zinsser once confessed to him that he -- Dr. Zinsser -- had not actually bothered to follow the methodological protocol with which he had been provided to carry out the process necessary to – potentially -- replicate the 1931 results concerning the capacity of bacteria to change their morphology and functional properties, and, yet, Dr. Zinsser went ahead and had been critical of those announced results nonetheless.

Apparently, many people in the audience at the May 1932 Association of American Physicians were influenced --- at least in a rhetorical sense -- by what Dr. Rivers had to say on that occasion. This outcome – to whatever extent it is true – might well have been because many members of the audience permitted themselves to forget about such matters as empirical evidence, methodology, and demonstrable results, and, instead became caught up in arguments from authority as well as the infamous capacity of Dr. Rivers to verbally and publically bully individuals in a manner that rarely had anything to do with the truth of an issue but was, instead, dedicated to Dr. Rivers need to satisfy the hungers of his own ego at the expense of the feelings and reputations of other individuals.

Several decades prior to the verbal brawl before the Association of American Physicians in 1932, Peyton Rous had, in 1911, established a strong case – strong enough to lead to winning the Nobel Prize for his work some 55 years later -- that the cause of cancer might have something to do with the presence of a virus -- in the original sense of the term ... that is, a poison or toxin of some kind that was capable of passing though a filter that was capable of separating out larger forms of bacteria. However, because, at the time of the foregoing discovery, the orthodox manner of depicting or framing the cause of cancer was considered to be a function of some sort of mutagenic change to the way in which DNA and/or RNA were being processed, and, therefore, such mutated cells became rogue centers of dysfunctional biological activity.

Later on, the work of Dr. Eleanor Alexander-Jackson established that the so-called Rous virus had been observed to generate both DNA as well as RNA sequences and since viruses in the modern sense only were supposed to contain either DNA or RNA but not both, the Rous virus was really more bacterial in nature. In a 1969 paper that was authored by both Dr, Alexander–Jackson and Dr. Virginia Livingston, the assertion was made that the reason why no one had been able to understand that the cause of cancer was due to the presence of a single Rous-like bacterial form was that most researchers had refused to be willing to entertain the possibility that the pleomorphic perspective -- which indicated that bacteria were capable of altering their morphology and functionality – might actually be correct. In short, researchers had been unwilling to undergo a process of de-framing in which various forms of fabrication which were shaping their perspective needed to be removed.

Five years later, in 1974, Dr. Lida H, Mattman, working out of the Biology Department at Wayne State University discovered the existence of what are referred to as "cell-wall deficient forms of bacteria'. For example, what are now referred to as mycoplasmas give expression to such entities, and the data surrounding cell-wall deficient forms tends to further corroborate the pleomorphic idea that began with Béchamp, and was further substantiated through the research of individuals such as Enderlein, Rife, Kendall, Alexander-Jackson, Livingston, Mattman, and others.

Unfortunately, the sorts of people who had control over much of medicine and biological research back then were being led around by the nose by people such as Morris Fishbein, Cornelius P. Rhoads, and Thomas Rivers. Rivers had not only been a member of the Rockefeller Institute for more than a decade, but in 1935 he became the Director of the Rockefeller Hospital and served in this position until1959, and, in addition, he became the Vice President of the Rockefeller Institute from 1953 until in his death in 1962, and throughout these decades he vigorously served, protected, and defended the interests of the Rockefeller approach to medicine which was rooted in: (a) The monomorphic theory of microorganisms that had been first proposed, sans evidence, by Pasteur in the late 1800s, as well as: (b) The commercially extremely profitable notation that petroleum-based pharmaceuticals were the key to 'doing no harm'.

Like Fishbein of the American Medical Association and Cornelius Rhodes of the Sloan-Kettering Cancer Center (which had some rather incestuous ties with the Rockefeller Institute), Thomas Rivers sought to disparage, if not destroy, anyone – such as Rife and Kendall – who championed a perspective other than the one to which Dr. Rivers was committed, As a result, the foregoing three individuals took active steps, each in his own inimical manner, to discredit, suppress, harass, and undermine a great deal of the research that, among other things, was able to evidentially show or strongly suggest that a monomorphic view of microorganisms was an untenable theory and that, instead, the pleomorphic approach to microbiology was – from the perspective of actual evidence -- far superior to the empirically challenged idea of monomorphism. Therefore, a great deal of the research that was published, taught, and applied throughout America during their tenures as directors of the previously noted powerful organizations (tenures which loomed over the first six-plus decades of the twentieth century) was forced to genuflect before the likes and dislikes of such power brokers and recite whatever catechism of medical theology and litanies of cognitive self-effacement that were called for by various sets of circumstances.

Fishbein, Rhodes, and Rivers were all following the "leadership" model that had been established by Louis Pasteur. In other words, they were all people who were more interested in power and self-serving ideologies than they were interested in the well-being of individuals, and, consequently, they leveraged power as well as were leveraged by that which made such access to power possible, and, in the process, they betrayed both the truth and their fellow human beings.

To somewhat paraphrase or re-phrase the words of Günther Enderlein that were quoted during the opening pages of the present chapter, the foregoing three individuals were people who might know a lot about disease but knew very little about the nature of life or what constituted health. Nevertheless, they considered themselves to be gods of medicine – if not more -- and, therefore, they set about creating servants in their own image, but there were those who followed the sound of a different drum.

In 1913, Royal Rife was a happily married, twenty-five year old man. He had moved to San Diego (from Nebraska) in order to further pursue his life-long interest in electronics, microscopes, inventions, as well as biology, and, ne was able to pursue a number of those interests when he worked for the Navy during World War I and had been sent to Europe by the US government in order – for reasons that are unknown and, perhaps, classified – to investigate various laboratories in different countries.

A few years following the end of the war, Rife became intrigued with the possibility of finding ways to use electricity in some fashion that might help cure diseases of one kind or another. More specifically, he began to explore the idea that different electrical frequencies might have different effects upon biological organisms.

He was able to secure funding from a couple of interested San Diego industrialists who were willing to bankroll his scientific, medical, and inventive pursuits. Rife put the money to good use during the 1920s, and, as a result, he successfully invented both an extraordinary microscope as well as certain frequency generating prototypes that seemed to be able to eliminate various kinds of pathogenic microorganisms.

Rife actually had begun work to construct the sort of microscope that he had envisioned in 1917. However, once his instrument had been built (and it consisted of thousands of parts), he proceeded to make a series of improvements to his novel form of microscope.

His microscope was unprecedented in a variety of ways. To begin with, at the time, the best microscopes of the day were capable of resolutions in the order of between 2,000 and 2,500 diameters, whereas Rife's initial microscope was capable of resolutions in the range of 31,000 diameters,

Piece by piece (eventually reaching a total of nearly 5,700 pieces), he expanded the original resolution capacity of his microscope to 50,000 diameters. As a result, he was able to observe the actual dynamics of life down to a size of $1/20^{th}$ by $1/15^{th}$ of a micron which enabled him to observe, among other things, the sorts of pleomorphic transformations in microorganisms that eluded normal light microscopes and which, for different reasons noted previously, could not be captured by electron microscopes.

The microscope contained a series of 14 lenses and prisms, together with an illumination unit, all of which were made from quartz materials that were transparent to ultraviolet light. These features enabled an observer to see objects that were invisible to normal light microscopes that did not use quartz lenses and which, therefore, framed or hid the presence of objects that were visible when one used lenses capable of transmitting ultraviolet light.

The Rife microscope had a second system of illumination that bent and polarized its light in a manner that could be controlled via the intricacies made possible by some 5,700 parts and which permitted the operator of the microscope to run through an array of very small changes in frequency gradation that were capable of bringing into focus those objects that had a chemistry which generated a frequency that interacted with whatever frequency of polarized, bent light which was being modulated within the microscope at a given time. In effect, the Rife microscope was able to paint microorganisms with frequencies of light to which such microorganisms responded in characteristic ways (such as color) and through which the microorganisms became visible as entities with specific, colors that was unique to the frequency that was characteristic of the chemical dynamics inherent in such microorganisms.

With the help of the foregoing capabilities of his microscope, Rife drew up a color-coding chart which enabled him to differentially and consistently identify numerous microorganisms as well as various stages of their pleomorphic life cycle. Each micro entity had a specific form of color emanation that never varied, and, therefore, if, after adjusting the microscope in certain ways, one observed a microorganism with a certain color emanation, then, one knew whether, or not, it was something that one had previously encountered or whether it emanated with a color that had not, yet, been catalogued and, consequently, constituted a new discovery of sorts.

Frequency not only played a role in enabling one to see, for example, certain kinds of microorganism in different stages of their pleomorphic life cycles, but frequency also played a role in the development of an instrument that was designed to terminate the existence of certain forms of microorganism. Through a process of trial and error, Rife was able to determine the MOR or Mortal Oscillatory Rate associated with any given microorganism that enabled one to disintegrate such entities into non-existence.

Rife's initial investigations in this regard involved a search for a frequency that would terminate the microorganism that was believed to cause tuberculosis. However, after he located the proper MOR frequency and disintegrated the entity, he found, nonetheless, that some of the test animals continued to die from some sort of toxic poisoning.

Rife was aware that during the late 1800s Robert Koch had had similar experiences during his experiments with anti-venom. In other words, despite giving the requisite anti-venom to animals, Koch discovered that some of those animals still died.

After some critical reflection, Rife began to suspect that in some of those perplexing cases it might be that before the targeted, pathogenic microorganism had been eradicated (the one that was believed to cause tuberculosis), Rife entertained the possibility that, perhaps, different editions of the targeted, pathogenic microorganism had either released, or been transformed into, some sort of virus – that is, a toxic or poisonous entity. If so, then, this toxin or poison (i.e., a "virus" in the original sense of the term) could be responsible for the death of some of the test animals that had died despite the fact that the original form of that microorganism had been treated with, or exposed to, an appropriate MOR.

If the foregoing conjecture were correct, then, Rife had to discover what the nature of such a "virus" was and, then, seek to determine what its MOR might be. Three years of intensive research and experimentation were needed for him to be able to resolve the problem.

Eventually, however, he found that two different frequencies were necessary. One MOR frequency was needed to terminate the original bacterial form which was capable of causing tuberculosis, but, as well, another MOR frequency was also needed to be able to terminate the "viral" form (in the original sense of "virus") of that same microorganism.

In other words, in order to properly treat tuberculosis once it has arisen, one had to learn how to simultaneously terminate two different pleomorphic stages or forms in the life cycle of a given microorganism. Yet, terminating the pathogenic stages of that microorganism's life cycle doesn't actually indicate what it is – or was -- in the terrain within which such a microorganism exists or existed that induced it to enter into those aspects of its life cycle that are pathogenic in nature rather than continue on in an apathogenic mode of existence.

One of the reasons why it took so long for Rife to find a solution to the foregoing quandary was that, initially, he had tried to find ways of staining the "virus" form of the microorganism in a traditional manner by using chemical dyes of one kind of another. After a considerable amount of unsuccessful trial and error, he came to the conclusion that the "virus" mode of the pleomorphic microorganism was too small to stain in a traditional manner (i.e., through the use of chemical dyes), and, as a result, he began to search for alternative methods of staining.

It was at this point in his explorations that the intuition came to him concerning the idea of using frequencies as a means of rendering such entities visible. Consequently, he set about building a microscope that had the capacity to use frequency as a way of inducing what had been invisible to become visible through the unique color emanation that arose when the microscope used a certain frequency of light in conjunction with a microorganism that had a sort of receptive frequency.

Although Rife's first practical breakthrough came in relation to his work on the tuberculosis problem, his original impetus fur undertaking such work had been a function of his ultimate desire to find a cure for cancer. In fact, his cancer research had begun in 1922, but he was having difficulty identifying the precise form of the microorganism that he believed might be the cause of cancer.

Therefore, in the meantime, he worked a problem about which he did have some knowledge since he knew (from the work of Robert Koch and others) what the identity of one of the primary culprits was that seemed to play a causal role in the onset of tuberculosis. When he discovered the MOR or frequency for terminating that pathogen, and, then, upon further research, discovered that there was a viral form of that same pathogen which also had to be identified as well as eliminated, he became caught up in the many tasks that were entailed by the process of updating his microscope so that it could paint microorganisms – and, thereby, make them visible – with appropriate frequencies that induced those microorganisms to become manifest or resonate with unique colors.

During the latter stages of the foregoing research, Rife's work was assisted considerably by the presence of Dr. Milbank Johnson and Dr. Arthur Kendall. Both Dr. Johnson and Dr. Kendall were well-regarded.

Dr. Johnson was a high-profile physician in Los Angeles who, among other things, was a member of the board of directors at the Pasadena Hospital in California. Dr. Kendal was the Director of Medical Research for the Evanston, Illinois-based Northwestern Medical School, and, was not only a well-regarded microbiologist but the inventor of a culturing medium that, among other things, would play a central role in helping Rife in his cancer investigations.

The culturing medium that was invented by Dr. Kendall was protein-based and devoid of living cells that were capable of sustaining the "viruses" (in the original sense of the term; that is, denoting a toxin or poison) which could not be filtered out of, or removed from, say, a blood sample, Nevertheless, the K-medium was able to sustain those viruses despite the absence of such cells and, therefore, as pointed out earlier, contradicted the 1926 claims of Dr. Thomas Rivers which conjectured that one of the distinguishing features between "viruses" and bacteria was that the former could not reproduce in the absence of cellular life.

Since the modern notion of a virus presupposes that the foregoing assertion of Dr. Rivers is true, and since Dr. Kendall's invention of the K-medium demonstrated that one of the supposed primary differences between viruses and bacteria (according to Dr. Rivers) -- which had to do with the alleged need of viruses to live off the avails of living cells --, was, actually, false, then, one comes to the rather startling conclusion that evidence has existed for more than 90 years indicating that the modern theory of viruses is incorrect because that theory relies on a perspective – namely, the foregoing conjecture of Dr. Rivers – which the existence of K-medium served to show was untenable. Nevertheless, the mythology of modern virology is unwilling to abandon its insistence on carrying on with its counterfactual façade that one can differentiate between viruses and bacteria because viruses need a cell host to be able to perpetuate themselves. As Dr. Kendall and Royal Rife had shown by the early 1930s, viruses are actually a bacterial-like form of organism that is capable of engaging in metabolic processes quite independently of the presence of cellular life.

The K-medium of Dr. Kendall helped Rife to be able to culture the viral form of the bacterial microorganism that, along with the latter bacterial form, was responsible for tuberculosis. Rife's new improvements to his microscope was capable of not only making such microorganisms visible in a manner that was capable of being replicated, but showed, as well, the nature of the pleomorphic dynamics that gave rise to different stages of the life cycle of a single microorganism as those entities transformed into one another.

On November 30, 1931 the *Los Angeles Times* carried a story about a meeting held several days previously that had been arranged by Dr. Milbank Johnson on behalf of more than 30 prominent members of the scientific and medical communities in California in order to provide those individuals with an opportunity to learn about the work of both Royal Rife and Dr. Kendall. A photograph of the two scientists juxtaposed next to the new microscope was featured some five days later in the same newspaper.

A month later, on December 27, 1931, the *Los Angeles Times* published another story on the work of Royal Rife. This time the article was about a gathering of some 250 scientists who had been invited by Royal Rife and his colleagues to learn about their research and inventions.

The research and work of Rife and his colleagues was given national exposure through the mainstream journal *Science*. Moreover, several weeks prior to the aforementioned Los Angeles Times article of December 27, 1931, an edition of *Science News*, a sort of supplemental magazine related to the journal *Science*, ran with a story about how filterable bodies – i.e., viruses in the original sense of the word of being toxins or poisons that could not be separated out by filters – had been viewable via the Rife microscope.

The foregoing kind of coverage and notoriety is what led to Dr. Thomas Rivers and Dr. Hans Zinsser trying to cancel the presentation of Dr. Andrew Kendall before the Association of American Physicists in May of 1972 that was to be held at Johns Hopkins. When they were not able to cancel the scheduled meeting, they wormed their way in to being allowed to make their own presentation and used that opportunity to engage in a series of attacks that were filled with rhetorical bombast and little more, but many members of the audience who were physicians seemed to find that sort of rhetoric to be comforting.

Apparently, only one individual in the audience is reported to have stood in defense of Dr. Kendall. However, what was missing in numbers was more than compensated for by the prestige of that speaker – namely, Dr. William H. Welch.

Dr. Welch was the individual who first began to introduce, and teach about, bacteriology in the United States. Moreover, his scientific stature was such that at one point in time the library at Johns Hopkins had been named in his honor.

The thrust of the remarks offered by Dr. Welch on the occasion of the May 1932 presentations was that the work of Dr. Kendall had served to advance the cause of medicine. However, unfortunately, rhetoric, verbal bullying and unpleasantness seemed to carry the day.

Notwithstanding the foregoing sort of setbacks, Royal, Rife, Dr, Kendall, and other individuals such as Dr, Edward C. Rosenow of the Mayo Clinic continued to move forward with their research concerning, among other things, the pleomorphic nature of microorganisms, as well as with a continued search for medical protocols that might successfully treat different kinds of pathology.

Dr. Rosenow was of the opinion that as impressive as the substantially increased capacity of the Rife microscope might be with respect to being able to resolve the details of living objects on the sub-micron level, nonetheless, as far as Dr, Rosenow was concerned the capacity of that same microscope to be able to make visible what previously had been invisible by means of its ability to paint those microorganisms with a resonance that induced the latter entities to emanate with a color that uniquely identified them as being one kind of organism rather another was of far greater importance. This is precisely the feature of that microscope that, along with the K-medium of Dr. Kendall, led, in 1932, to the discovery of the microorganism that appeared to be the cause of cancer.

Through a series of fortuitous but unintended consequences, Rife discovered that when he took a cancer culture and sustained it with K-medium and, then, exposed that culture for approximately 24 hours to the lighting frequency of an argon gas-filled tube that had been heated by 5000 volt electric current, and, then, followed the foregoing processes by exposing the culture to a combination of water and vacuum for another 24 hours that was maintained at 37.5 degrees

Centigrade, he was able to see that for which he had been looking for nearly a decade, In other words, after being exposed to the aforementioned sequence of methodological steps, he observed a significant change in the cancer culture as part of it was induced to emanate at a frequency that was visible through his microscope as being purple-red in color.

The size of the particle was sub-micron in dimensions – namely, $1/20^{th}$ of a micron by $1/15^{th}$ of a micron. According to Rife, the cancer microorganism had four different pleomorphic stages.

The smallest of the discovered microorganisms was labeled "BX" and seemed to be responsible for inducing carcinomas and melanomas involving different kinds of skin cells. A slightly larger version of the same underlying microorganism was referred to as "BY" and it seemed to be related to the emergence of sarcomas (a form of cancer involving connective tissue such as: Fat, cartilage, and bone as well as vascular and blood stem cells). The other two forms of the cancer-related microorganism were a monococcoid form which has been observed to be present in the blood of roughly 90% of all cancer patients, as well as a fungal form of that same underlying microorganism.

All three of the latter forms of the same underlying microorganisms were capable of being transformed into the smallest form of the microorganism – that is BX -- within a period of 36 hours. Once such a transformation had taken place, the resulting BX microorganism was shown to be capable of inducing tumors to develop with all of the attendant pathological characteristics of such tumors, and, in fact, Rife and his colleagues had been able to demonstrate this more than 300 times with precisely the same set of results.

Rife indicated – without necessarily knowing or understanding – that what induced the foregoing transformations to occur had something to do with the nature of the biological terrain in which those forms had been placed, Consequently, the actual cause of cancer was a function of the way such different forms of the same underlying microorganism interacted with or were engaged by the biological terrain in which they were placed.

While Rife maintained that when the terrain of a human body was properly balanced it was not susceptible to any of the foregoing sorts of cancer-related transformational activities taking place, nevertheless, what precisely constituted the character or nature of a properly balanced biological terrain was not clear or necessarily known. In a sense the four forms of the pathogenic microorganism served as the toxic or poisonous inflammatory dynamic that appeared to constitute what might be referred to as necessary conditions, that lacked the sufficient wherewithal to be able to cause cancer, but the precise nature of the conditions that needed to be present in the biological terrain to enable such toxicity to take hold and come to dominance were somewhat elusive.

Once Rife had identified the pleomorphic forms of the underlying microorganism that played a role in the onset of cancer, he went in search of the MOR or specific frequency that was needed to terminate those forms. Through trial and error, he discovered the requisite MOR and proceeded to show that he could terminate such entities irrespective of whether they existed in isolation (that is, outside some sort of biological terrain), as well as when those microorganisms were located within test animals, and, in fact, during the course of his experiments, he was able to accomplish the foregoing process of termination in tests animals more than 400 times.

When the appropriate terminating frequencies were applied, the test animals became free of all cancerous dynamics. They were pathology free – that is, they had been "cured"

The next step involved human trials. While the complete story encompassing the cancer clinic that was held at the University of Southern California in 1934 might never be known because, in one way or another, all of the notes and documents were lost or mysteriously disappeared, nonetheless, there are enough eye-witness accounts of competent and trained observers to provide an overview of what appeared to have taken place.

The frequency treatments did not destroy tissue but only affected the pathological forms of the underlying microorganisms. Moreover, the treatment was found to be completely painless.

Initially, a patient was exposed to the frequency machine for a period of three minutes every day. However, subsequently, Rife and his colleagues discovered that applying the three-minute treatment every third day led to better results.

Apparently, the staggering of the treatment protocol to every third day seemed to provide a patient's body with the time it needed to be able to detoxify (via the lymphatic system) and get rid of the dead carcasses of the pathological microorganisms that were being terminated by the frequency treatment. When the frequency protocol was run every day, this tended to lead toward the detoxification system becoming overwhelmed and, as a result, could lead to problems of toxicity of one kind or another if a given patient's body was not provided with enough time for the build-up of dead microorganisms to be eliminated.

A total of 16 individuals exhibiting an array of cancerous conditions were treated at the University of Southern California in 1934. All of the foregoing individuals had been diagnosed by various medical officials as suffering from conditions of incurable forms of cancer.

Following 3 months of the frequency protocol that had been developed by Rife, 14 of those individuals were pronounced as having been cleared of all traces of cancerous activities, and among the individuals who provided such a clean-bill-of-health determination were a number of prominent pathologists, physicians, microbiologists, and other people who were well-versed in the sciences.

Were any follow-up studies done with the foregoing individuals? I have not come across any evidence indicating that this was done, and, so, of course, there are unanswered questions concerning what the ultimate health status of those individuals might have been 5 or 6 years after the clinic ended in 1934.

Irrespective of what might have been happening with those individuals in relation to the issue of cancer later on in their lives, the purpose of this section of the present chapter has been to not only (a) provide an overview of a very exciting but, unfortunately, an almost completely unknown (save for the research efforts of individuals such as Barry Lynes and Christopher Bird) period of medical history in America, but, as well, (b) for the purposes of the present book, to indicate that Rife and his colleagues had established, once again (following in the empirical footsteps of Béchamp and Enderlein before them) that microorganisms operate in accordance with pleomorphic principles rather than the monomorphic ideas of Pasteur, and, as a result, because the scientific and medical communities in the United States have permitted the dogmatic evangelical, power-seeking ideologues of monomorphism to take control of how biology and medicine are: Taught, researched, written about, and practiced, many pathological conditions – cancer among them – continue to be improperly understood, and, therefore, improperly treated, and it is the public that suffers from such intransigence.

Like Rife, Gaston Naessens (1924 – 2018) was a genius who had: An abiding interest in science; a capacity for incredible inventiveness, as well as a commitment to discovering ways that might either cure an array of pathologies or, at least, help improve the quality of people's lives in substantial ways. Furthermore, like Rife, Gaston Naessens was harassed by medical authorities (e.g., Dr. Augustin Roy) who lacked his intelligence, character, talent, and success.

While still in his twenties (which would have been some 20 years, or so, after Rife had constructed his own ground-breaking microscope in the late 1920s and early 1930s), Naessens – completely independent of Rife's work -- invented a microscope that was as revolutionary in its own way as was the earlier Universal microscope of Royal Rife. The Naessens microscope – which came to be known as the "Somatoscope" – was capable of resolutions down to 15 nanometers. (150 angstroms), and like Rife's Universal microscope, but unlike the electron microscope, the Somatoscope enabled one to observe actual living organisms as they went about their lives and pleomorphic transformations.

The Somatoscope employed principles of optics and physics that still are not completely understood. However, less one suppose that the microscope was an exercise in trickery of some kind, one might note that individuals such as Rolf Wieland, who served as the head of microscopy for the internationally acclaimed German optics firm Carl Zeiss indicated in 1989, after having had an opportunity to work with the Naessens instrument, that he considered the Somatoscope to be a significant improvement in light microscopy.

One might also note that the Somatoscope was capable of resolutions that were far superior to microscopes that were being constructed some forty years later than the time in the 1950s when

Naessens came up with his invention. For example, the World Research Foundation announced in 1990 that it was releasing the Ergonom-400 microscope that was capable of magnifying objects some 25,000 times (which was actually less than the what had been achieved by Rife's Universal microscope) and which had a capacity to resolve objects down to 100 nanometers (1000 Angstroms) ... some 85 nanometers (and 850 Angstroms) less than what Naessens microscope was capable of achieving.

The reason why the Somatoscope carries the name it does is because of the ultramicroscopic entities that Naessens discovered through the use of his optical invention. More specifically, in the blood of human beings as well as in the sap of plants, Naessens had observed a subcellular microorganism that was capable of reproduction and whose existence was entirely unknown prior to Naessens discoveries. Naessens referred to this organism as a "somatid" (tiny body).

Somatids were capable of being cultured independently of a host body or cell. In addition he found that they were pleomorphic in character – that is, they were capable of changing their forms of morphology and functioning during the course of their life cycle.

In fact, he determined that in healthy individuals, the somatid only underwent the first three pleomorphic transformations of a total of some 16-plus possibilities. However, in sick individuals, one could observe one or more of the other 13, or so, possible transformations, and which of these possibilities became manifest was functionally dependant on the condition of the biological terrain in which they existed.

Notwithstanding the importance of discoveries made by Béchamp, Enderlein, and Rife, Naessens, brought a level of detail to the study of pleomorphism and its varied roles within the lives of human beings (both apathogenically as well as pathogenically) that had not been attained by any of his predecessors. Naessens not only was confirming the earlier work of Rife, Enderlein, and Béchamp while also disconfirming the "research" of Louis Pasteur, but, he also was adding significant, additional information.

The pleomorphic life cycle of the somatid involved such entities as: Spores, double spores, bacterial forms, double bacterial forms, rod forms, microbial globular forms, yeast forms, fungal forms, mycelial forms, and fungal filaments – each of which had different morphological features as well as different biological functions. Naessens maintained that if one knew how to read the somatid cycle in the blood of an individual, one could determine what manner of pathology was likely to emerge up to 18 months in advance of overt symptomology.

Naessens considered the microzymas that had been discovered and observed by Béchamp to be larger "cousins" of the much smaller somatid. Presumably, Enderlein's notion of spermits, protits, or endobionts might also be close relations, of one kind or another, to the primordial somatid.

Naessens ran the somatid through a number of experiments, and it seemed to have a relatively indestructible nature. For example, acid seemed to have no effect on somatids, and, furthermore, the outer aspect of a somatid seemed to be impervious to a diamond-tip drill.

Somatids also appeared to be capable of withstanding, without adverse effect, normally lethal exposures of as high as 50,000 rems of radioactive exposure. Moreover, somatids also seemed to be able to retain a full range of functionality after having been heated to temperatures such as 200 degrees Centigrade (392 degrees Fahrenheit).

Like Béchamp's microzymas, somatids are believed to survive the decay and decomposition of a biological organism. Thus, just as Béchamp discovered microzymas in limestone samples taken from the Earth that were gauged to be some 60 million years old, and just as he detected the presence of microzymas in samples of street dust and chimney soot, so too, somatids are believed to be present in every part of an ecological system.

Nonetheless, the origins of both microzymas and somatids, along with the spermits/protits of Enderlein are unknown. Moreover, what kind of dynamics transpires within such entities is largely unknown.

According to Naessens, somatids exhibit electrical properties. More specifically, the inner dimension of the particle appears to be positively charged, whereas the exterior portion of that particle is negatively charged.

When somatids are immersed within a liquid environment such as blood plasma, the particles repulse one another. This resonates with the behavior of healthy cells within a similar sort of liquid environment – namely, the cells tend to repel one another,

However, Naessens indicates that the charge associated with a somatid is actually much larger than what one finds in conjunction with cells. In fact, Naessens considers somatids to be energy condensers that might be able to underwrite, or make possible, various kinds of energy dynamics.

Naessens believed that the possibility of life was dependent on the presence of somatids. He maintained that while somatids could exist independently of life, he did not believe that life could exist independently of somatids, but what the precise nature of that relationship actually might be appears to be, at the present time, shrouded in mystery.

He contends that for each organ of our bodies, there are somatids that are unique to, and which service, that organ and only that organ. Furthermore, all of the different kinds of somatids that are dedicated to various kinds of organs are simultaneously present in either the circulatory system and/or the lymphatic system.

Experiments have been conducted by Naessens in which he has extracted the somatids from a white-furred rabbit and transferred those somatids at the rate of one cubic centimeter per day for two successive weeks into the bloodstream of a rabbit with black fur. Within a period of about a month, Naessens indicates that the hair of the formerly black-furred rabbit will become lighter as roughly half of the hairs making up the fur continue to be black while the other half of the hairs making up the fur of the previously black-furred rabbit will have turned white.

Naessens indicates that the reverse of the foregoing transformation can also take place. All one has to do is start with the somatids from a black-furred rabbit and transfer those somatids to the bloodstream of a white-furred rabbit in accordance with the indicated rate and for the designated length of time, and one will end up with a gray-colored rabbit with half of the hairs of the previously all white rabbit continuing to remain white while the other hairs that make up the fur will have become black.

As interesting as the foregoing experiment is, it is not the most interesting discovery that was made in conjunction with such experiments. If one cuts roughly the same size patch of skin from rabbits that have undergone the aforementioned process of somatid transfer, and, then, one takes the skin patch of the rabbit from which somatids have been extracted and, then, grafts its patch of skin onto the body of the rabbit to which somatids have been transferred, the graft will exhibit none of the traditional signs of rejection.

If the foregoing experiment can be verified and expanded upon, the implications for the whole issue of organ transplants and accompanying rejection issues might become a thing of the past. Unfortunately, because medical orthodoxy has been so resistant to Naessens research and his discovery of the pleomorphic nature of the somatid life cycle, such orthodox practitioners seem willing to place their patients at risk so that such practitioners can save their own vested interests.

Somatids are viral-like in size. Yet, given the right kind of biological conditions, they are capable of all manner of pleomorphic transformations, and, therefore, they were not viral-like in functionality. In other words, they could survive and function independently of host cells, and, furthermore, during certain stages of the somatid cycle they were capable of exhibiting bacterial-like properties despite being able to resist the process of being filtered from a given sample.

From the perspective of toxicity or exhibiting poisonous properties, many stages of the somatid cycle resonate with the original etymological sense of the term "virus". In other words, many of those somatid stages give expression to entities or forms that have toxic properties or potentials, but all of those somatid stages exhibit a capacity for independent activity and, therefore, are not dependent on the cellular mechanisms of other organisms to carry out those activities as is required by viruses in the modern sense of the word.

Consequently, while somatids are capable of assuming morphological forms on the sub-micron or nano scales, and while they have the capacity to give expression to toxic/poisonous properties under certain condition, nonetheless, somatids are not viruses in the modern sense of the term. As such, they are a non-viral form of microorganism, because no viral species – theoretical or otherwise – has the properties, potentials, and capabilities of somatids.

Naessens refers to somatids as being precursors to DNA. However, what this means or entails is not at all clear.

In fact, the notion that somatids are precursors to DNA raises at least one important question. Given that the 16-plus stages to which the aforementioned pleomorphic cycle of a somatid gives expression, and given that RNA and DNA capabilities are present in the entities that are present in the bacterial, fungal and other kinds of biological forms that make up the components of that cycle, then, exactly how does such DNA/RNA capability arise if somatids – in their most primordial form -- are said to be precursors to DNA?

During a relatively brief discussion encompassing issues of viruses (in the modern sense of the term), evolution, and somatids that takes place fairly early in the book by Christopher Bird entitled: *The Persecution and Trial of Gaston Naessens*, there is reference to a report in the August 10th, 1989 edition of the British journal *Nature* concerning the alleged discovery – apparently for the first time – of large quantities of viruses (some 2.5 million such entities per liter) in unpolluted seawaters. Prior to the appearance of the Nature article by Ovind Bergh and his colleagues at the University of Bergin in Norway, biologists, apparently, had always believed that seawater contained extremely low concentrations of viruses.

According to the *Nature* article, the entities that were found by Bergh and his colleagues were less than 1.2 micros in size. This is roughly equivalent in size to some of the larger somatid forms that been discovered and observed by Naessens.

There are several problems with the foregoing considerations. For example, although the entities that were found in the seawater were referred to as viruses, how were the identities of the entities confirmed to be viruses? Were they dismantled, sequenced and demonstrated to consist of only DNA or RNA encapsulated within a protein package of some sort and nothing more?

How can one be sure that whatever entities were found in the unpolluted seawater weren't somatids or endobionts (e.g., spermits or protits) of some kind? Perhaps, they were maybe even samples of microzymas.

How does one know that what had been discovered by the Norwegian research group were viruses? Were all 2.5 million entities per liter examined?

Furthermore what is the basis of the supposed claim by biologists that prior to the Bergh "discovery", unpolluted seawater was believed to contain only small amounts of viral entities? Does such a prior belief give expression to an actual empirical determination or is it just an unsupported conjecture that is awaiting empirical confirmation, and, if so, then, in point of fact, the alleged discovery of Bergh and his colleagues actually suggests that whatever the supposed empirical basis is for claiming that seawater was believed to contain low amounts of viruses is, obviously, actually wrong and had no real empirical basis.

The Norwegian researchers that wrote the *Nature* article are excited – and Christopher Bird is including reference to that study in his book with a similar sort of curiosity -- because they all believe they might have opened up a theoretical possibility which accounts for how DNA or RNA might have become dissolved in seawater in large amounts and, thereby, become sources for subsequent genetic experimentation in the open waters. However, to put first things first, before one begins to calculate the genetic possibilities that might come in the form of dissolved DNA from alleged viral entities in seawater, perhaps, one might explain how such a complex molecule as DNA was able to arise and find its ways into such an encapsulated particle. Furthermore, without being able to rigorously prove that one is, in fact, dealing with viruses -- rather than, say, somatids, spermits, protits, or microzymas -- in the unpolluted seawater samples one is examining, then one might want to exercise a bit more scientific caution concerning what one believes one has found and what the theoretical ramifications of such a "finding" might be.

One might note in passing – although this is hardly the sort of thing that ought to be dismissed so quickly – that Naessens had discovered a formula that was capable of treating, among other things, an array of pathological disorders, including cancer. The compound, was given the name "714-X" (the "7" stood for the 7th letter of the alphabet -- "G," the first initial of his first name -- while the 14 stood for the 14th letter of the alphabet – "N," the first initial of his second name, and the X stood for the 24th letter of the alphabet and symbolized his year of birth – 1924).

Just as Rife ran into trouble with medical authorities as a result of his successes – rather than failures – in treating cancer, and just as Dr. Frederick Koch had been harassed by the American Medical Association for having developed a treatment for cancer -- namely, glyoxylide (an article – "Glyoxylide: A Cure For Cancer" appeared in the December 3, 1936 edition of the *New England Journal of Medicine*) and, subsequently, in the 1940s was forced to migrate to Brazil (a situation that national columnist Drew Pearson referred to as one of the biggest scandals in the history of American medicine), and just as Dr. Stanislaw Burzynski has been harassed constantly for more than 50 years by medical authorities in both federal and state governments as a result of having had success using antineoplaston (amino acid-based) compounds in the treatment of cancer, and just as Dr. Nicholas Gonzalez was harassed by an array of medical authorities for having developed a diet and supplement-based way of successfully treating various kinds of cancer, so too, Gaston Naessens was harassed by Canadian medical authorities (Dr. Augustin Roy among others) for his success, rather than failures, in treating cancer – and many of the cases he treated were diagnoses as being terminal in nature.

What Rife, Koch, Burzynski, Gonzalez, and Naessens (there also are others who could be added to this list) all shared in common was the development of a form of treatment – although the nature of the protocols being used as different for each of those individuals – which was capable of achieving successful outcomes in conjunction with the treatment of, among other kinds of maladies, cancer. What the opponents of the foregoing individuals all had in common was an inability to cure cancer, and in fact, their legacy of a "cut, burn, and poison" approach to cancer has been, for the most part an abject failure, wasting billions of dollars and costing millions of lives across more than a hundred years.

As far as the current book is concerned, rather than becoming entangled in issues of cancer treatment, I am most interested in the way in which one can go from the research of Béchamp, and, then, proceed on through the research of Enderlein, Rife, and Naessens and be able to empirically substantiate the existence of a long-standing scientific tradition that is not only capable of demonstrating how microorganisms are pleomorphic in nature, but, as well, can show that the theory of germs introduced by Louis Pasteur and adopted by much of subsequent science and medicine is without reliable foundation. However, to the extent that cancer treatments have been mentioned in the present chapter, this has been done to indicate that while some individuals (Enderlein, Rife, and Naessens – among others) have had success in the treatment of cancer, nonetheless they have been harassed because of that very success by a cadre of authorities who insist – for ignoble reasons – on working against the former individuals , and, therefore, one is confronted by a very fundamental issues – namely, the kind of theory of medicine that one uses to frame experience can have a huge impact – both constructively and destructively – on how one engages the idea of pathology and, therefore, how patients are treated.

To whatever extent one wishes to frame the world of microorganisms through the monomorphic lenses of Pasteur's theory of germs, one is introducing frames of obfuscation that are hiding, if not distorting, information which alters what one sees and how one sees that which one is permitted to see. To whatever extent one wishes to engage the world of microorganisms through the pleomorphic lenses of Béchamp, Enderlein, Rife, and Naessens, one is being introduced to forms of framing that disclose a great deal more accurate information than is available through the lenses of a monomorphic approach to microbiology.

I remember watching a video featuring Dr. Barre Lando in which he was discussing different facets of his medical training background. He indicated that at one point during his development as a would-be healer he had gone to Canada to study with Naessens and that, from time to time, symposia of one kind or another would be organized by Naessens and his associates for purposes of, among other things, providing interested or curious individuals with an opportunity to be exposed to, in a hands-on manner, concerning the power and capabilities of the Somatoscope, as well as to offer them a chance to explore the world of somatids, the somatid cycle, and other facets of pleomorphism,

On such occasions, Dr. Lando indicated that a variety of people with medical backgrounds from Canada and/or the United States would attend those gatherings. They would be instructed in the use of the Somatoscope and be shown, among other possibilities, some of the dynamics of pleomorphic transformations that could be observed with that instrument. However, even though, invariably, those individuals would marvel at what they, via the Somatoscope, were seeing and, therefore, were unable to deny what their eyes and minds were showing them to be real phenomena, nonetheless, they also indicated that they would never be able to divulge what they were seeing when they returned to their respective practices because they would be running the risk of promoting a perspective that countermanded medical orthodoxy and, as a result, this would likely open themselves up to the possibility of being sanctioned or penalized in one way or another by members of that orthodoxy.

Chapter 6: **The Great Influenza**

Having read John M. Barry's book: *The Great Influenza: The Story of the Deadliest Pandemic in History*, I must admit that I was somewhat confused when, subsequently, I reflected on the many laudatory blurbs that prefaced the pages of his publication. For example, the person who reviewed the book on behalf of the *Journal of the American Medical Association* stated that: "I loved the range of this book, how it directs a searchlight on science and scientists ...."

The foregoing sort of statement confused me because I didn't feel the book in question had all that much science in it and, furthermore, most of the so-called "scientists" that were mentioned and discussed in Barry's book were, for the most part, individuals who were part of the power structure in allopathic medicine that – thanks to Rockefeller -- was imposing itself on America during the time of the supposed 'great influenza' in 1918-1919, Unfortunately, during that power grab, many of those individuals rather vigorously suppressed, as well as oppressed, a great deal of science along with a variety of alternative approaches to medicine that were present in America at, and prior to, the aforementioned period of time.

Presumably, any person who wishes to be referred to as a scientist ought to be someone who actually is open to looking -- in an objective and critical reflective manner -- at all of the available evidence that might be entailed by a given topic. Yet, the vast majority of the individuals being placed in such a glimmering manner through the alleged spotlight shining forth from Barry's aforementioned book were individuals who had uncritically adopted Pasteur's perspective concerning a monomorphic theory of germs without, apparently, having any direct understanding with respect to what the quality, or lack thereof, in Pasteur's work and character might have been.

There is not one mention of either Antoine Béchamp or Günther Enderlein in Barry's book, despite the fact that Béchamp completed his research in bacteriology more than a decade before the so-called 'Great Influenza' and, in addition, Enderlein had started to expand upon the work of Béchamp approximately four years before the so-called 'Great Influenza'. On the other hand, the name Pasteur appears at least 34 times during the course of Barry's work.

In addition, neither the terms: "pleiomorphic" ("pleomorphic") nor monomorphic seem to occur within the pages of Barry's book. However, the phrase: "germ theory" occurs 28 times in that same book but the phrase is presented entirely without any historical, scientific, or medical context that indicates there were two entirely different approaches to the nature, function, and significance of bacteria.

In other words, no indication is given that there is a significant difference between, the perspectives of, as well as evidence concerning, Pasteur and Béchamp. On the one hand, based on very little and often questionable data, Pasteur presents a monomorphic theory of germs in which bacteria and other possible microbiological entities supposedly invade human beings (and other organisms) from without (i.e., the surrounding environment) and infected the latter in a manner that led to the emergence of some sort of pathology of varying degrees of severity within the invaded organism. On the other hand, based on a great deal of quite substantial evidence, Béchamp's pleiomorphic/pleomorphic account indicates that bacteria are capable of changing their morphology and function according to the nature of the conditions in which they existed.

Therefore, when the biological terrain of, say, a human being changed due to exposure to some form of toxicity or poisoning, such changes are capable of inducing pleiomorphic/pleomorphic organisms to undergo morphological and functional changes. These sorts of changes sometimes exacerbated the pathological changes that already had occurred in the biological terrain of a given human being independently of such pleiomorphic/pleomorphic transitions.

Enderlein had been expanding on and developing Béchamp's pleiomorphic/pleomorphic perspective for some four years before the so-called 'Great Influenza" struck. Yet, as indicated previously, Barry's book is devoid of any reference to that research.

Just as Béchamp had been able to generate, in his own methodological manner, a considerable amount of concrete evidence in support of the reality of pleiomorphism/pleomorphism, so too, Enderlein had managed, through the use of darkfield microscopy, to contribute a great deal of evidence in support of the idea of pleiomorphism/pleomorphism. However, Pasteur had produced no real hard, concrete evidence to indicate that bacteria were inherently monomorphic and, therefore, were incapable of changing either their morphology or their function in response to changing conditions within the biological terrain in which they existed, nor did Pasteur have any actual evidence to demonstrate that microbiological entities invaded human beings from without or used that process of invasion to, first, infect and, then, generate symptoms within an invaded host.

Furthermore, Pasteur had claimed that the blood of healthy human beings was sterile and, therefore, contained no microorganisms. Yet, both Antoine Béchamp as well as Günther Enderlein had published work indicating that the blood of even healthy human beings was not sterile when it came to the presence of microorganisms of one kind or another.

A reviewer of *The Great Influenza* wrote in *Nature* that: "Barry's writing ... manages{s} to capture the science of virology ...," while another individual proclaims in a *New York Review of Books* entry that: "The fact is that flu is one of the most formidable infections confronting humankind. The virus mutates constantly as it circulates among birds, pigs, and human beings, so each new flu season now challenges experts." Perhaps, *Nature* and the *New York Review of Books* should have selected other people to write their respective reviews of Barry's book because, as will be shown in a number of subsequent chapters, virology is not, and has never really been, a science, and, in addition, there actually is no concrete evidence to demonstrate that flu, or any disease, is caused by viruses.

Both of the foregoing reviewers have confused the notion of theoretical narrative with the idea of scientific facts. This is because they seem to have failed to understand that Barry's book is largely an exercise in framing in which a narrative about a medical theory is portrayed as being an expression of actual science when this is not the case.

In many ways, although I am sure that John Barry would disagree with the following characterization, his book on the 'Great Influenza' is actually an account of the manner in which there was a complete failure among the practitioners of allopathic medicine to deal with a crisis in public health in 1918-1919. Moreover, perhaps the primary reason for such a failure is that they had little understanding of the way in which living organisms actually work – as Enderlein had once said: "Medicine knows a lot about diseases but nothing about life."

I believe one would be well-advised to engage Barry's book through the following orientation. In 1918-1919, viruses did not exist in the modern sense.

In other words, viruses at that time were not considered to be sequences of either DNA or RNA – but not both – which are encapsulated within a glycoprotein coating (amino acid sequences –- protein aspect –- with oligosaccharide chains –- the 'glyco' aspect). Viruses at the time of the 'Great Influenza" were believed to constitute poisons or toxins of an unknown nature that were capable of by-passing the filtration processes that were known to be able to remove bacteria-sized entities from a given fluid sample such as blood.

Therefore, although there were certain experiments that had been conducted prior to 1918-1919 that seemed to suggest the possibility of something like a virus in the modern sense, nevertheless, the notion of a virus a hundred years ago was largely theoretical in nature, and it was used as a way of accounting for certain kinds of pathological conditions in those instances when all known bacteria were believed to have been removed from a fluid or tissue sample related to such pathology.

Given the foregoing considerations, one cannot automatically suppose that the medical practitioners back in 1918-1919 should be understood as individuals who were heroically trying to deal with the impact of a virus in the modern sense but who, unfortunately, were hamstrung, so to speak, because the electron microscope and the molecular biology of the gene had not yet been invented, and, therefore, they just couldn't understand what it was that they were dealing with or how to engage it. While medical practitioners back in those days did have a few theories about what might cause influenza-like pathologies, the reality of their situation is that they were flying blind and had no idea what was causing the phenomena they were encountering in their patients in 1918-1919.

Furthermore, one also might be well-advised to avoid trying to engage the events about which Barry is writing through the lenses of modern virology in an attempt to make sense, retroactively, of what might have been happening in 1918-1919. While using the modern theory of virology to, supposedly, illuminate past events might help one to create a narrative that seems to enlighten one with respect to what might have been taking place over a hundred years ago, one should be sure that the light one is using to accomplish such a task is reliable and does not distort what one is trying to see, and as subsequent chapters of the present book will attempt to demonstrate, the modern theory of virology is anything but reliable when it comes to providing a scientifically demonstrable way of understanding what happened over a hundred years ago, let alone necessarily being a medium that is capable of accurately reflecting what might be transpiring today.

Clearly, on the basis of what John Barry has written in his book *The Great Influenza: The Story of the Greatest Pandemic in History*, he does appear to believe that everything which supposedly occurred in 1918-1919 can only be properly understood when engaged through the lenses of modern virology. In other words, he believes that the plethora of illnesses and deaths which occurred a little over a hundred years ago was the result of a flu virus that had mutated in a way to which human beings had not, yet, adapted and, therefore, to which they were highly vulnerable or susceptible.

Yet, oddly enough, the foregoing perspective is unable to make sense of a crucial and central series of experiments that had been run during the period 1918-1919. More specifically, several groups of "volunteers" (prisoners) were selected, first in Boston, and, then, subsequently, in San Francisco (100, or so, people were in each group).

Those individuals were exposed to different fluids and tissues from patients who, supposedly, had the flu and who were described as being in various stages of the disease, ranging from mild to severe. They were described as exhibiting an array of symptoms associated with what was being referred to as, or which had been diagnosed as, cases of influenza.

Materials from ill people were gargled by volunteers, and the latter individuals also were coughed on, as well as breathed on, for extended periods of time at close-quarters, and also doused with a variety of bodily fluids of the aforementioned influenza patients. Not one of the volunteers ever became sick.

So, if "the" cause of the pathologies that were occurring in 1918-1919 were due to a mutated virus that was highly infectious, virulent, and lethal for human beings who, supposedly, were particularly susceptible to those "germs" because people had not encountered such a germ previously or had not, yet, become adapted/immune to it, then why did none of the volunteers become sick with "influenza" or come down with any other pathological condition during the aforementioned experiments? On the basis of the foregoing series of experiments that took place on both coasts of the United States, whatever seemed to be taking place in 1918-1919 did not appear to be spread through exposure to the bodily fluids and other biological samples emanating from ill people, and, therefore, one has to seriously question whether a virus of some kind was responsible for what took place during the so-called Spanish Flu.

There are ways of accounting for what might have transpired in 1918-1919 other than by means of the idea of an infectious, lethal virus of some kind. For example, as was indicated in an earlier book if mine – *Observations Concerning My Encounter with COVID-19 (?)* – how Arthur Firstenberg put forth a great deal of evidence in his book *The Invisible Rainbow* to support the idea that many people in 1918-1919 might well have been suffering the effects of radio frequency poisoning that was due to the newly developed, and recently deployed, military radio transmitters that were able to project, powerful signals over vast distances ... signals which could be detected in many locations around the world.

The sorts of debilitating conditions that can ensue from exposure to electromagnetic poisoning have been shown to be very much like the kinds of pathological conditions that are attributed to the effects of alleged viruses. Since evidence indicates that some individuals are much more susceptible to experiencing adverse biological effects due to the presence of those kinds of transmissions than are other individuals (it is estimated that some 5% of the population are quite sensitive to the presence of such transmissions), then, perhaps, many of the people who became ill, and died, during the period of 1918-1919 might have been from among the aforementioned vulnerable group of radio frequency sensitive individuals.

Furthermore, one might note that environmental forms of poisoning – such as that which might be produced through exposure to radio frequencies -- generate results that are easy to mistake for, or confuse with, the phenomena of contagion. In other words, when a group of people in a given area are exposed to an environmental poison of some kind, a fair number of them might become ill, and, as a result, a medical observer might interpret such a cluster of illnesses to constitute evidence that a contagious disease of some kind is present and is being passed from person to person when, in reality, the illnesses that are occurring are because a group of people were exposed – perhaps at different times and, consequently, not everyone will necessarily become ill at the same time – to a toxic agent of some kind in their environment.

Furthermore, given the proven pleiomorphic/pleomorphic nature of microorganisms that are present in the body (something that was demonstrated again and again by both Antoine Béchamp as well as Günther Enderlein long before the advent of the so-called Spanish Flu) -- and given the proven manner in which the morphology and function of those organisms can be induced to change as a result of certain kinds of shifts in the biological terrain in which they exist (for example, the tissues and organs of a human being – and, again, this is something that was demonstrated again and again by Antoine Béchamp as well as Günther Enderlein long before the events of 1918-1919), then, one also should take into consideration the possibility that exposure to certain kinds of radio frequencies can poison the biological terrain of a human being, and, therefore, perhaps, the presence of such toxicity could induce microorganisms that are normally in a constructive, symbiotic relationship with a given biological terrain to change and become pathogenic in one way or another.

If someone is unaware of, or does not understand, the nature of the pleiomorphic/pleomorphic cycles that occur in microorganisms within the human body, then, such an individual might identify the microorganisms that have been induced to change their morphology and function as a result of the toxicity that has been introduced into the surrounding biological terrain by something such as radio wave poisoning as being responsible for the pathology which is occurring.

An alternative possibility, however, is that the poisoning of the biological terrain of an individual by a certain kind of electromagnetic toxicity might have induced those normally symbiotic microorganisms to become pathogenic.

Not all people are highly sensitive or vulnerable to the presence of radio frequency poisoning, and, therefore, not everyone will necessarily get sick. Perhaps the biological terrain of some individuals is better able to detoxify -- and, therefore, eliminate in one way or another -- the toxic ramifications which may follow from radio frequency poisoning.

There are additional possibilities beyond the idea of radio wave poisoning which are also able to account for at least some of the substantial death tolls that appear to have taken place in 1918-1919. For instance, aspirin was a common treatment for individuals with flu-like symptoms, but there is also considerable evidence to indicate that aspirin was often administered in toxic doses that either killed the recipient of those dosages or sufficiently debilitated them so that they became vulnerable to an array of other pathologies that might arise in a biological terrain that had been poisoned through the administering of excessive doses of aspirin.

One also needs to consider the possibility that American and European communities were not properly prepared or equipped to deal with a public health crisis of the magnitude that supposedly occurred during 1918-1919. There simply were not enough competent doctors, nurses, and/or support staff to look after the people who became ill, nor were there adequate sets of facilities, equipment, supplies, medicines, and/or food available in many communities to be able to provide what was needed to properly attend to the ill and dying.

Anyone who has researched the events of 1918-1919 will have come across photos of huge rooms or spaces that were filled with rows and rows and rows of beds occupied by sick individuals. Anyone who supposes that those people were all receiving the very best of care and that such overcrowded conditions were conducive to recovery from whatever was ailing them has not grasped the many logistical and medical problems that permeate those sorts of settings, and consequently, affect the quality of medical treatment – or lack thereof -

-- problems that also must be taken into consideration as a potential source of lethality in the lives of many people during the period 1918-1919.

There are still other ways to account for many deaths during the so-called "Spanish Flu". For instance, one of the hallmarks of allopathic medicine is its inclination to inject people with all manner of materials irrespective of whether anyone knows what will happen in the short or long run as a result of those sorts of injections. Thousands of the patients in 1918-1919 were military people who had been mandated to receive a multiplicity of anti-venom and serum injections.

Many of those anti-venoms and serums already had proven to be highly toxic for various people when taken individually. Unfortunately, there was little, or no, evidence to determine what the effect would be when such materials were received in the form of a series of injections given one after the other.

It is the nature of the allopathic mentality to claim credit whenever its medical experiments seem – however debatable this might be -- to lead to positive outcomes. However, another facet of the allopathic mentality is to exercise considerable denial and engage in the dynamics of blame shifting whenever medical experiments have tragic results.

Inadequate personnel, supplies, equipment, facilities, and medicines, as well as problematic forms of medical treatment, could all have come together in a perfect storm of tragic circumstances and caused the death of thousands of people in 1918-1919. All of the foregoing factors would have been capable of introducing additional forms of toxicity into the biological terrains of already ill patients, and this would take place quite independently of whatever the nature of their illness or illnesses might be that original caused people to seek out medical care.

The foregoing dynamics of deterioration within the biological terrains of patients would have induced microorganisms that were present in such toxic terrains to enter other morphological and functional stages of their pleiomorphic/pleomorphic cycles. However, doctors, nurses and other medical personnel who were operating out of the allopathic sphere of influence – with its monomorphic presuppositions -- would not permit themselves to accept the idea that microorganisms were capable of changing their morphology and functioning at different stages of their pleiomorphic/pleomorphic cycles. Consequently, they would have had absolutely no understanding of why certain forms of microorganisms were suddenly appearing in their patients or what the significance of the presence of those sorts of microorganisms might be.

For example, without even knowing what he actually might be saying, Barry's book actually makes an oblique reference to the foregoing considerations when it indicates: "... bacteria that almost never caused pneumonia were now making their way unopposed into the lungs, growing there, and thriving there" (page 317 of the Kindle edition of *The Great Influenza*). A monomorphic approach to microorganisms would tend to struggle to try to explain in any sort of plausible fashion what the sorts of bacteria to which Barry is alluding in his book were doing in the lungs. On the other hand, a pleiomorphic/pleomorphic account of that same information would engage it from the perspective of anticipating that there would be transitions in the morphological and functional nature of a given microorganism as a result of having been induced to enter into a particular stage of its pleiomorphic/pleomorphic cycle due to the toxicity present in a patient's biological terrain which could have been caused by any number of possibilities (From: EMF poisoning, to: inappropriate treatments such as toxic doses of aspirin or the toxicity introduced into someone's biological terrain as a result of an array of anti-venoms and serums, along with inadequate treatment protocols and facilities).

Much of the first hundred pages, or more, of John Barry's book are either about the people and circumstances that assisted allopathic medicine to become the dominant approach to engaging pathology in America, or are about some of the politics and ideological orientations that shaped the mood and mentality surrounding the war that was present in the world leading up to and including the period 1918-1919. I'll have a little more to say about the relevance of the 1910 Flexner Report in relation to the rise of allopathic medicine in America toward the latter part of the present chapter, but, for now, I would like to take a look at some of what Barry has to say about the nature of influenza and pneumonia.

Barry begins by indicating that pneumonia tends to be described as a condition of inflammation within the lungs that if it is permitted to progress unopposed will tend to lead to a consolidating sort of dynamic in which lung tissue that is generally soft and elastic, becomes hardened and inelastic. He goes on to indicate that while the foregoing sort of definition does not mention the idea of infection, nonetheless, he contends that most instances of pneumonia are the result of some kind of microorganism that has invaded and infected the lungs.

While I have no doubt that any number of medical personnel would agree with Barry's characterization concerning the nature and cause of most pneumonia, I would like to offer a counter possibility for consideration. To begin with, for example, one might note that there are, in fact, a variety of forms of pneumonia that are not causally attributed to the presence of microorganisms of any kind, and given this piece of information, one might revisit Barry's characterization of pneumonia as primarily being due to the presence of invading bacteria and ask the following question: Namely, are the microorganisms that are found to be present in cases of pneumonia the cause of the pneumonia or is the presence of those microorganisms caused by the condition of pneumonia?

If one accepts the monomorphic theory of microorganisms along with its accompanying theory of germs that was postulated by Pasteur in the late 1800s, then, the answer to the foregoing question is that the microorganisms are present because they somehow were able to successfully invade the biological terrain of a human being and subsequently set about generating the infection that leads to the condition of inflammation that is known as pneumonia. However, if one accepts the pleiomorphic/pleomorphic account of microorganisms, then, it is possible that something of an unknown nature (e.g., some sort of environmental toxin, poison, or pollutant, including radio wave toxicity) caused the initial inflammation or irritation that set in motion a series of bodily defenses, one of which involves a toxic-terrain induced transduction of one, or more, pleiomorphic/pleomorphic microorganisms that is – are -- present in that terrain but which (as a result of the dynamics of the microorganism's pleiomorphic/pleomorphic cycle) is transformed into a bacterial form that might be at the scene of the inflammation for known or unknown reasons – some of which might be pathogenic in nature -- but the presence of such microorganisms does not necessarily prove that they are the cause of the initial inflammation that led to condition of pneumonia.

To be sure, the presence of such transduced microorganisms might give rise to certain kinds of symptoms, and, conceivably, the introduction of, for example, antibiotics might result in the reduction or disappearance of those sorts of symptoms. However, unless one had an understanding of pleiomorphic/pleomorphic dynamics with respect to such a microorganism, one might not actually know why such changes occurred when they did or what the significance of those changes might be and whether, or not, there might be alternative ways of treating the symptoms that might arise when such microorganisms are present ... forms of treatment that did not involve antibiotics.

One might keep in mind how in the previous chapter Gaston Naessens was described as someone who believed that each kind of organ or tissue had its own modality of somatid with a concomitant pleiomorphic/pleomorphic cycle. Moreover, such cycles had as many as 16 or 17 stages.

According to Naessens, only the first three stages of that cycle occurred in healthy individuals, but when a person's biological terrain became toxic for whatever reason, then, a relevant somatid particle would undergo – according to the condition of the surrounding biological terrain – some mode of transformation into one, or another, of the other pleiomorphic/pleomorphic stages. Which form of microorganism manifested itself under those circumstances would dictate what kind of treatment would be used to respond to the morphological and functional transitions that were taking place in the somatid cycle.

In the previous chapter it was also indicated that Günther Enderlein had developed his own understanding of the pleiomorphic/pleomorphic cycle of microorganisms. According to Enderlein, the changes that a given microorganism underwent, would determine the aspect of Sanum Therapy that would be followed and which was intended to deal with various kinds of transitions in the endobionts that were present ... treatments which helped the individual to work her or his way back to, or be helped to be brought back to, a state of well-being in which all forms of toxicity would have been removed from the biological terrain of that person and endobionts would return to their normal, symbiotic forms of functioning.

John Barry claims that: "Influenza causes pneumonia either directly, by a massive viral invasion of the lungs, or indirectly – and more commonly – by destroying certain parts of the body's defenses and allowing so-called secondary invaders, bacteria, to infest the lungs virtually unopposed." (Page 152 of the Kindle edition of: *The Great Influenza*). However, if – as I believe the next four chapters will demonstrate – viruses do not actually exist, then, Barry's foregoing statement will have to be altered because there actually is no evidence to indicate that something called a "virus" in the modern sense actually exists and is capable – outside of theory – of invading the lungs or destroying certain parts of the body's defenses, and, in the wake of such destruction, open up an individual's body to secondary infections from bacteria.

If viruses do not exist, then, the cause of the sorts of pneumonia to which Barry is alluding is actually idiopathic in nature. In other words the actual cause of the sort of inflammation that is called pneumonia is not known, although one might keep in mind that radio frequency poisoning is capable of interfering with and undermining lung functioning.

Moreover, given the foregoing considerations, then, whatever bacterial forms of microorganism might show up at the site of that sort of inflammation is not necessarily because there has been some massive invasion from an influenza virus which has destroyed important facets of a person's defense network but, rather, this is because the presence of the inflammation in the aspects of the biological terrain that are known as the lungs has induced changes in the pleiomorphic/pleomorphic cycle of whatever microorganism, microzyma (Béchamp), endobiont (Enderlein), or somatid (Naessens) that is present in, or which arrives in response to, the inflammation that exists in the lungs. Understood from the foregoing perspective, influenza is not a viral infection, but, rather, it is an idiopathic condition that often is accompanied by symptoms of respiratory distress which, if severe enough, might be diagnosed as constituting a form of inflammation that is referred to as pneumonia or a condition that is pneumonia-like. Moreover, the presence of bacterial forms of microorganism at the site of inflammation does not necessarily indicate that the inflammation was caused by such microorganisms but, instead, the presence of those microorganisms might just have been a matter of having introduced an added layer of complexity to the condition of inflammation that could be treated in a variety of ways.

Chapter Fourteen of John Barry's book begins with an account of how influenza might have emerged at Camp Funston, a US Army training facility located on Fort Riley, southwest of Manhattan Kansas. According to Barry, although the evidence in support of such an account is circumstantial, nonetheless, he believes the case is strong.

Barry cites the names of three individuals – John Bottom, Dean Nilson, and Ernest Elliot – who travelled from Haskell County, Kansas to Camp Funston during late February or early March of 1918. Apparently, a virulent form of influenza had taken hold in Haskell County, and, according to Barry, one, or more, of the aforementioned individuals might have transported the alleged influenza-causing virus to Camp Funston.

By introducing the term "virus" into his account and by claiming that influenza is caused by a virus, Barry is not reporting circumstantial evidence but is actually creating the illusion that such evidence is present. While it might have been true that some sort of influenza-like malady was widespread in Haskell County (although Barry provides no data to document such a claim), one can legitimately contend that such influenza was caused by a virus only if one has proof that that is the case.

The evidence or data needed to prove the foregoing kind of claim did not exist in 1918. Moreover, unless Barry can demonstrate that viruses actually exist, then his foregoing claim concerning the alleged underlying cause of influenza is nothing more than a theory that gives expression to the idea that viruses in the modern sense of the term are believed to exist and are believed to be capable of causing influenza, and, then, such a theory is used as a hermeneutical lens through which to engage and interpret certain events in February of 1918.

This is nothing more than a narrative. It is not evidence – circumstantial or otherwise.

Whether, or not, one should accept such a narrative as a valuable way to hermeneutically engage the events of 1918-1919 depends on the viability of the viral theory of influenza. However, as previously noted, the next four chapters of the present book will explore the possibility that the notion of virus in the modern sense of the term is not necessarily all that viable, but until one works her or his way through the promised material, then, for the time being, all one can do is to leave open the issue of whether influenza viruses, or viruses of any kind, actually exist because, as already has been indicated in the present chapter, there are heuristically valuable ways of understanding the information which Barry is presenting in his book that are not tied to the issue of viruses.

Even if one were to accept the viral theory of influenza as being true, Barry provides no evidence to indicate that any of the three men that he identified in the opening paragraph of Chapter Fourteen in his book were actually sick or that they were carriers of the alleged virus. Although many people in Haskell County, Kansas might have been sick, this does not mean that everyone who lived there was either sick or would become sick or that they were necessarily sick with influenza, and, furthermore, there is no information that is provided by Barry concerning where in Haskell County the three people which he mentioned were from and whether, or not, that part (or those parts) of Haskell County was (were) as hard hit with influenza as other parts of the county might have been.

Barry notes that the three men from Haskell County arrived at Camp Funston somewhere between February 28 and March 2, 1918. Since the first cases of influenza emerged at the camp on March 4th, he goes on to suggest that such a timeline is very compatible with influenza's supposed period of incubation.

He further indicates that 1100 troops were hospitalized within three weeks following those initial cases. However, he does not say whether any of the three men that he had identified by name were among either the first cases of illness on March 4, 1918 or were among the 1100 individuals who were hospitalized subsequently.

Moreover, Barry offers no account concerning how whatever was transpiring in Haskell County actually began. In other words, he provides no explanation about how or why the people of Haskell

County supposedly contracted such a lethal, virulent strain of the alleged influenza virus or from where that alleged virus might have come.

He does note a little later in his book that individuals with expertise in epidemiology scoured the health records of both civilian and military populations that led up to the events at Camp Funston. Nonetheless, no discovery had been made within those records which were capable of demonstrating that some sort of anomalous kind of influenza outbreak had taken place prior to the events at Camp Funston, and the absence of such evidence tends to make one somewhat more cautious concerning whether, or not, whatever might have been happening in Haskell County was actually related in some causal manner to what transpired at Camp Funston.

As far as the notion of an incubation period for influenza is concerned that was mentioned by Barry in conjunction with the events at Camp Funston, there are a few possibilities that one might want to reflect upon before reaching any conclusions. To begin with, since the alleged influenza virus that supposedly led to the so-called 'Spanish Flu' pandemic has been described as being unique in its virulence, lethality, and extent to which human beings were said to be highly susceptible to its presence, one can't possibly know what the incubation period of such an entity might have been.

Supposedly, what took place at Camp Funston was out of the ordinary. Consequently, one cannot assume that ordinary or usual notions of incubation periods will necessarily apply.

Furthermore, by introducing the idea of an incubation period into the discussion, Barry is framing the discussion in terms of a germ theory which requires the existence of viruses that take a certain amount of time to begin to properly incubate and infect an organism. This is a perspective in need of the sort of evidence that Barry does not ever supply in his book but, instead, throughout the pages of that book, he simply presupposes that such viruses exist and, therefore, are capable of accounting for what transpired in February/March 1918 and beyond.

Secondly, one doesn't actually know what the nature of the relationship is between the initial hospitalizations of March 4, 1918 and the subsequent 1100 cases that required hospitalization. While

Barry identifies the March 4th cases as constituting instances of influenza, he doesn't say what the nature of the malady is, or maladies are, that subsequently waylaid those other 1100 hundred soldiers, and if the incubation period for influenza was supposedly just a matter of a few days, why did it take three weeks for 1100 people to contract that disease … if that disease is what they had?

Given the 1918-1919 mandates concerning the injection of a multiplicity of anti-venom and serum injections into the bodies of military personnel, how can one be sure that a substantial portion – if not most -- of the 1100 individuals who were hospitalized over the next three weeks were not just exhibiting the adverse effects that might be entailed by those jabs? Alternatively, given the make-shift and rather primitive conditions that tended to be characteristic of facilities like Camp Funston that were preparing men for war and given that February/March weather in Kansas can be pretty brutal, how can we be sure that a lot of the aforementioned 1100 soldiers weren't just succumbing to a set of conditions that were not necessarily conducive to the continued well-being of many of the people at that camp? Moreover, perhaps the 1100 illnesses were a synergistic interaction of a negative kind involving both the multiplicity of toxic jabs that were received together with the primitive living conditions present at the camp.

How long does it take for a person to break down from the impact of a multiplicity of jabs and primitive living conditions? How long does it take for the biological terrain of different individuals to begin to become toxic in one way or another as a result of exposure to such conditions and especially if they were receiving inappropriate or inadequate forms of treatment from medical personnel who had no idea what it was that they were dealing with? How long does it take for microorganisms within an individual -- that, under normal conditions, might have a symbiotic relationship with that individual -- to become induced to change their morphology and functional properties as a result of the presence of a failing biological terrain (due to a cocktail of toxic jabs and living conditions, and, possibly, inappropriate forms of treatment) which caused those microorganisms to move through various stages of their pleiomorphic/pleomorphic cycle and create additional problems for the ill individuals?

The time it takes for someone's biological terrain to become toxic as a result of problematic environmental conditions might, like the so-called incubation period of an allegedly infectious virus, be just a matter of days. How does one distinguish between the two?

John Barry further develops his narrative by stating that on March 18, 1918 – just several weeks removed from the time when the first cases of influenza supposedly emerged at Camp Funston -- two other camps in Georgia (Camp Greenleaf and Camp Forrest) recorded a substantial number of hospitalizations. He goes on to indicate that approximately ten percent of the personnel at each camp became sick.

Leaving aside the issue of what, if any, evidence actually ties the events at Camp Funston to the events at the other two camps, let's consider another issue. More specifically, depending on how many individuals were present in each of the foregoing camps, 10% of that total might be an impressive number.

Nonetheless, irrespective of how many people make up that figure of 10%, one can't help but begin to ask questions along the following lines. If the putative influenza virus that supposedly was circling Earth was so unique, virulent, infectious, and lethal, and if human beings were allegedly unprepared for it because they, supposedly, had never encountered it before, then, why did only 10% of the personnel in those camps become sick?

Barry concludes the foregoing discussion by indicating that 24 of the 36 largest training camps reported substantial case numbers that, apparently, had been diagnosed as suffering from influenza. What permitted the other 12 camps to escape seemingly unscathed by the ravages of that influenza?

He also adds that: "Thirty of the fifty largest cities in the country, most of them adjacent to military facilities, also suffered an April spike in 'excess mortality' from influenza." (Page 169 of the Kindle edition) Aside from asking about what happened in the 20 largest cities that did not experience an April spike in excess deaths, one might also like to critically reflect on the following consideration -- namely: Given that earlier in the present chapter mention had been made of Arthur Firstenberg's book *The Invisible Rainbow* and its thesis that the maladies of 1918-1919 might have been the result of radio wave poisoning due to the roll out by the military of an array of powerful radio transmitters and receivers that were capable of sending and receiving such signals over considerable distances and which had been deployed during the period of 1918-1919, then, one might want to entertain the possibility that since many of the cities that experienced spikes in excess mortality were situated near military facilities, is it possible that the excess death spikes in those cities might have been the result of radio wave poisoning from the near-by military bases and that the people who died were individuals who might have been particularly sensitive to the presence of those kinds of transmissions. Furthermore, although such deaths were diagnosed as having been due to influenza, it is possible that given the previously noted capacity of radio wave poisoning to induce symptoms in human beings that are like those that are attributed to influenza, then, is it possible that while those individuals might have died of an influenza-like illness, the actual nature of that illness could have been due to radio wave poisoning rather than being due to the presence of a virus whose actual existence is (as I will attempt to show in a number of subsequent chapters) subject to considerable doubt?

As noted previously, much of the first third of John Barry's book is a sort of hagiography concerning the architects of the allopathic medical system that began to dominate the United States from about 1910 onwards. For instance, not only does he dedicate his book to the "spirit" of Paul Lewis, but he begins the prologue for his book with a description of the problem for which the assistance of Paul Lewis had been sought – a problem that, presumably, helps set the stage for the topics that are explored in the rest of his book.

According to Barry, although Lewis was a physician, he never actually served as a practicing doctor. Instead, he was committed to doing research in the laboratory.

During the latter part of the opening decade of the 20th century, Lewis had been working at the Rockefeller Institute in New York and, supposedly, had been able to prove that a virus caused polio. That discovery was considered by many scientists of the day, and later on, to constitute a significant discovery for the fledgling science of virology.

Since Barry does not provide any of the details concerning the aforementioned work of Lewis, one has no way of knowing what the nature of the proof might be that, to which Barry is alluding with respect to the discovery of Lewis concerning the alleged nature of polio. The matter is further complicated by the fact that the electron microscope had not, yet, been invented, and, viruses – at that time – were treated as poisonous or toxic entities of an unknown nature that were capable of escaping the process of filtration and, yet, such entities somehow seemed to be capable of inducing disease, and, so, the idea that someone had proven that an entity which couldn't be seen was actually a virus in the modern sense and was responsible for causing polio tends to give rise to a variety of questions that tend to continue to hover over Barry's description of the alleged discovery by Lewis.

Barry also mentions that Lewis had developed a vaccine which was capable of immunizing monkeys against polio with nearly complete effectiveness. However, although I realize that for some individuals the following subjunctive possibility is something that those individuals believe should be engaged with considerable caution if not skepticism or rejection, nevertheless, **if** the arguments of the next four chapters are successful and, as a result, evidence can be shown which indicates that the idea of viruses in the modern sense might not actually exist (that is, entities might not exist which consist of a sequence of DNA or RNA molecules – but not both sets of those molecules at the same time – and which are encapsulated within a glycoprotein package and which are capable of infecting, if not causing some sort of pathogenesis in the infected organisms), then, whatever it is that might have been discovered by Lewis in the opening decade of the twentieth century and whatever it might be that Lewis was protecting monkeys against, those discoveries might have had nothing to do with viruses in the foregoing modern sense of the term -- although what took place in the laboratory might have had something to do with viruses in the original sense of the word ... that is, a way of referring to toxins or poisons of an unknown kind that were capable of by-passing the process of filtration and which could not be detected or identified by the technology of those times.

In passing, one also might raise what would seem to be a relevant question with respect to the polio treatment devised by Lewis. If his treatment was virtually a 100% effective way of helping monkeys to defend against polio, then, why were another 40 years required to develop a treatment for polio in human beings that often was not only ineffective but also was actually responsible for spreading the disease to other human beings in various instances that have been documented and which will be explored in a later chapter of the present book?

Notwithstanding the foregoing considerations, the aforementioned problem for which the assistance of Dr. Lewis was being sought had to do with a malady that was affecting a number of sailors. One of the primary symptoms of the illness had to do with a hemorrhagic-like condition that was present in the affected individuals.

The patients were bleeding in a variety of ways – from the nose, through the throat, as well by way of the ears, and sometimes from their eyes. In certain instances only one of the foregoing pathways might have produced profuse forms of bleeding, while in other cases there were individuals who were shedding blood through several orifices at the same time.

In addition to the hemorrhagic-like conditions, many of the sailors complained of severe headaches as well as pains in their bodies which were so intense that it seemed to the ones who were experiencing the phenomena that it was as if their bones were breaking.

Another aspect of their symptomology had to do with the color of skin in a number of the patients. Some of them seemed to have a certain trace of blueness in their fingertips and in their lips ... possibly indicating the presence of some sort of cyanotic or oxygen-deprived condition, while the skin of some of the sailors had become so darkened that one could not tell if the sailor was black or white.

According to Barry, Dr. Lewis could recall only one other instance in which he had encountered something that was somewhat similar to what he was seeing in conjunction with the sailors he was examining. On that earlier occasion a number of sailors had been removed from a British ship and moved to an isolation unit in a local hospital in Philadelphia.

All of those sailors eventually died. However, there had not been any ramifications ensuing from that event which suggested that contagion of some kind might have played a role in, or been a part of, the form of pathology from which they were suffering.

Following the deaths of the British sailors, autopsies were performed. Apparently, those autopsies showed rather stark evidence that in the case of all of those sailors a great deal of damage had taken place in their lungs.

While the evidence before us is of a very limited nature, nonetheless, there are several observations that might be made. To being with, there is considerable evidence which has been accumulated over the last hundred years, or more, that is capable of lending support to the idea that when EMF-sensitive individuals –- and even individuals who are not as biologically sensitive -- are exposed to non-ionizing forms of poisoning that can be caused by radio waves, then extensive damage has often been observed to occur in conjunction with neurological functioning, as well as in relation to both the respiratory system and the circulatory system, including the condition of cyanosis.

Secondly, in both of the situations to which Barry is alluding at this point in his book, the personnel being described were all from the military. Since – as I noted previously in the current chapter -- it was the military which had been deploying an array of powerful new forms of radio transmission and reception during this same period of time perhaps, there are good reasons for entertaining the possibility that the sailors in each case might have been suffering from EMF-poisoning rather than from the effects of viral infection.

Thirdly, the fact that a number of individuals in each set of the foregoing circumstances which are being described by Barry had become ill does not necessarily indicate the presence of a contagious disease. The phenomenon of clustering which occurs in cases that involve a variety of people who have been exposed to some sort of environmental toxin and become ill will, on the surface, exhibit some of the characteristics of a contagious disease because a number of people are all becoming ill within a given overlapping framework of time and space, but the pathology in question is not affecting a number of people at the same time because some sort of contagious entity is being passed from one person to another but, rather, illness exists because all of those people have been exposed to the same environmental poison or toxin.

Barry's account of the British sailors who died tends to lend some degree of credence to the idea that, conceivably, those individuals had all been exposed to some sort of environmental toxin and, as well, might have been individuals who were particularly sensitive to the potential adverse events that can arise from having been exposed to the presence of radio waves. After all, as Barry points out, apparently, no one besides the sailors who died had become ill, either in conjunction with the ship from which those individuals had been taken or later in conjunction with any of the individuals (medical personnel or otherwise) who were present at the Philadelphia hospital to which they had been taken.

Barry mentions in passing that a number of people who had either known or worked with Dr. Lewis considered him to be one of the smartest people they had ever known. Nonetheless, if one's thinking and creativity are hemmed in by the theoretical lenses through which one engages the world, then, how smart one might be is often irrelevant.

One will not be able to grasp the nature of something if one is prevented from having access to all relevant information -- either actively (through, say, censorship), or passively (through, say, the theoretical perspective that might be framing everything one engages). On the basis of the information which is present in Barry's book, there is absolutely no indication that any of the individuals that he mentions in that book – such as Dr. Paul Lewis – had any appreciation for, or awareness about, the possibility that Pasteur's theory of germs could not be reconciled with the sorts of scientific discoveries concerning the pleiomorphic/pleomorphic nature of microorganisms that had been made by researchers such as Béchamp and Enderlein. Furthermore, as Arthur Firstenberg makes quite clear in his work *The Invisible Rainbow,* there has been a great deal of evidence which has been established prior to 1918-1919 that was capable of demonstrating the pathological potential which EMF phenomena might have, and, apparently, neither the military nor most of the scientists and doctors who were operating out of the allopathic system of medicine had bothered to consider the possibility that, maybe, the powerful new forms of radio transmission that were being deployed might have deleterious consequences for, at least, some individuals.

Ten days prior to the circumstances during which a number of British sailors were isolated at a Philadelphia hospital, Barry describes how there had been a similar set of events which had transpired in Boston in conjunction with navy personnel. While arrangements had been made in Philadelphia to isolate any individuals who might become ill in an attempt to curtail the impact of whatever contagious elements might be present, nevertheless, four days following the arrival of a detachment of sailors arrived from Boston, 19 sailors seemed to come down with the same sort of illness as had surfaced in Boston earlier.

All of the aforementioned ill individuals were isolated. Yet, despite the use of the isolation protocols that were intended to contain the problem, a further 87 sailors became ill the following day.

Moreover, additional countermeasures were taken and not only were those sailors placed in isolation, but all the people with whom those individuals had had contact were also placed in isolation. Yet, within several days, an additional 600 sailors were hospitalized with what appeared to be the same sort of disease that was affecting all of the individuals who previously had been placed in isolation.

If the cause of the illnesses that were being observed in the various groups of sailors were due to an environmental toxin or poison – such as non-ionizing forms of EMF radiation like radio waves -- then, isolating people is not going to be able to stop what is taking place. In such cases, people are not infecting one another but, instead, they are all being poisoned by exposure to same sort of toxin or poison.

In addition, one should keep in mind an issue that was discussed earlier. More specifically, experiments were conducted which indicated that no matter how subjects were exposed to the fluids and detritus of people who supposedly were sick with influenza, none of the subjects got ill, and, therefore, whatever was happening was not due to contagious infection.

After describing the heroic efforts of Dr. Paul Lewis and a number of other scientist/physicians to deal with the form of pathology that was rapidly spinning out of control before their very eyes, John Barry proceeds to make a few comments about the extent of the death toll associated with the events between 1918 and 1920. At one point, he indicates that the disease which reared its ugly head during the aforementioned period of time was the most prolific terminator of human life of any disease known to have occurred up to that time.

He goes on to mention a low-ball estimate that was made concerning the death toll and which totaled some 21 million people, but, then, quickly, dismisses that estimate as being "almost certainly wrong." He follows up the foregoing low-ball estimate with allusions to calculations that, supposedly were made by various epidemiologists which have placed the death toll of the so-called Spanish Flu as being, perhaps, as many as 50 million deaths, and, maybe, even as much as 100 million individuals.

Unfortunately, Barry provides no real analysis that would provide one with a persuasive set of reasons why one should accept any of the foregoing estimates, or why one should suppose that the initial low-ball estimate is "almost certainly wrong." Nothing is said about methodology or any of the problems that might have existed in relation to determining the reliability of whatever metric or set of metrics which might have been used to tabulate body counts or to verify that people who died during that period of time actually died of a viral-caused influenza.

For example, if someone gets sick and, as a result of iatrogenic mistakes that might be made by doctors, nurses, or health care workers, receive forms of treatment (such as toxic amounts of aspirin) that are the actual cause of death, then, who gets to state what the cause of death was in such circumstances. Or, if because of inappropriate forms of treatment, a sick person's biological terrain becomes even more toxic and such toxicity induces microorganisms to enter into problematic stages of their pleiomorphic/pleomorphic cycles, and, as a result, the patient dies from a form of pathology that arises out of such events – events that the attending doctors do not understand and, therefore, cannot treat properly because they operate out of a monomorphic theory of germs introduced by Pasteur that completely fails to understand the pleiomorphic/pleomorphic properties, stages, and significance of microorganisms -- can one really say that this kind of patient died of influenza? Or, alternatively, if an individual who has an EMF-sensitivity and actually dies from the damage which non-ionizing radiation can inflict upon the human body – via, say, powerful new forms of military radio transmitters -- but because the symptoms of that death seem to be influenza-like in nature, can one actually say that those individuals should be counted as having died from some sort of infectious disease during a world-wide pandemic?

Despite the glowing tributes that have been paid by a variety of reviewers to Barry's book *The Great Influenza* (a few of which have been mentioned during the opening pages of the present chapter) concerning the alleged scientific qualities of that book, there does not seem to be any actual science that is present within the pages of his work. Instead, he merely appears to put forth a hermeneutical narrative which frames the events of a certain period of history in a way that might serve the interests of those who are busily, if not frantically, promoting the idea that events like the misleadingly-named 'Spanish Flu' of 1918-1919 constitute instances of dangerous, life-threatening pandemics that are being caused by infectious agents which continue to threaten the well-being of people today and tomorrow –- unless drastic steps of a questionable nature are taken that will profit certain corporations and enable governments to oppress people for reasons that cannot necessarily be justified.

However, Barry's book fails to present any evidence – or provide the reader with a rigorous examination of that evidence -- which is capable of substantiating the tale that he is spinning. Rather, his writing appears to be filled with sounds of virological fury that don't seem to signify much of anything.

There are 350 mentions of the name Flexner that occur in Barry's aforementioned book. The extent to which that name is present in his book goes a long way toward helping to provide some insight into the nature of the perspective out of which Barry seems to be operating.

The Rockefeller Institute for Medical Research was established on January 2, 1901. Several years later it developed a well-equipped and well-staffed research laboratory, and, then, seven years later opened a hospital.

The task of heading the Institute was offered to William Henry Welch. He was a Yale graduate whose undergraduate degree was in the classics, but he eventually changed course in his life when he, first, apprenticed with his father to become a physician, and, then, subsequently, began to study chemistry, as well as travelled to Europe later on —especially to Germany and Austria -- in order to learn about, among other things, laboratory science – a profession that was largely non-existent in America.

However, Welch turned down the position at the Rockefeller Institute offer and, instead, recommended that his protégé be given that position. His recommendation was pursued, and Dr. Simon Flexner was appointed to become the first director of the Rockefeller Institute of Medical Research –- although, in many respects, at least during the early years of the Institute's existence, Welch exercised considerable control over much that what took place there.

Flexner had travelled a somewhat twisted road to become a physician. Eventually, however, he distinguished himself in a variety of ways and not only studied at Johns Hopkins – a school that had been established to, among other things, bring rigor to the teaching of science and medicine, but later on, he also added a top tier position in the medical school at the University of Pennsylvania before moving on to the newly-created Rockefeller Institute in Medical Research.

Although, from time to time, the Institute would seek to spearhead research into such areas as surgery, its primary focus was on infectious diseases. Barry notes that one of the early "accomplishments" of the Institute had to do with establishing links between viruses and cancer. However one might put an asterisk next to that "achievement" because, as has been mentioned several times previously in the current chapter, the next four chapters of the present book will demonstrate, hopefully, that the notion of viruses – whether in connection to cancer or other sorts of infectious disease – is not necessarily the slam dunk that Barry – and so many others -- seems to suppose is the case.

While establishments such as John Hopkins and the Rockefeller Institute were beginning to rival the quality of research and instruction that was available at prestigious universities and laboratories in Europe, the vast majority of medical preparation in

America was considered by some to be abysmal. For example, Barry notes that in 1904 the Council on Medical Education was created by the American Medical Association and began to gather data on some 162 medical schools in both Canada and the United States.

Before proceeding to further examine the transformation that was about to take place in medical education in America, one might offer the observation that there is no end to the irony that appears to be at play in the early twentieth century desire of the American Medical Association to improve the quality of medical education in the United States. This is because the head of the AMA at that time was George H. Simmons who had begun his adult life as a journalist and, then, through an apparently fabricated process -- since there is no hard evidence which is capable of substantiating his claims -- he began presenting himself to the world as a medical doctor.

After Simmons had begun practicing medicine in Nebraska, he, apparently, obtained some sort of degree from Rush Medical College in Chicago which was nothing more than a money-making diploma mill for those who wanted to be called doctor without actually ever engaging in an educational process that might merit such a title. So, the decision of the AMA to begin pushing for more rigorous standards in medical education was set in motion while the head of the AMA was using questionable credentials to lend legitimacy to his alleged status as a "doctor".

Simmons tenure as head of the AMA was immediately followed by another medical imposter in the form of Morris Fishbein who, like Simmons, also picked up a piece of paper from the aforementioned Rush Medical School diploma mill and later admitted in a 1938 trial that he had never treated a patient in his life. Both Simmons and Fishbein exploited the AMA and its membership in order to advance their own self-serving financial interests and so that each of them could seek to enhance their respective spheres of influence, if not control, over the practice of medicine in America. Under the guidance of Simmons and Fishbein, the AMA used to offer to give its 'seal of approval' to various products and treatments ... not on the basis of research but on the basis of having received money in exchange for the AMA's seal of approval, and this is because the AMA had few, if any, laboratories of their own,

While much could be said about their self-promoting and self-enrichening tenures as heads of the AMA, I will just remind the reader that some of the exploits of Morris Fishbein already have been encountered in an earlier chapter (4) of the present book. If one will recall, Fishbein sought to ruin the life of Royal Rife and bury all knowledge concerning Rife's incredible Universal Microscope, as well as to censor information concerning Rife's discovery of a way to successfully treat, among other things, cancer simply because Fishbein's desire to be given a piece of the financial pie that was beginning to accrue in conjunction with Rife's frequency treatment had been thwarted.

Notwithstanding the fact that the head of the AMA at the time of its push for improvements in medical education in North America was a charlatan – indeed, something of a quack -- the push continued toward establishing what were being claimed to be more rigorous standards in medical education, but which also could be understood to be motivated by the desire of some individuals – such as Simmons, Fishbein, the Rockefellers, and those who were being subsidized by Rockefeller money -- to take control of medicine in order to be able to dictate what, supposedly, constituted proper medical knowledge and/or approved ways of treating patients ... and what was considered to be acceptable medical practice usually meant some sort of profit to corporations run by, or controlled by, the Rockefellers or which were run by those funded by Rockefeller money.

The practice of allopathic medicine had taken root in Europe. As more and more individuals from the United States travelled overseas in order to be able to study the European method of engaging medicine – which gave heavy emphasis to surgery, injectable medicines, pharmaceuticals, and the sort of research that could help extend and enhance those sorts of medical practice -- then when such academic explorers returned home from their studies, the observance of allopathic medicine not only began to spread but, as well, that orientation began to dominate how medicine was taught and practiced through places such as John Hopkins and the Rockefeller Institute of Medical Research.

To a considerable degree, the allopathic approach to medicine was being shaped by names such as Pasteur. Consequently, while the questionable character of Pasteur's monomorphic theory of germs was being featured among some of the most fundamental shaping influences in allopathic medicine, unfortunately, there was little, or no, room for the much more thoroughly scientific ideas concerning pleiomorphism/pleomorphism which had been advanced by Béchamp. In fact, as was documented to a degree in the last chapter, the ideas of Béchamp were far more scientific than anything that Pasteur had to offer -- and, as a result, allopathic medicine tended to be skewed or biased in a problematic manner from almost its very inception as a way of understanding and practicing medicine.

In 1907 the AMA issued a report that was quite critical concerning the alleged state of medical education in North America. However, at the time of the report's release, the AMA represented less than ten thousand medical doctors and because there were more than a hundred thousand doctors who were practicing in North America, the AMA did not promote its own report – fearing, perhaps, that a considerable amount of its revenues might disappear if doctors became angered by the contents of the aforementioned report and, as a result, would no longer be interested in paying money to have products and treatments receive the AMA's seal of approval.

Consequently, the AMA turned over its report to the Carnegie Foundation in a search for some sort of assistance with respect to furthering the potential influence of that report, The Carnegie Foundation, with assistance from the Rockefeller Institute, decided to commission Abraham Flexner, Simon Flexner's brother, to write a report concerning the status of medical education in North America.

Three years later, in 1910, Abraham Flexner – who was not a medical doctor but who had been educated at John Hopkins -- issued a report entitled: *Medical Education in the United States and Canada*. Subsequently, the report was usually referred to as 'The Flexner Report' by most individuals.

Before writing the foregoing report, Abraham Flexner returned to John Hopkins. He talked with, among others, William Henry Welch who had so much to do with establishing the Rockefeller Institute of Medical Research, including putting forth the name of Simon Flexner to be its first director. By Abraham Flexner's own admission, his perspective concerning medicine was shaped by what he had learned through his conversations with people such as Welch, and, as well, his perspective was shaped by the nature of his own experiences while attending John Hopkins which was a stronghold in the United States for teaching the precepts of allopathic medicine.

Flexner was of the opinion that at least 120 of the existing 162 medical schools should be closed. While his criticisms of some of the schools he took to task for their supposed inadequacies and incompetence might have been warranted, the impact of 'The Flexner Report'– which would be backed and promoted by such institutions as the Carnegie Foundation, the Rockefeller Institute, and John Hopkins, along with various other proponents of allopathic medicine – had an array of consequences that might, or might not, have been intended.

All forms of medicine other than allopathic medicine were to be cast aside, and this was to be done without any real objective examination of what might be of value – and, therefore, worth retaining -- with respect to medical approaches such as homeopathy, or naturopathic, chiropractic, and indigenous forms of medicine, not to mention Chinese approaches to well-being and disease, as well as the ayurvedic system of medicine. Moreover, and to reiterate the point once again, allopathic medicine is rooted in the work of, among others, Pasteur who promoted a monomorphic theory of microorganisms in which infectious diseases arose through the invasion of an organism by external germs that were claimed to be incapable of changing either their morphology and/or functioning during their life-cycles -– all of which had been, was being, or would be directly contradicted by the considerable research of Antoine Béchamp, Günther Enderlein, Royal Rife, Gaston Naessens as well as many other researchers.

In addition, Abraham Flexner wanted to make medical education a more time-consuming, and, therefore, more expensive process in which candidates for medical school would have to possess college degrees in order to be able to have an opportunity to enroll in an additional multi-year program of education focused on medicine. This sort of requirement would make it very difficult -- even more difficult than already was the case, -- for women, people of color, and those who were poor to have any chance of obtaining a medical education.

'The Flexner Report' was not just about trying to improve the quality of medical education. That report was framed in a way that was intended to promote a particular kind of medicine – namely allopathic medicine. Furthermore, whether intended, or not, that report was also about excluding certain kinds of people and ideas from being a part of medicine ... principles of exclusion that have continued to varying degrees to the present day and principles of exclusion that have adversely affected the quality of medicine that is being taught and practiced in North America.

The American Medical Association, under the leadership of its fraudulent doctor-director, began to rate schools of medicine. Those schools that were awarded an 'A' by the AMA were schools that implemented all, or most, of the recommendations that had been made in 'The Flexner Report', not only with respect to requirements concerning the quality of their laboratories and technical equipment, but, as well, in relation to whether, or not, those schools were teaching the right kind of ideas or whether, or not, those schools were hiring individuals who would promote the 'right' way to engage issues concerning the nature of disease, health, and well-being ... ideas which had to comply with various core principles of allopathic medicine. Schools that failed to meet the foregoing standards received ratings of 'C' or 'D' – not necessarily because they didn't have qualities of value to offer their students but because they did not conform to the narrow confines of the paradigm of allopathic medicine and, as a result, were soon forced, in one way or another, to close their doors.

John Barry's book, *The Great Influenza*, is actually one of the ramifications or consequences of 'The Flexner Report'. This is because Barry has framed his book according to the principles of allopathic medicine that 'The Flexner Report' helped to establish and which entailed the exclusion of so many other potentially legitimate considerations concerning disease, health, and well-being ... and one of those considerations has to do with the possibility that viruses in the modern sense of that term might not exist, and if it should be the case that viruses in the modern sense do not exist, then, much of Barry's book is rather worthless if not counterproductive.

John Barry's book *The Great Influenza* is not only part of the intellectual progeny that has, to a degree, been engendered by 'The Flexner Report', but, as well, his book is also tied to Rockefeller Medicine (The name Rockefeller appears 181 times in Barry's book).. This is not all that surprising because 'The Flexner Report' is, itself, also a function of, and in the service of, Rockefeller medicine

Rockefeller medicine gives expression to the activities of all those individuals, institutions, hospitals, universities, governments, and corporations that seek to commercialize, as well as have substantial influence over – if not control of – the process of limiting the practice of medicine to the allopathic paradigm. This kind of medicine is often referred to as Rockefeller medicine irrespective of whether, or not, at the present time, the Rockefellers, or their corporate heirs, still are running the show.

Since, on the one hand, allopathic medicine tends to stress the importance of surgery, injections, and pharmaceuticals as being the best way to treat most medical problems, and, on the other hand, since allopathic medicine also gives emphasis to the importance of laboratory research, and given that the purpose of such laboratory work is, hopefully, to advance -- in some, often arbitrary, manner -- the development of surgical procedures/techniques, injections, and pharmaceuticals, then, Rockefeller medicine is really about the attempt (irrespective of who does it) to commercialize the products that are generated through laboratory research, especially in conjunction with the invention of vaccines, injections, and pharmaceutical pills that, at least in the beginning often were derived from petroleum-based materials which, of course, were controlled to a considerable degree by the Rockefellers.

Rockefeller medicine played a major role in the rise of the Drug Trust that, in many ways, dominates and controls much of what happens in Western medicine today. More specifically, before the emergence of what has come to be known following World War II as the "Drug Trust" (a collection of major pharmaceutical companies that substantially influence much of modern, western medicine), the world of pharmaceuticals in the United States was controlled prior to the war by I.G. Farben in Germany (a chemical company ... among other things) and Standard Oil – the Rockefellers – in the United States. However, when World War II ended, a variety of political and legal actions were taken at different times in an effort to counter monopolistic cartel practices involving the aforementioned two, companies and, as a result, both Standard Oil and I.G. Farben were broken up into three companies, each.

Nonetheless, notwithstanding such political and legal actions, the Rockefellers maintained substantial control of the oil industry, and, consequently continued to have considerable influence in the commercialization of pharmaceuticals and injections. This latter sort of influence is demonstrated by, among other things, the fact that, for a time, BASF (one of the three companies that emerged from the break-up of I.G. Farben) was legally represented in the United States by a Rockefeller law firm, namely, Shearman and Sterling for which William Rockefeller was a partner.

Moreover, many of the drug companies that arose in America thereafter frequently included – either directly or indirectly – someone connected to the Rockefellers. For example, such connections were often in the form of individuals who would serve on the Boards of Directors for those kinds of companies, along with representatives from an array of influential institutions and corporations involving the media, universities, the military, defense contractors, the intelligence agencies, insurance, medicine, ex-government employees, and bankers in order to maximize their exposure to the ways of power in society.

In many ways, Rockefeller medicine was, and is, a more sophisticated, corporatized, commercialized, institutionalized and, perhaps, equally manipulative updating of the activities of the father of John D. Rockefeller – namely, William Rockefeller. The latter Rockefeller used to take bottled concoctions of oil that came from wells that were discovered close to Pittsburg, Pennsylvania in 1842 and sell the bottled contents, at inflated prices, as an alleged – but unproven -- cure for cancer -- much as many modern promoters of cancer treatments do.

Unfortunately, none of the current heirs to Rockefeller medicine appear to have any knowledge of, or understanding concerning, the discoveries of Béchamp, Enderlein, Rife, or Naessens that have revealed many facets of the pleiomorphic/pleomorphic life cycles of various microorganisms and all of which carry important implications for the treatment of a variety of diseases that afflict human beings. Consequently, the heirs to Rockefeller medicine seem to have little, or no, insight into the possible ways that the practice of allopathic medicine – which is, in part, based on Pasteur's deeply flawed notion of a germ theory that is rooted in the empirically-challenged notion of monomorphism -- might actually be undermining the ability of the human body to re-establish a condition of well-being because the pharmaceuticals and vaccines that are used in Rockefeller medicine could be interfering with the pleiomorphic/pleomorphic cycle of the microorganisms that -- according to Béchamp, Enderlein, Rife, Naessens, and many others -- are natural, symbiotic participants in human existence and which have different roles to play in helping to maintain, or to restore, proper functioning in the biological terrain of human beings..

John Barry's book –– *The Great Influenza* – appears to suffer from the same sorts of empirical and conceptual blind spots as does Rockefeller medicine and its allopathic counterpart in which his book is rooted. In other words, the aforementioned work of Barry appears to show a general lack of understanding of, or insight into, the work of Béchamp, Enderlein, Rife, and Naessens, and, therefore, his perspective seems to have rendered him unable to provide a viable explanation for what might have happened in 1918-1919 since he ignores a pleiomorphic/pleomorphic approach to disease or wellbeing and, consequently, tries to engage those events through the flawed lenses of Pasteur's theory of germs which has problematically biased his entire presentation.

Chapter 7: **Piecing Together the Alleged 1918 Virus**

Before being employed by the National Institute of Allergy and Infectious Diseases, Jeffrey Taubenberger used to work for the Armed Forces Institute of Pathology (AFIP). The Institute has been in existence for about 130 years and began its operations during the Civil War as the result of an executive order by Lincoln which instructed the Army Surgeon General to study diseases that were connected to the battlefield.

The foregoing executive order was issued because more people were dying from various forms of pathologies that arose in conjunction with military conflicts than actually died as a result of the weapons that were being deployed during those engagements. Consequently, the Institute became a venue for collecting and studying samples taken from surgery as well as data from autopsies involving both human beings and animals that had roles of one kind or another within the military.

Taubenberger is a specialist in molecular pathology. This discipline develops methods for making diagnoses based on changes in genetic composition rather than -- as is the case in conjunction with traditional methods of pathology -- using microscopic examination of biological samples to do so.

Pathology samples are generally fixed in chemicals such as formaldehyde, and, then, embedded in wax. This makes the process of isolating DNA and RNA difficult to accomplish because the genetic material found within the samples that are fixed in the foregoing ways tends to become quite degraded over time.

RNA is much more fragile than DNA is. However, Taubenberger indicates that researchers have developed techniques which permit pathologists to help optimize – as much as possible – recovery efforts concerning the two aforementioned molecules, and, consequently, the alleged 1918 flu virus served as an opportunity for using, exploring, and developing the kind of recovery techniques to which Taubenberger was alluding earlier that involve various kinds of molecules which might be of interest to researchers.

Nevertheless, whatever the nature of the foregoing sorts of recovery techniques might be, unless one can show how those protocols are capable of zeroing in on RNA that is uniquely from alleged viral bodies rather than from other biological sources (such as cells) which also are capable of serving as sources of RNA, then one is faced with a problem. More specifically, why should one suppose that whatever RNA is recovered through the techniques to which Taubenberger is alluding can be said – with a high degree of confidence – that such molecules come from viral bodies rather than from other biological components – such as tissue cells that have died and released their genetic contents into the samples that have been preserved?

Taubenberger said his recovery project was intended to "get a first direct look at the virus." However, for a number of reasons (some of which are noted in the following discussion), one might wish to question whether, or not, his research group actually ever came in contact with the alleged virus, and, therefore, in order to investigate such a possibility, let's take a look at various facets of Taubenberger's research that are touched upon in the 1998 PBS Taubenberger interview.

According to him, there were some 70 samples that were present in the Institute's archives that had been drawn from people who supposedly died from the influenza in 1918. These samples had been fixed in formalin and paraffin, and half of them were selected arbitrarily or randomly for purposes of study.

People died in different ways during the so-called Spanish Flu event of 1918. Some individuals died very quickly following the onset of symptoms, and this was quite different from the way people were believed to normally succumb to past cases of influenza.

Given that there were differences in the length of time that passed between, on the one hand, instances in which symptoms first began to appear, and, on the other hand, the point when life processes ceased in various patients, one query that could be explored is whether all the people who were dying in 1918 were necessarily dying from the same underlying pathology. For example, over the years, there have been a number of theories based on various kinds of evidence which suggest that whatever deaths occurred during 1918 might have been due to something other than -- or, perhaps, in addition to -- a suspected influenza virus.

Among the theories which have arisen over the years, are the following possibilities. (1) The forms of vaccines and medical treatments that were in use in 1918 often were injurious to patients in one way or another and, as a result, people might have died from the medical treatments they received rather than from a virus; or, (2) what had been diagnosed as cases of influenza were, instead, actually due to the work of the bacteria that is responsible for tuberculosis – a disease that was endemic in many places during the era of the "Spanish Flu and which can give rise to symptoms that are very similar to ones that are present in cases of influenza and, consequently, medical practitioners might have improperly diagnosed the nature of the problem with which they were dealing; or, (3) many people might have been developing bacterial infections of one kind or another due to the masks that were being worn to (supposedly) protect them against the alleged virus; or, (4) the pathology that was being referred to as the Spanish Flu might, actually, have been a form of poisoning that occurs when susceptible people are exposed to excessive amounts of certain kinds of electromagnetic radiation; or, (5) conceivably some combination of the foregoing possibilities came together in a sort of perfect storm of lethality, but, subsequently, were all subsumed in an undifferentiated fashion under the category of "death due to influenza" (much as has been, and is being, done, in conjunction with alleged COVID cases over the last several years).

To be sure, the aforementioned observed differences concerning the time intervals between symptom onset and death might have been a function of the extent to which individuals within the affected population could have possessed varying capacities of resistance to the forms of pathology to which they might have been exposed. Nonetheless, as intimated previously, another way of accounting for the foregoing kinds of differences in temporal intervals between symptom onset and death is that an array of lethal causes might have been involved in the events of 1918, and some of those maladies might have been more lethal than others, and, if this were the case, then this might explain why some individuals died far more quickly than other individuals did.

Besides the issue of rapid rates of morbidity, another oddity concerning some of the people who became sick during 1918 had to do with the onset of pulmonary edema in which the lungs of patients would fill up with fluids generated by, among other things, the blood from hemorrhaging tissue. Such people died by drowning in their own fluids.

What was odd about the foregoing feature is there was very little, if any, inflammation which had been observed prior to, or during, the rising, deadly onslaught of such bodily fluids. The presence of pulmonary edema together with the absence of inflammation was not ordinary when compared with cases of influenza that had occurred in past years.

A third, somewhat unique aspect of the patient histories that were being studied by Taubenberger in conjunction with the 1918 "Flu" had to do with the age of the individuals who were succumbing to whatever the pathology might have been that was stalking people during that time. Most of the cases he studied involved people who had been healthy and were young adults rather than consisting of the sorts of elderly individuals who normally fell victim to influenza.

Therefore, in summary, there were at least three properties associated with some of the 70 cases that had been archived from 1918 that distinguished those cases from what might be considered to have been "normal" instances of influenza based on past clinical experience. First, the time interval between the onset of symptoms and the occurrence of death was extremely rapid in various cases; secondly, many of those cases involved pulmonary edema without being accompanied by any kind of inflammation, and, finally, many of the people who were dying were much younger in age than the individuals who normally were vulnerable to the ravages of influenza.

So, presumably, any explanation that proposes to account for what is transpiring in cases such as some of the ones that were occurring in 1918 will entail putting together a causal framework that might be capable of providing a degree of insight with respect to those cases that were exhibiting properties or characteristics that departed from what previous clinical experience had indicated was the normal course of events involving influenza. Such an explanation would need to answer at least the following questions – namely: Why was pulmonary edema showing up in 1918 patients without simultaneously being accompanied by inflammation, or why were some people succumbing quickly in 1918 relative to what seemed to have happened in the past with cases of influenza, and, finally, why did whatever was happening in 1918 seem to affect – in atypical fashion relative to "normal" cases of influenza in previous years -- young people rather than the elderly?

The foregoing questions will be re-visited toward the end of this chapter. However, let's leave aside -- at least for the time being -- the foregoing considerations and continue on with exploring the information that is being transmitted through Taubenberger's 1998 PBS interview.

For instance, according to Taubenberger, influenza viruses are believed (this is based on theory and conjecture rather than being based on actual empirical evidence) to replicate very quickly. Yet, why – or how -- the foregoing characteristic is made possible is not addressed by Taubenberger.

What is said is the following: The process of rapid replication allegedly takes place within the cells of lung tissue, and, then, in about five day's time, viral bodies are hypothesized to be withdrawing from the foregoing cells and moving on to infect other cells and/or individuals. Consequently, according to virologists, after about a week one will not find any viral bodies present in lung tissue cells that had been infected previously by those alleged viral bodies.

As a result, Taubenberger wanted to examine samples of "influenza" patients who died in 1918 that -- according to the archived medical records -- had died within one week, or less, from whatever pathology had befallen them. In theory, such samples might provide him with an opportunity to access some of the replicated RNA material before it disappeared from a cell's interior during the process of cellular degradation.

One of the cases that met the foregoing conditions was accompanied by a sample that displayed strong histological features. In other words, when one looked at the tissue sample with a microscope, one could detect evidence that had been interpreted by some to have been the result of primary influenza pneumonia.

Virology theory contends that the influenza virus consists of eight RNA fragments. These fragments supposedly vary in length, and are believed to run from approximately 1000 to 2500 base pairs per fragment.

In his PBS interview, Taubenberger indicates that the sizes of the fragments that he was able to recover from the 1918 patient lung tissue sample were only about 150 to 160 base pairs long. He admits in the interview that his research project consisted largely of trying to find ways to piece together different RNA fragments that were recovered from the sample being studied and, then, eventually, he hoped to arrive at a stage of research through which he would be able to come up with a model for the entire genome of the influenza virus.

Taubenberger's research is, to some extent, based on assumptions concerning the number and type of genes that are contained in different kinds of alleged influenza viruses. In other words, the number of genes (supposedly eight) is based on a theory about gene structure and function rather than being based on discoveries concerning the actual number, structure and function of genes "in the wild" that have been isolated, characterized, and sequenced in a rigorous methodological manner.

In the PBS interview, Taubenberger indicates that his research group first looked at segments of five different genes in order to attempt to develop a sense of what the overall genomic properties of the influenza virus might look like. However, given what has been said earlier in this chapter, Taubenberger and his associates weren't necessarily looking at subsections of the actual genes of an alleged influenza virus, but, instead, might only have been looking at theoretical constructions of those genes ... theoretical constructions that might, or might not, accurately reflect the structure of certain facets of the contents that could have – possibly -- originally existed within the cell tissue samples being studied.

Taubenberger states that after completing the foregoing sorts of preliminary studies, his group began to narrow its focus on what was considered to be – at least theoretically -- one of the hypothesized primary surface proteins of the alleged influenza virus. The aforementioned protein supposedly is coded for by the hemagglutinin gene, and virologists believe (but have not proven) that the hypothesized hemagglutinin protein is the means by which alleged influenza viruses gain access to the interior of a host that supposedly is being infected by such a theoretical agent.

Nonetheless, once again, all Taubenberger -- as well as his research associates -- might have accomplished is to have engaged reality through the lenses and filters of the theoretical framework to which virology gives expression. After all, among other things, no one, yet, has been able to capture the dynamics of an actual virus entering a cell through the activity of the hypothesized hemagglutinin surface protein.

Consequently, one cannot be certain that the aforementioned sorts of cellular access events actually take place. Alternatively, if the foregoing dynamics actually do occur, one still does not know the details of those dynamics and whether, or not, the character of that activity accurately reflects the theory which virologists have put forth concerning how they believe influenza viruses are structured and function.

Notwithstanding the foregoing considerations, Taubenberger maintains that his research group has succeeded in putting together the genetic sequence that is alleged to code for the hemagglutinin protein. The sequence is said to be about 1800 bases in length.

However, as noted earlier, all one can really say is that the research group has come up with a "possible" sequence which is highly theoretical in nature. This is because Taubenberger and his associates have never actually isolated an influenza virus but, instead, have put forth various hypotheses concerning the nature of those sequences that is based on various theoretical principles for which there is a consensus, of sorts, by a certain number of practitioners within the field of virology.

Yet, science requires more than consensus. One must be able to empirically demonstrate that the working hypothesis which is being used to explain – at least tentatively -- certain kinds of phenomena can be verified independently by means of real world data that is capable of being replicated in a variety of experimental circumstances.

Unfortunately, in many respects, virology gives expression to a set of theories concerning the way its proponents believe (rather than know) certain dimensions of reality operate. As a result, virology doesn't necessarily accurately capture the facet of reality to which its theories are alluding.

As an addendum to the foregoing claim, one might note in passing that despite a lot of early hype on the matter, nonetheless, virology failed miserably to come up with a defensible viral theory of cancer during the 1970s and 1980s. Moreover, as the Perth Group in Australia -- along with Peter Duesberg, Kary Mullis, and others -- has shown, through a variety of empirical venues, virology also struck out with respect to being able to provide a verifiable explanation for precisely how HIV causes AIDS, and, yet, despite such a monumental failure, many virologists continue to engage life through their best, blustery, Wizard of OZ, knob turning, lever pulling, smoke generating, pay no attention to the man behind the curtain modes of behavior.

Furthermore, since the HIV causes AIDS debacle (which led to the deaths of millions of people in Africa and elsewhere through the ill-advised use of poisonous anti-viral medicines such as AZT), many virologists have been making a very good living promoting various modalities of fear-porn as they sought to transmit their alleged concerns to fellow human beings with respect to all manner of alleged imminent viral pandemics [such as: West Nile Virus (1999), SARS (2003), Swine Flu (2009), MERS (2012), Avian Flu (2013), Zika Virus (2015-2016), and COVID (2019)] that, supposedly, were, or are, invading humanity. Moreover, virologists and other researchers were not shy to recommend that everyone urgently needed to be treated by means of one brand, or another, of virology-based vaccinations and pharmaceuticals despite the fact that none of their pronouncements – either with respect to the alleged pandemics or the proposed treatments for those putative pandemics – could be proven to be able to accurately reflect what actually transpired in the real world during the aforementioned time periods.

During his PBS interview, Taubenberger stated he felt that the complete reconstruction of the entire set of genetic instructions for the influenza virus (and not just the hemagglutinin gene on which he was focused prior to 1998) is likely to take years to complete since the fragments being studied are so small that the process of reassembling them is very time intensive. One should point out once again, however, that the foregoing sorts of efforts will not necessarily involve reassembling the actual genetic sequence of some viral entity (For example, the next chapter of the present book consists of a critical reflection concerning a CDC paper that purports to provide an account of the subsequent work of Taubenberger and others concerning their contention that they have "discovered" the viral agent that, supposedly, was responsible for the 1918 flu).

Instead, as intimated previously, he appears to be interested in developing a theory about what he and his associates believe such a sequence might look like, and this assumes, of course, that such an entity actually exists. In short, Taubenberger's research group is engaged in a process of interpreting certain kinds of data and, therefore, the group is not necessarily pursuing a course of research that is capable of uncovering the actual nature of the dynamics that give expression to the 1918 phenomena which they are seeking to explain.

In many respects, Taubenberger and his associates appear to have become entangled in a game of conceptual will-o'-the-wisp. If so, then the foregoing sorts of understanding which are guiding his research team could be nothing more than a series of variable glimpses into a mist of elusive data that is heavily shaped by theoretical, if not completely arbitrary, considerations that could be distorting the nature of what actually might have happened in 1918.

According to Taubenberger, his research group believes that it can assert, with some degree of definitiveness (a definitiveness which the current chapter, as well as the next several chapters are seeking to challenge) that the entity which they believe they have been studying is an actually existing influenza virus. More specifically, they claim that the agent they have been studying is a type A influenza and belongs to the subtype H1N1 where H and N stand for proteins that supposedly permit such an alleged virus to, respectively, be able to gain access to (i.e., infect), as well as to be able to exit (and, thereby supposedly kill), a given cell on its way to infecting other cells or organisms.

Virologists maintain that there are three types of influenza viruses – namely, A, B, and C. These types of influenza are further sub-categorized according to the kind of hemagglutinin (H) and neuraminidase (N) proteins that are believed to be present on the surface of any given influenza virus.

While such influenza types and subtypes give expression to virology theory, nonetheless, no one has seen viruses entering or exiting cells via, respectively, H and N proteins. Therefore, there appears to be an absence of the requisite kinds of data which might be able to definitively verify any of the aforementioned theoretical pronouncements of virology.

Currently, virologists claim there are 14 different kinds of hemagglutinin protein subtypes and nine different subtypes of neuraminidase proteins which differentiate one type of influenza from another type of influenza. The alleged virus that is believed to have been present in the lung tissue samples from patients who died during 1918 is thought to be the H1N1 subtype, and this belief rests on the sorts of antibodies which were found in people who had been alive during 1918 but were able to survive whatever took place at that time.

Although there are theories within virology and immunology about how, and why, antibodies emerge, there is no reliable empirical data which actually captures the process of antibodies coming into existence. The evidence all has to do with finding antibodies at one point in time but not another, and, then, coming up with a theory for why such antibodies are found at one time but not another, or why those antibodies exist in some people but not others (further discussion concerning such issues will appear in the chapter on immunology).

Virologists not only believe that influenza viruses infect human beings, but, as well, such individuals also are of the opinion that those presumed viral agents are able to infect chickens, ducks, and a variety of birds as well as pigs and horses. Furthermore, based on the study of serum drawn from human beings who lived during 1918 and were able to survive whatever transpired during that year, virologists maintain that the antibodies in circulation in those individuals are a closer match to alleged swine influenza bodies that virologists believe were discovered in the 1930s than the aforementioned 1918 antibodies were a match to the human influenzas that were supposedly discovered in the 1930s.

Unfortunately, during the interview, Taubenberger does not spell out what is meant by the idea that the so-called "matches" between certain types of influenza and antibodies circulating in the blood stream are a better fit when considered in conjunction with alleged swine influenza bodies of the 1930s rather than in relation to presumed human influenza bodies of the 1930s. Antibodies can be quite promiscuous with respect to the kinds of entities with which they manifest some degree of affinity, and, therefore, one cannot be certain – as some virologists seem to be -- that the reason why there is a some amount of affinity between antibodies from 1918 and swine influenza bodies from the 1930 is necessarily because the 1918 antibodies were formed due to, or response to, an encounter with some sort of swine flu entity either just prior to, or during, the events of 1918.

In fact, if -- contrary to current theories and models of virology -- one were to entertain an hypothesis that the 1918 influenza virus did not necessarily exist, then, one would have to come up with a different theory to account for why antibodies of a certain kind might exist at one time rather than another. After all, if the 1918 influenza virus did not exist, and if influenza was caused by something other than a virus, then, making the sort of claims that some virologists seem inclined to make concerning the alleged significance that is supposedly demonstrated through the presence of alleged matches between particular kinds of antibodies and certain kinds of alleged swine viruses becomes something of a problem.

Among other things, the foregoing conceptual crisis would force one to search for some alternative reason or set of reasons to account for why antibodies of a particular kind can be found in the serum of some people but not others. In other words, one would have to ask: Why do certain antibodies arise if this is not in response to the presence of some sort of viral agent?

Notwithstanding the foregoing considerations, Taubenberger and his research associates believe that the aforementioned purported antibody-swine flu match indicates that the 1918 flu did not come directly from avian sources but, instead, arose through some sort of mammalian connection. In other words, they believe that the path of viral transmission might have started with avian organisms, and, then, emerged, at some point, within mammalian organisms -- such as swine -- and, then, somehow, got passed on to human beings.

However, at the present time, there is no detailed account that is capable of providing a viable explanation for the supposed process through which various genetic fragments might be able to make the jump from avian hosts to swine hosts, and then, subsequently, to human hosts. Although, in general terms, the foregoing sorts of transition phenomena is presumed to have transpired through some modality of recombinant DNA or RNA processes, nonetheless, this presumption is unaccompanied by any sort of account concerning a demonstrable, step-by-step dynamic that gives expression to the proposed series of transitions in genetic material that runs from avian vectors, through swine vectors,, and, eventually to human beings.

The foregoing issue is crucial. In other words, based on antibody data (which, as previously suggested, does not necessarily mean what some virology researchers believe that data signifies), Taubenberger stipulates that prior to 1918, viruses supposedly had been circulating within human populations in a relatively non-lethal form except in conjunction with a small fraction of individuals who, for various reasons, might have been susceptible to those kinds of influenza agents, and, therefore, one needs to ask the following questions: How did the 1918 influenza virus acquire its alleged lethality, and what was the nature of the biological or molecular mechanism that underlies such supposed lethality?

According to Taubenberger, viruses – which are theoretical entities whose actual, real world existence has yet to be proven -- tend to be genetically unstable, and, as a result, are hypothesized to undergo regular transitions with respect to certain aspects of their structure and function. Taubenberger describes such hypothetical transitions as "... presumably an adaptation of the virus, to evade the host immune response, so that the influenza virus that was circulating last year is not the same as the influenza virus that is circulating this year" and concludes by saying: "So they're very clever in that sense."

To be sure, changes in genetic sequences might -- at least theoretically speaking -- give expression to some form of genetic instability, but determining the cause of those changes tends to be quite another matter. One cannot assume – as Taubenberger seems inclined to do -- that changes in the genetic sequence of a virus are due to some sort of, apparently, intentional or logistical viral strategy which seeks to adapt to a host's immune response by bringing about changes that enable successive generations to evade that same kind of immune response.

Viruses are not necessarily "very clever" in the foregoing sense." More specifically, if one were to assume that changes in genetic sequence occur among viruses, then, although some of those changes might confer a "novel" advantage of some sort, nonetheless, other changes might not necessarily confer any kind of advantage, or those changes could introduce something that is decidedly a disadvantage to the alleged virus.

Therefore, whether or not a presumed virus acquires some sort of new "trick" that permits the immune responses of a host to be evaded will depend on the nature of the changes in genetic sequence that either do, or do not, occur. Yet, such changes do not necessarily have anything to do with some kind of adaptive strategy of 'cleverness' that is supposedly actively transpiring within a given viral entity.

In other words, changes in genetic sequence within a proposed virus could be a reflection of nothing more than – to use Taubenberger's way of stating things -- the inherent genetic instability of those entities. If so, then, as previously indicated, whatever changes occur in such genetic sequences do not necessarily have anything to do with cleverness or adaptive, evolutionary strategies but merely give expression to the alleged virus's on-going susceptibility to genetic instability which arbitrarily moves the genome of the alleged virus in one direction rather than another ... sometimes with, possibly, felicitous results, and sometimes with problematic results, and, sometimes with the sort of variance that has no appreciable impact at all as far as issues of adaptability are concerned.

Taubenberger maintains that while mutations do tend to occur on a regular basis, most of these changes will not lead to substantially different structural or functional forms. However, he believes (in other words he hypothesizes) that every so often, substantial changes do occur, and this takes place, he supposes, as a result of some sort of recombinant exchange dynamic that is hypothesized to take place between two different species.

As a result, he maintains that the foregoing sorts of recombinant changes could give rise to a form of virus that has not previously been encountered. Furthermore, he believes that this sort of theoretical virus might pose a threat for any species that did not have the capacity to defend against the presence of that kind of an agent.

Of course, not all changes in genetic sequence will necessarily give rise to a variant that carries potential lethal implications in conjunction with human beings. Moreover, for a virus, the essence of adaptation is a function of being able to replicate and continue on, and such a capacity is quite independent of any potential that might bring about biological mayhem in the organisms that are being engaged by the virus.

In short, the capacity of an alleged virus to inflict pathology on its host – or, in conjunction with some degree of vulnerability or susceptibility in a host to the properties of a virus that will generate a dynamic that results in death or disease -- is not necessarily adaptive. On the other hand, the capacity of a virus to be able to replicate is quintessentially adaptive in nature.

Although there is considerable evidence indicating that recombinant processes do occur, nonetheless, the notion that those recombinant processes will necessarily give rise, at some point, to something that is, on the one hand, capable of evading the capacity of organisms to defend against the presence of such entities, and, on the other hand, will be capable of being highly lethal in relation to its impact on a given organism is really nothing more than a conjecture. Consequently, even though Taubenberger – along with other researchers -- has put forth a hypothesis which contends that the foregoing sort of 'substantial' recombinant event occurred in connection with 1918, nonetheless, he has not provided evidence which demonstrates that such an event or series of such events actually occurred.

In fact, during the PBS interview, he indicates that he actually is searching for the foregoing sort of evidence. Consequently, although – as noted earlier -- he does refer to a certain amount of data involving antibody titers in blood serum that had been drawn from people who lived during -- but survived – the 1918 event, nevertheless, at best, that sort of data is only suggestive – and can even be ambiguous with respect to its significance concerning the possible relationship between alleged swine influenza viruses and human beings -- and, therefore, given the aforementioned degree of promiscuity that often characterizes the activity of many kinds of globulin proteins – i.e., antibodies -- the presence of the sorts of antibody data to which Taubenberger is alluding does not necessarily support his contention that the existence of those antibodies means that they came into existence as a result of earlier encounters with swine flu antigens.

During the PBS interview, Taubenberger refers to three alleged pandemics – namely, events in 1918, 1957, and 1968 – which he believes give expression to the possibility that some sort of recombinant set of events occurred which gave rise –or, so, the theory goes -- to novel viruses of one kind or another that had lethal properties in all three of those instances. However, in each case, Taubenberger fails to put forth any evidence to persuasively demonstrate that what he believes was responsible for those three events – namely, changes in genetic sequence due to recombinant dynamics – is what actually happened.

Furthermore, one might note in passing that there is a certain amount of evidence to indicate that the events of 1918, 1957, and 1968 might not have been due to a viral agent at all. For example, in the book: *The Invisible Rainbow: A History of Electricity and Life*, Arthur Firstenberg puts forth considerable evidence in support of the possibility that the three "pandemics" cited by Taubenberger (as well as a number of other outbreaks of "influenza" that occurred prior to 1918 and after 1968) might have been due to various kinds of changes in electromagnetic radiation that were being introduced into the Earth's environment at those times.

For example, numerous new sources of powerful radio frequencies had come on line in many geographical locals just prior to and during 1918 and were being beamed throughout the world. Or, in the case of the 1957 pandemic, there were many powerful radar facilities that were being deployed in various parts of the world. Moreover, in the case of the 1968 pandemic, numerous communication and intelligence satellites had been, and were being, launched by various military groups as well as by an array of corporations and, as a result, such technology was bathing the Earth – and its life forms – in an array of electromagnetic radiation that had not previously been encountered by human beings to that degree.

Radiation poisoning has been demonstrated to be capable of producing many of the same sorts or symptoms that are present in cases of influenza ... symptoms that, for nearly a hundred years, have been attributed to a viral agent of some kind. In fact, although abundant evidence currently exists which is capable of demonstrating that electromagnetic radiation can bring about flu-like symptoms as well as many other kinds of pathological conditions (see the work of, among others, Samuel Milham, Olle Johansson, Martin Pall, and Devra Davis), nonetheless, to date, no one has been able to properly isolate an influenza virus which can be shown to be infectious or lethal (and the notion of "isolates" that appears in the virology literature is a bastardized version of the sort of rigorous methodologies that are needed to properly isolate, sequence, and demonstrate that such isolated agents actually exist as well as that they are actually infectious and lethal).

The foregoing considerations give expression to a very critical issue. If viruses, of one kind or another, cannot be shown (following proper isolation and sequencing) to be the cause of, say, influenza, then, one must look to some other sort of environmental trigger (e.g., chemical, electromagnetic, and/or biological) to account for the existence of those maladies.

Yet, if something other than a virus plays a role in the onset of influenza, then, the nature of the dynamic with which human beings are presently faced changes in substantial ways. For instance, instead of trying to come up with some kind of virology-based vaccine or virology-based pharmaceutical elixir, and, then, insisting that people – as a matter of public health – must become vaccinated with, or must ingest, such an anti-viral concoction, then, perhaps, the proper way of treating such maladies lies in another direction.

More specifically, if viruses do not have a causal role to play with respect to the occurrence of diseases such as influenza (and, to date, the viral theory of influenza rests on evidentially problematic grounds), and if, furthermore, viruses do not have a role to play in pathologies like SARS, MERS, Zika, COVID, and so on (and, once again, there has been no proper process of virus isolation that identifies different kinds of viruses as causing the foregoing maladies), then public health in those circumstances need not depend on discovering and mandating certain kinds of virology-based vaccines or pharmaceuticals.

Instead what is required is a shift in the nature of the paradigm through which those diseases are explored. In other words, if the nature of the problem with respect to the foregoing sorts of maladies is not a function of the role that different kinds of infectious agents of a viral nature play, then, perhaps the problems associated with, for example, influenza, might be better resolved if one were to suppose that the diseases mentioned previously might be due not to viruses but, instead, could be due to, for example, the impact that different kinds of electromagnetic and/or chemical poisoning are having on the environment along with the ecologies that reside in the environment.

If the latter possibility were the case, then the onus of responsibility for combating those pathologies would no longer be a matter of trying to foist off some sort of mandated vaccine or pharmaceutical program onto the people and, then, proceeding to try to argue that resolving those health crises requires individuals to do their civic duty and take their medicine in order to protect others. Instead, the responsibility for combating the aforementioned diseases shifts to those who are poisoning the environment through chemical, electromagnetic, and/or biological means, and, therefore, what must be mandated are not various kinds of vaccines or pharmaceuticals but, rather, mandates should be issued which require various environmental polluters to cease and desist with respect to the activities which are poisoning human beings.

Toward the latter part of his 1998 PBS interview, Taubenberger returns to the idea of evolutionary adaptation. For example, after mentioning how there are many bacteria which can be found on our skins and within various parts of the gastrointestinal tract that are well-adapted to the surrounding biological environment and which actually perform many useful functions for their hosts – such as generating vitamin K – he goes on to allude to different kinds of bacteria and viruses that are not well-adapted to their hosts and, as a result, those entities take on what Taubenberger believes to be is an adversarial relationship with their hosts.

Taubenberger does not explain how bacteria and their hosts came to work out adaptive solutions which serve their mutual interests – or how they discover ways that, at least, do not adversely affect one another. Furthermore, he does not mention the fact that there are many different kinds of agents that have been found on, say, human skin – such as staphylococcus aureus – that, under the right circumstances, are potentially harmful but which, for unknown reasons, are not always active, and, therefore, contrary to what Taubenberger claims, do not automatically take on an adversarial relationship with their hosts ... perhaps because of the nature of the pleiomorphic/pleomorphic life cycle stage through which such a microorganism is going.

In any event, Taubenberger indicates that if an agent -- virus 'x' -- were to behave in an overly aggressively manner with respect to their hosts, then, the infected individuals will die too quickly. As a result, this sort of aggressive activity would tend to prevent that virus from being able to move on to other hosts.

Taubenberger alludes to the idea that the alleged 1918 virus seems to have avoided the foregoing sort of problem and, instead, was able to work out a good evolutionary strategy. In other words, although he believes that the virus killed a lot of people, nevertheless, it somehow managed to constrain its activities in ways that only lethally affected somewhere between 2 and 5 percent of the population.

According to Taubenberger, by behaving in the foregoing manner, such a strategy provided the alleged virus with an opportunity to move from host to host and, thereby, spread all over the world since only a relatively small percentage of the host population succumbed to the alleged onslaught of that virus. One wonders, however, whether the aforementioned 2-5% solution is the product of an evolutionary strategy that emerged in some inexplicable manner or whether that percentage merely reflects the possibility that 2-5% of the population is, for whatever reasons, vulnerable to the presence of certain kinds of agents and, therefore, the 2-5% figure might have nothing to do with some sort of viral evolutionary strategy but, instead, just gives expression to the manner in which alleged viral agents with certain kinds of properties interact with susceptible biological systems in a given set of contingent circumstances and, in certain instances, leads to a series of complex interactions that result in the demise of some of those organisms.

Taubenberger maintains that as a virus is transmitted from locale to locale in different regions of the world, people eventually would have developed an effective immune response to the virus. He further contends that such a state of affairs of general immunity would have placed the alleged virus under "enormous pressure" to undergo mutation so that it could change some facet of its genetic composition – such as the part of the genome that gave expression to one or another protein on its surface – in order to be able to find new ways of supposedly infecting human hosts.

Notwithstanding Taubenberger's foregoing account, one might note that mutations either occur, or they don't. One does not need to assume that there is some sort of "pressure" that is present which induces a given virus to mutate in certain directions.

Taubenberger's use of the term "pressure" might merely be his way of framing the discussion by means of a theory which seeks to advance the possibility that there is some kind of "force" in existence which is capable of inducing organisms to move in – or mutate in -- new directions that will prove to be adaptive. However, over a period of several billion years, the primary lesson of life on Earth would seem to be that, sooner or later, almost all species tend toward extinction irrespective of whatever changes might, or might not, take place with respect to their genomes.

As far as we know, to whatever extent alleged viruses exist, they consist only of a glycoprotein coating which houses either an RNA or DNA-based genomic reservoir which codes for a small number of genes that, under the right circumstances, supposedly enable those alleged viruses to, supposedly, go about the business of replicating themselves by hijacking the machinery of a host cell or organism. Whether the foregoing entities can be considered to be alive in some sense is a debatable issue, but irrespective of their existential status, there is nothing in their molecular or genetic composition which would seem to suggest that there is some underlying force or pressure within them, or working through them, that requires mutations of a certain kind to emerge ... namely, mutations that would allow those entities to find new ways to infect and/or inflict damage on a host.

However, Taubenberger resorts to the idea of viruses operating under an 'extreme pressure' to bring about adaptive mutations of certain kinds in order to account for why, after 1918, the alleged pandemic did not continue on but, eventually, petered out. Presumably, the hypothetical virus had undergone some sort of mutation that would permit it to continue to circulate within the human population but, in the process, had – due, perhaps, to the immune responses of host organisms – lost the ability to have anything more than a limited capacity for lethality with respect to all but a small percentage of human beings who were somehow vulnerable to such a viral presence.

Yet, to suppose, as Taubenberger does, that an alleged virus must mutate if it is to continue on is not necessarily true. Indeed, until one knows why some people are either more vulnerable than others -- or vulnerable at all -- to the presence of a viral agent, one cannot necessarily suppose that such an alleged virus will have to mutate in order to continue to be able to infect a host.

Thus, irrespective of whether, or not, antibodies arise in conjunction with the presence of a given viral agent -- and leaving aside the issue of whether, or not, the presence of those antibodies helps confer sufficient immunity to prevent all of an alleged virus's genetic potential from being able to express themselves -- it might be that some small percentage of a previous, hypothetical viral population will continue to exist even if such entities were to have lost their capacity to act in a lethal manner with respect to most individuals within a host population. A virus – to whatever extent it exists – has certain capabilities that (given the right opportunity) will be expressed, but in other circumstances might just remain inactive.

If the right kind of conducive circumstances do not arise, then, even if the alleged virus was not able to fully express itself, nonetheless, it might continue to exist for an indeterminate or indefinite period of time quite independently of whether, or not, a host actively engages – or is engaged by -- such an agent. The entity just wouldn't replicate, and since viruses – to whatever extent they exist – are not necessarily "alive," then whether or not replication continues to occur is not necessarily a matter of "life and death" for such an entity.

The life cycle of a virus – to whatever extent it exists -- is digital in nature. It is either on or off ... that is, it either replicates or it doesn't.

Whatever else happens with respect to such an entity – in the way of lethality or infectivity or pathology – will be a matter of the particular manner in which a given hypothetical virus and a given host interact with one another during the time in which the two supposedly are in contact. Conceivably, a hypothetical virus could remain inactive or dormant even though the circumstances that are necessary for replication are not present, and, yet, such a body might still continue to inhabit a host just as bacteria like staphylococcus aureus can be found in human beings in a non-active or non-problematic state.

Consequently, Taubenberger's notion that viruses – to whatever extent they actually exist -- must mutate in order to continue their existence is little more than a conjecture. While the possibility that he mentions is consistent with the theory of viruses as well as an evolutionary framework, there is not any evidence which is capable of definitively demonstrating the truth of the conceptual thrust of his conjecture concerning the existence of some sort of pressure that induces a virus to continue to mutate in ways that are increasingly adaptive in some sense of the word.

Indeed, one might suppose that developing some sort of capacity for lethality is actually counterproductive for a virus's continued viability. Viruses appear to complete their life-cycle via replication and not through inflicting pathology.

There is no evident evolutionary purpose that appears to be served by enhancing the capacity of a virus to inflict pathology. Being able to gain access to the interior of a cell or to be able to find a way out of that cell or to be able to borrow some of a cell's potential to replicate does not necessarily require the virus to be able to "infect" that cell in pathological manner and, thereby, cause some sort of disease anymore than DNA or RNA needs to inflict damage on a cell in order to be able to replicate.

Taubenberger's 1998 PBS account of the 1918 pandemic leaves unanswered a number of questions. For example, what was the specific nature of the recombinant event(s) involving -- at least, possibly, initially -- birds and mammals (such as swine) and, then, how did the process of species jumping continue on by, allegedly, making the transition from the foregoing sorts of mammals to human beings? One also would like to know the precise character of the dynamics of lethality that supposedly arose in an unknown manner, and, therefore, one might ask whether the lethality came from birds, or mammals, or, in some unanticipated way, emerged during the time when the jump was made to human beings? Finally, one might also ask why and how such a lethal agent suddenly appeared to vanish.

Apparently, Taubenberger is putting forth nothing more than a narrative which has been woven from various assumptions and conjectures based on a hermeneutical engagement of different kinds of empirical data. Indeed, in many respects, virology – and any discipline (for instance, molecular pathology) that has a potential for contributing to the development of virology -- appears to be nothing more than a theoretical narrative which seems to be masquerading as a set of scientific discoveries.

Taubenberger states that: "Historically, it seems that most new influenza viruses emerge in Asia, in the Far East, which is another thing that's unusual about the 1918 virus because everything we know historically suggested that it actually originated in the United States." One might wonder, however, about why different kinds of influenza supposedly have such an inclination to begin in Asia.

Could the foregoing sort of asymmetry in racial or ethnic susceptibility be a function of certain kinds of environmental conditions (e.g., electromagnetic, chemical, as well as biological)? Or, could such a racial or ethnic asymmetry be due to some sort of genetic vulnerability that is more pronounced in Asians relative to other racial and ethnic groups? Or, perhaps such an asymmetry might be due to some sort of systemic iatrogenic issue in which various kinds of pneumonia and respiratory diseases are being misdiagnosed as, or confused with, influenza, and, as a result, one is being given a distorted impression of what is actually taking place or whether there is any actual kind of asymmetry in susceptibility to influenza that is present.

Nonetheless, notwithstanding the foregoing sorts of considerations, Taubenberger's claim that the 1918 event started in the United States is not necessarily capable of being verified. More specifically, there is a considerable body of evidence (e.g., see *Virus Mania* by Torsten Engelbrecht and Claus Köhnlein, as well as *The*

Invisible Rainbow by Arthur Firstenberg) indicating that large numbers of people were dying all over the Earth from influenza-like maladies at roughly the same time in 1918, and, indeed, even Taubenberger states during the PBS interview that the spread of influenza took place with an incredible rapidity that occurred "within a period of a month or so in the fall of" that year.

Consequently influenza-like deaths were taking place in many locations around the world in a fashion that seemed to be faster than could be accounted for by any possible route of surface transmission that was available at that time (e.g., horses, automobiles, trains, or ships). On the other hand, the seemingly inexplicable rapidity of disease transmission in 1918 would be quite consistent with the possibility that the deaths being attributed to the "Spanish Flu" were actually due to the generation of electromagnetic frequencies that were poisoning people all over the world in a, more or less, simultaneous fashion at roughly the speed of light.

The explanation which Taubenberger offers as a way of trying to account for why influenza tends to emerge in Asian societies rather than in Western nations is zoonotic in nature. In other words, he contends that the cultural eating habits of many Asians involves going to so-called wet markets where various exotic life forms are available for purchase and consumption.

Presumably, somewhere along the line -- during or following the aforementioned visits to the so-called wet markets -- influenzas supposedly made a species jump from birds to mammals of one kind or another, or, a species jump allegedly transpired between mammals of one kind to other mammals such as human beings. Yet, as intimated previously, Taubenberger really doesn't appear to have any concrete evidence that is capable of demonstrating the validity of his zoonotic hypothesis.

Taubenberger goes on to indicate that during the 1950s "influenza viruses could be cultured and characterized in the laboratory." Technically speaking, however, viruses are not living and, therefore, do not need to be cultured. Indeed, short of a fully functioning host, there is no medium in which one could place an alleged virus in order to help it grow and replicate.

In fact, if a given virus is functional, then, one does not need to place such a virus in some sort of medium culture. All one has to do is take a virus that has been properly isolated – and, therefore, separated from everything else including a culture medium of some kind – then, expose a potential host to that isolated virus and, finally, just wait to see what takes place.

This is what transpires in the wild, so to speak. Introducing cultured mediums into the research process merely obfuscates the character of whatever pathogenic dynamics might follow.

According to Taubenberger, various attempts were made to exhume bodies of individuals in Alaska and elsewhere who supposedly died of influenza during 1918. However, while those exploratory expeditions were able to bring forth live bacteria through the use of various kinds of culture mediums, no one had been able to induce influenza viruses to surface.

In passing, Taubenberger mentions the work of a Canadian researcher, Dr. Kirsty Duncan, who has been attempting to locate the bodies of individuals who had died from influenza in 1918 but who had been buried in very cold – i.e., frozen – conditions. He notes that she is hoping to be able to uncover functional viruses from the foregoing sorts of cold storage exhumations.

Taubenberger contends that he feels the aforementioned research venture is not likely to succeed. He goes on to indicate that influenza viruses are quite fragile and that although bodies frozen in permafrost might retain some fragments of viral RNA, nonetheless, those samples would be unlikely to contain "live" or viable viral entities because of – as previously noted -- the fragile character of the influenza virus.

While Taubenberger mentions the extremely fragile nature of influenza viruses in the foregoing overview, nonetheless, he doesn't actually go into any sort of detail about the kind of environmental conditions that are necessary in order for a virus to be able to "survive" – i.e., be in a position to replicate when conditions are right. Presumably, the understanding which the aforementioned sort of missing information might help engender would be of value if one wanted to try to figure out the nature of the dynamic through which alleged influenza viruses and human beings tend to engage one another, and, furthermore, such information also would be of value if one wished to determine what kinds of conditions might be more conducive or less conducive to such alleged viruses becoming active within a host – human or otherwise.

Taubenberger believes that, generally speaking, societies in 1998 are in a much better position than they were in 1918 to be able to deal with potential pandemics. He feels this is the case because, among other things, "...we know that influenza viruses exist, and we can analyze them and watch their emergence and evolution." In addition, Taubenberger maintains that societies also are better prepared to deal with potential forthcoming pandemics due to (1) advancements in medical treatment such as drugs that, supposedly, are able to thwart the capacity of influenza viruses to, for example, replicate, as well as due to (2) the emergence of influenza vaccines which Taubenberger claims "are obviously the most important factor of our current armamentarium against influenza viruses."

However, as noted previously, neither Taubenberger, nor anyone else, has actually gone through the necessary set of rigorous procedures which are capable of properly isolating, characterizing, or sequencing the alleged 1918 influenza virus, nor, in addition, has he or other researchers also been able to go on to reliably demonstrate that such isolated virus are both infectious as well as lethal. Moreover, the antiviral treatments that are used to treat various viruses have proven, quite frequently, to be quite hazardous in their own right (for example, consider the deadly impact that the use of AZT had on the treatment of alleged cases of HIV or the impact that remdesivir is having on the people to whom it is administered).

Finally, notwithstanding Taubenberger's foregoing claim to the contrary concerning the alleged essential role of vaccines, there is considerable evidence that flu vaccines (e.g., see *Jabbed* by Brett Wilcox; *The Vaccine Court* by Wayne Rohde; Dissolving *Illusions: Disease, Vaccines, and the Forgotten History* by Dr. Suzanne Humphries and Roman Bystrianyk; *Vaccines: A Reappraisal* by Dr. Richard Moskowitz, Vaccine Epidemic, edited by Louise Kuo Habakus and Mary Holland, as well as *What Really Makes You Ill? – Why Everything You Thought You Knew About Disease Is Wrong* by Dawn Lester and David Parker) are neither safe nor effective. In this respect, one might consider, among other possibilities, the fiasco that arose in 1976 with respect to so-called swine flu in which hundreds of cases were documented in which human beings suffered from Guillain-Barré Syndrome, instances of transverse myelitus, or death as a result of the flu vaccines that were given in 1976.

One might also note in closing – and as was intimated to be a topic that would resurface toward the beginning of this chapter -- that early in the PBS interview Taubenberger listed a number of features that were atypical with respect to cases of influenza that had been encountered prior to the 1918 event. More specifically, he indicated that: (1) the death of many individuals took place very rapidly following the onset of symptoms; (2) a substantial number of the cases that occurred in 1918 exhibited signs of pneumonia edema without any accompanying inflammation; (3) a large proportion of the cases he studied involved individuals who had been healthy and were young, rather than the sort of elderly people who, in the past, normally fell victim to influenza; (4) the "influenza" that occurred in 1918 seemed to emerge, more or less, simultaneously in different parts of the world rather than following some sort of epidemiological path that moved from one location to the next via individuals who were traveling by foot, or via horses, trains, or ships.

Nothing which Taubenberger stated in the 1998 PBS interview is capable of providing an answer to any of the foregoing anomalies that he, himself, introduced into the discussion and which seemed to differentiate the 1918 event from previous bouts of influenza. While he offers a lot of conjectures during his interview, nevertheless, he does not provide much in the way of substantive, definitive information that is capable of addressing the four aforementioned anomalies that apparently were uniquely characteristic of the 1918 "influenza" event and do so in a satisfactory manner.

Finally, as indicated earlier in this chapter, during the 1998 PBS interview, Taubenberger attempted to describe some of his research concerning the hemagglutinin gene and, in the process, sought to link that work to the events of the 1918 "Flu". However, at best, his research only appears to advance a theoretical narrative, of sorts, concerning what he believes transpired in 1918 rather than giving expression to a fully delineated account of the 1918 phenomenon that is capable of being empirically substantiated.

Chapter 8: Virology -- The Game Is Afoot

Since the work of John Enders in the 1950s, virologists have been engaging in a fraudulent game (maybe, in some cases, intentionally or, maybe in other cases, because they have never bothered to really critically reflect on what they were doing) in which virologists attempt to give the impression that they have discovered the basic structure and nature of a given entity (e.g., virus) when all they have really done is reify some theoretical abstractions by running through a algorithmically-driven process of computer modeling in which everything that is generated through that process is nothing more than a conceptual placeholder which virologists seek to instantiate with actual existential qualities that are not theoretical in nature – as Geppetto did (at least in fictional terms) with Pinocchio and Dr. Frankenstein sought to do with his own creation – and, therefore, virology is, to a considerable degree, just a matter of fictional pretense.

For instance, Jeffrey Taubenberger's alleged "discovery" concerning the genetic sequence and structural character of the H1N1 virus that, supposedly, was at the heart of the 1918 Spanish Flu epidemic follows a script similar to that of Landt and Drosten with respect to the issue of using PCR to allegedly detect the presence of SARS-CoV-2 [see Chapter 6 of my book: *Observations Concerning My Encounter With COVID-19 (?)*]. In lieu of having access to a real, concrete, material virus with a specific sequence of DNA or RNA molecules that underwrites the functioning of real genes, Taubenberger, like those who worked before him as well as those who have come after him, constructed a set of artificial, synthetic genes based upon arbitrary, entirely theoretical considerations and, as a result, the entire structure of the H1N1 genome – like that of SARS-CoV-2 -- is an invented, fictional, computerized structure, and hopefully, the remainder of the present chapter, along with several of the following chapters will lend credence to the foregoing claim and fulfill the promise that was repeatedly made in the previous chapter.

The CDC article: "The Deadliest Flu: The Complete Story of a Virus Pandemic Influenza" -- begins with a Transmission Electron Micrograph of the alleged virus that, supposedly, caused the 1918 pandemic known generally as "the Spanish Flu" despite not necessarily having its origins in Spain. However, the aforementioned micrograph does not constitute proof that the bodies depicted in the image are either infectious, lethal, or even a virus.

A micrograph, after all, is a static rather than a dynamic depiction of something about which interpretive claims are being made. This remains the case even if one were to concede that the bodies being depicted in the micrograph actually constitute a virus or even if one were to concede that the entities in the image constituted the same virus that many individuals believe was so lethal in 1918, and neither of these latter two contentions are necessarily foregone conclusions.

The CDC article at issue here operates on the assumption that the proper explanation for the 1918 phenomenon has to do with a viral agent that was both highly infectious and highly lethal. As a result, the CDC article argues that the 1918 event provides valuable data and insights concerning how to prepare for future viral pandemics, and, hopefully, as will become clear over the net several chapters of the present book this latter assertion is not necessarily tenable either.

Early on, the aforementioned CDC article maintains that "an unusual characteristic of the alleged 1918 virus was the high death rate it caused among healthy adults 15 to 34 years of age." Such a statement makes a number of assumptions.

For example, the foregoing statement presupposes – but does not prove -- that the people who died in 1918 all died from the Spanish flu virus. However, there is considerable evidence to indicate that this might not have been the case if one were to factor in such issues as the widespread practice of using toxic/lethal doses of aspirin to treat 1918 patients as well as the many pathological problems generated – such as an array of adverse effects – due to the multiplicity of horse serums that were being mandated and injected into members of the military during that period of time. Moreover, the aforementioned claim in the CDC article also operates on the assumption that the people who died were actually healthy individuals ... as opposed to individuals who were outwardly apparently healthy but who might actually have had underlying health problems of one kind or another which had not, yet, shown up in the form of symptoms, and, therefore, while an agent of some kind might have played a role in the demise of certain individuals, there may have been a number of factors aside from the presence of a putative virus that, supposedly, was responsible for the death of various people.

For instance, we should not dismiss the extent to which iatrogenic forces might have been at play during the events of 1918-1919. John Barry's book, *The Great Influenza*, quite clearly documents that the doctors and other medical practitioners in 1918-1919 had no idea what they were dealing with, and, therefore, they had no idea how to successfully treat whatever malady or maladies with which they were confronted. Therefore, one cannot discount the possibility that through ignorance, incompetence, or some combination of those two qualities, a lot of people might have died as a result of the kind of medical treatment that they received.

According to the CDC article, a dedicated group of researchers were able to: "... search for the lost 1918 virus, sequence its genome, recreate the virus in a highly safe and regulated laboratory setting at CDC, and ultimately study its secrets in order to be able to better prepare for future pandemics." As the previously noted title indicates, the CDC article being explored here purports to be a "complete" account of the history to which the foregoing process of research gives expression ... but let us put this claim to the test.

The story provided by the CDC paper begins with a small, ocean-side Alaskan village known as Brevig Mission. In 1918, the village contained approximately 80 adults, consisting mostly of Inuit indigenous people.

The article goes on to say that there has been some degree of controversy concerning just how the inhabitants of that village became infected. Some individuals believe that a presumed virus was transmitted by a local member of the postal service, while others contend that the alleged virus arrived in the village through one, or another, trader who travelled to Brevig Mission via dog sled.

Notwithstanding the foregoing considerations, if one doesn't know how the alleged virus was introduced into a community, then, one can't necessarily be sure that a virus is what killed those individuals. All one can say is that something happened in 1918 which resulted in the death of 72 of the 80 inhabitants of that village, and one does not necessarily know why the 72 individuals who died seemed to be particularly vulnerable to whatever happened, while eight people were able to survive.

One also one does not know if the latter eight individuals got sick and, then, recovered, or whether they ever became ill. Furthermore, if the latter possibility is the case, then, why didn't they get sick?

What one does know is that all of the deaths took place within a six day period, lasting from November 15th to November 20th in 1918. The bodies were all buried in a mass grave near the village and remained that way until 1951.

In 1951, Johan Hultin, a Swede, was doing doctoral research in microbiology at the University of Iowa. He sought, and received, permission from village elders in Brevig Mission to excavate the bodies from 1918 because he believed that he might be able to find remnants of the 1918 flu in tissues of the bodies that had been buried and preserved in a frozen state and had been entombed in the permafrost for more than three decades.

Hultin was able to procure lung tissue samples from five of the excavated bodies. Nonetheless, back in his laboratory at the University of Iowa, he was unable to induce what he believed or assumed were viral entities to become active when he injected his collected lung tissue samples into chicken eggs in order to try to get the alleged virus to grow.

In 1997, nearly a half century later, Hultin read an article by Jeffrey Taubenberger, and others, that appeared in the journal *Science*. The article was entitled: "Initial Genetic Characterization of the 1918 'Spanish' Influenza Virus."

Taubenberger is a molecular pathologist who, at that time, was working within the Armed Forces Institute of Pathology in Washington, D.C. He, together with other members of his research team, had been able to obtain a lung tissue sample from an apparent victim of the 1918 flu who had been stationed in Fort Jackson, South Carolina at the time of the alleged pandemic.

The soldier had been hospitalized on September 20, 1918 with a diagnosis of influenza and pneumonia. However, whether, or not, that diagnosis was accurate is a separate issue (more on this shortly), and even if the diagnosis were correct, there are a variety of causal possibilities besides viral infection which might account for the presence of such flu-like or pneumonia like symptoms.

In any event, less than a week later -- on September 26, 1918 – the soldier died. A sample of lung tissue had been taken from him and stored for possible subsequent examination.

Making a clinical diagnosis of influenza or pneumonia gives expression to a judgment that is made by a physician with respect to various symptoms that are being observed. What is causing those symptoms is a separate, although, obviously, not necessarily an unrelated issue.

However, electron micrographs that would be capable of capturing images of possible viral-like entities would not be possible for over a decade and a half. Consequently, to maintain in 1918 that symptoms of influenza or pneumonia were caused by a viral infection would be an entirely speculative perspective (This is a point that is touched upon in passing toward the latter part of the CDC article being discussed here.).

Physicians tend to treat symptoms. The cause of those symptoms might not ever be known until an autopsy is performed, and, perhaps, not even then.

Furthermore, the issue of autopsy findings is somewhat of a moot point in 1918. Very few autopsies were performed in conjunction with determining the cause of whatever might be bringing about the deaths that transpired in 1918.

Putting the foregoing considerations aside for the moment, Taubenberger's research group had been able to sequence nine relatively small remnants of single-stranded RNA chains from the aforementioned soldier's lung tissue sample. Those nine fragments were alleged to be from four of the purported eight gene segments that were theorized to make up the genome of the 1918 influenza.

One problem with the foregoing account is that since human cells – including samples from the lungs – often contain single-stranded RNA sequences of many different kinds, one cannot necessarily be sure that any given RNA fragment which one is able to acquire from human tissue is necessarily from a virus. Moreover, even if the single-stranded RNA sequence were from a virus, there is no guarantee that the segment will be from one particular kind of virus (i.e., 1918 Influenza) rather than from some other virus that might have been in the lung tissue of the soldier who died in 1918.

Virologists contend – on the basis of purely theoretical and often arbitrary considerations -- that the Influenza A viral genome consists of eight, single negative-strand RNAs that are between – again, according to purely theoretical considerations -- 890 and 2340 nucleotides long. Each RNA segment is believed (believed, not known) to encode one to two proteins ... including the glycoproteins -- hemagglutinin and neuraminidase – which is where the 'H' and the 'N' come from in the H1N1 subtype that is believed (again, believed and not known) by many virologists to constitute the 1918 influenza virus.

There are thousands, if not millions, of RNA fragments that are to be found within the conglomeration of materials that, supposedly, are being used to culture the foregoing sort of virus. So, the question becomes, how does one know that the "nine relatively small remnants of single-stranded RNA chains from the aforementioned soldier's lung tissue sample" actually constitute fragments from an alleged 1918 influenza virus?

Notwithstanding the foregoing fundamental question, Taubenberger's research group maintained that the RNA which it had sequenced constituted a novel form of influenza A – namely, H1N1. This virus was alleged to belong to a subgroup of viruses that tended to inhabit pigs and human beings rather than birds (and one should note that the aforementioned subgroup of viruses is, itself, a purely theoretical concoction based on arbitrary considerations that have been developed through speculative computer programs rather than having been discovered as a result of actual empirical analysis involving a real world entity that, through independent scientific means, has been proven to be a virus containing sequences of such and such nature.

After reading the Taubenberger article in *Science*, Johan Hultin, wrote to Taubenberger and inquired about whether, or not, Taubenberger would be interested in what might be discovered if Hultin returned to Brevig Mission and, once again, tried to obtain some lung-tissue samples from the interred bodies that had died during the 1918 phenomenon. Taubenberger said he would be interested in such a venture, and, consequently, Hultin returned to the village which he had visited in 1951.

During this return journey, and after, once again, receiving permission from village elders, Hultin unearthed the body of an Inuit woman who was buried some 7 feet deep in the mass grave. Her lungs had been extremely well-preserved due to the permafrost in which they had been entombed.

After placing the lungs in an appropriate kind of preserving fluid, Hultin later sent the excavated biological materials to Taubenberger. Word subsequently came back to Hultin from Taubenberger "that positive 1918 virus genetic material had indeed been obtained from" the lung tissues that had been sent."

Nothing is said in the CDC article at this point about what made the RNA sequences from the Inuit woman's lungs positive with respect to the 1918 virus. In other words, one does not know whether the RNA sequences from the Inuit woman's lung tissue cells were from a virus, and, moreover, one does not know what those sequences of unknown origin are being compared against in order to permit someone to be able to conclude that, in fact, some of her RNA had come from the 1918 Influenza virus that supposedly had caused the woman's death.

Putting aside the foregoing sorts of issues for the moment, the CDC article proceeds to state that in February of 1999, a paper entitled: "Origin and evolution of the 1918 'Spanish' influenza virus hemagglutinin gene" appeared in the *Proceedings of the National Academy of Sciences*. The article was written by, among others, Anne Reid, who was part of Taubenberger's team of researchers and Johan Hultin had been given credit as being one of the co-authors of the article even though he had no role in the actual writing of the paper.

The Hemagglutinin gene is hypothesized to help make possible the entry of the influenza virus into the interior of a healthy cell within the respiratory system of a human being and, thereafter, enable the virus to go about replicating itself. The foregoing claim is actually only based on a theory about how a virus gains access to the interior of a cell since no one has actually seen or proven how the breeching process take place, just as -- once a virus is alleged to have gained entry to the interior of a cell – no one has seen, or knows how, an alleged virus is able to take control of the cell's replication machinery or how it supposedly sets in motion a series of events that lead to the death of an allegedly infected cell. Everything which is said about such a virus – or viruses in general -- is part of an elaborate theoretical framework that is based, in large part, on computer-generated data, and, to a considerable degree, is also based on speculations concerning how to interpret that data or organize it.

At this point, the CDC article offers an illustration of what virologists believe the influenza virus looks like. One needs to understand that the illustration in the CDC article is someone's rendition of the virus since there are no electron micrographs that are capable of verifying that such an illustration accurately depicts something that – via independent means – has been proven to be a virus.

The hemagglutinin – HA – protein that was the subject matter of the aforementioned Reid article is -- according to theory -- a surface protein which is believed (not known) to aid the virus to gain access to the interior of a human cell. Once inside a cell, the virus supposedly proceeds to infect a healthy respiratory tract, but, so far, nothing has been said in the article to indicate how this infection process takes place or why it can be so lethal.

The fact that an entity of some kind might be able to gain entry into the interior of a human cell doesn't, in and of itself, prove anything. One needs to understand the dynamics taking place within human cells, but this is difficult to do in conjunction with objects that are the size that viruses are said to be (on the scale of 50 to a couple hundred nanometers), and, therefore, such accounts tend to be heavily theory-laden.

The aforementioned HA component is one of the features of the virus that is believed (but not actually known) to be targeted and tagged by antibodies (as will be developed in a later chapter, the whole idea of what antibodies do is actually largely theoretical in nature). One theory underlying flu vaccines is built around the idea of finding a way to target, and, then, neutralize, the HA surface protein of that virus, and, in the process, undermine the putative means by which such viruses are believed (not known) to gain access to the interior of human cells..

The CDC article goes on to indicate that the 1999 Reid (et. al.) study was able to put together a proposed sequence structure for the hemagglutinin surface protein. This structure was based on combining fragments from the lung tissue samples drawn from the woman unearthed in Brevig Mission, as well as from the soldier who had died at Fort Jackson, along with remnants from a service member who had been stationed – and who died -- at Camp Upton in New York in 1918.

The foregoing amalgamation of data constitutes a theoretical construction. The aforementioned study did not isolate such a protein in any of the bodies, but, instead, inferred its possible existence on the basis of genetic data drawn from three different people – genetic data that, at no point, had been shown to be viral in origin.

According to Reid and others, the 1918 virus had initially invaded human beings sometime between 1900 and 1915. Since the HA gene was believed (not known)to have various mammalian – as opposed to avian – adaptations, and, therefore, was theorized to be more human-like or swine-like --"depending on the method of analysis" -- the virus was, for theoretical reasons, placed within a mammalian clade.

More specifically, Reid and Taubenberger maintain that the purported 1918 virus sequence that had been constructed is most closely related to the oldest classical strain of swine influenza – namely, "A/sw/Iowa/30. Moreover, they note that the former viral sequence seems to be quite different from current avian influenzas but, also add that no one is certain about what avian influenza viruses might have looked like back in 1918.

How closely related the purported 1918 virus sequence is to the oldest classical strain of swine influenza is not specified. Furthermore, precisely what the considerable differences are that differentiate current avian influenzas from the alleged 1918 viral sequence that was constructed is also not spelled out in the CDC article, and, even if such differences were spelled out, nonetheless, one must keep in mind that those differences in alleged sequences of genetic materials are entirely theoretical in nature since nothing that is being claimed has been shown or proven to have come from an actual virus.

Nonetheless, Reid and Taubenberger believe (but do not know) that the HA component of the virus originated from an avian viral source. However, they are uncertain about the extent to which the virus might have been undergoing changes within a mammalian evolutionary framework before it assumed (allegedly) the form that supposedly led to a pandemic.

There are a number of points to note with respect to the foregoing claims. First, one might highlight the acknowledgment by Reid and Taubenberger that whether a researcher considered the HA component to be swine-like or human-like depended on the nature of the method of analysis which was used, and, therefore, one needs to recognize that conclusions concerning the alleged mammalian nature of the HA protein might be more a reflection of a given method of analysis than any sort of "intrinsic" feature of a theoretical HA protein.

Secondly, because Taubenberger and Reid are uncertain about how long the HA component of the virus might have been, allegedly, undergoing evolutionary changes within a mammalian environment before emerging as something capable of, supposedly, bringing about a pandemic, they are not certain about how the virus came to possess its – presumed -- lethal qualities ... and they are not certain about what the nature of such lethality actually involves. In fact, they can't even be certain if the virus is what was actually responsible for the deaths of so many people.

In addition, although they believe (and do not know) that the HA component of the virus ultimately came from an avian source, they have no data to demonstrate how the virus component might have been able to jump species. The alleged link between an avian source and a mammalian version of the virus is entirely speculative.

Finally, the so-called mammalian adaptations to which Reid and her associate authors allude are not necessarily expressions of evolutionary change. Those differences might be nothing more than artifacts of computer programming dynamics that occur during the process of algorithmically constructing different versions of the alleged HA protein, and, as such, is entirely theoretical in nature.

In other words, since the computer programs that are used in such research are run a number of different times, the available base pairs and fragments that have been detected in a given culture (but whose origins have not been established) are put together according to an underlying pre-fabricated template for – in this case – a given protein. Consequently, differences will show up during each computer run as a function of the program and, therefore, one cannot suppose that differences which show up in a computer constructed model of a protein are due to evolutionary changes over time and, instead, just might be expressions of the way a computer program constructs things on any given occasion or run.

Reid and her fellow authors also indicate that the alleged 1918 virus' HA1 protein exhibited four glycosylation sites. Virologists believe (but do not know) that glycosylation sites play a critical role in influenza viral functioning, but one should probably keep in mind that the foregoing belief is part of a theoretical framework in which the notion of "an influenza virus" is embedded within a theory about viruses rather than being an expression of having experimentally observed an actual in-cell performance involving those glycosylation sites.

According to the theories of virologists (rather than established actual empirical facts that are known by them), current HA proteins that are – according to theory -- associated with human beings exhibit anywhere up to five additional glycosylation sites when compared with the alleged (but yet to be proven) 1918 virus's HA1 protein. These extra sites are believed (not known) to be the result of a process of "antigenic drift" which, according to theory, constitute small changes that are introduced into a component – in this case a protein – that occur as a result of errors that, supposedly, take place during the process of being copied to form the next generation version of that component.

These instances of antigenic drift are believed (not known) to be adaptive in nature as a given kind of alleged virus supposedly adjusts to its animal hosts. However, the foregoing perspective is somewhat presumptuous because one cannot automatically assume that any particular copying error that might occur will necessarily give rise to a functional adaptation.

Such instances of theorized antigenic drift are cited as being one of the reasons why there is a new flu season every year or why someone might be able to become infected with an alleged influenza virus on more than one occasion. Nonetheless, once again, this is like putting the cart before the horse because one cannot be certain that any given case of influenza that might occur in the future is necessarily infectious as a result of such changes.

Perhaps, somewhat more importantly, Reid and the other authors of the aforementioned article did not come across any sequence changes for the HA protein that might account for why the 1918 influenza virus was, supposedly, so virulent. For example, unlike modern theorized versions of avian influenza A viruses involving H5 or H7 variants which, supposedly, exhibit "cleavage site" mutations that are associated with added virulence due, allegedly, to the way in which those sites theoretically permit a virus to grow in tissues outside of its usual host cells through the alleged insertion of amino acids in the aforementioned cleavage sites, the 1918 virus theoretical construct did not contain any alleged sequences that coded for amino acids which could become inserted – at least theoretically -- into the cleavage sites in its alleged HA proteins.

Because Dr. Reid and her associate researchers could not identify any biological markers associated with the theoretically constructed HA protein that might have been capable of generating the sort of enhanced virulence that supposedly was exhibited by the 1918 influenza virus, the researchers maintained that there were probably a number of factors which might have synergistically interacted with one another to give expression to enhanced virulence, and, therefore, lethality during the 1918 pandemic. However, the foregoing claim concerning the multifaceted nature of virulence really amounts to little more than an admission that the researchers actually had no idea why the 1918 influenza might have been capable of doing the damage that it was perceived to have done, and also had no idea about whether, or not, that alleged virus was even responsible for what took place in 1918.

The aforementioned research group wrote a second paper in June of 2000. That article focused on the alleged or theoretical neuraminidase gene which supposedly codes for a surface protein known as NA and was entitled: "Characterization of the 1918 'Spanish' Influenza Virus Neuraminidase Gene."

The NA protein is believed (not actually known) to enable an alleged virus to escape from a, supposedly, infected cell, and, therefore, according to theory, helps the alleged virus to spread to other cells.

According to the theories of immunologists, antibodies arise in conjunction with the theorized NA surface proteins of viruses, and while such antibodies do not prevent infection, such antibodies are believed (but not necessarily known) to help stem the tide of supposed viral spread from taking place within human beings.

Unlike the genetic sequence for the theorized hemagglutinin surface protein (HA) which was pieced together using data from tissue samples that came from three different human bodies, the research group that was working with the tissue samples that had been sent to them by Hultin and which had been obtained from an excavated cadaver of a woman in Alaska, the researchers exploring the theoretical NA protein were able, supposedly, to work out a genetic sequence for the neuraminidase molecule by using tissue samples from just one body. Nonetheless, whether one is working with tissue samples from three bodies or from one body, the process of generating a genetic sequence from such samples is pretty much the same and, consequently, such a process depends on using a computer program (set of algorithms) involving, oftentimes, a theoretical template that is believed (not known) to be related to whatever alleged viral component in which one is interested, in order to be able to make educated guesses about whether the, say, RNA fragments that are present in a given tissue sample contain a sufficient number of the right kind of fragment sequences that might have underwritten the expression of a certain kind of surface protein ... in this case, the neuraminidase protein.

In short, the hypothesized genetic sequence for the theoretical neuraminidase protein that many virologists believe (but do not know) was present in the 1918 influenza virus – along with the computer generated genetic sequence for the theoretical hemagglutinin (HA) viral surface protein -- is a conceptual construct. Neither the protein nor its purported genetic sequence was found intact on the surface of, or inside of, an actual, concrete, existential virus that had been properly isolated but, instead, such models of a virus were put together by running a variety of RNA fragments (of unknown origin) that were present in tissue samples through a computer program to see whether, or not, those fragments could be put together in a way that was capable of matching -- to varying degrees of homology – the theoretical template being used in the underlying computer program.

This is like taking the scattered letters of an alphabet that are within a sample of some sort and, then, running those letters -- along with various fragmented, short combinations of those letters -- through a computer program containing templates of certain words – say, the words: "hemagglutinin" and "neuraminidase" – in order to see whether, or not, one might be able to come up with a set of possible alphabet sequences that were capable of matching up with the program templates. One's understanding is being filtered through the lenses of a theoretical framework, and, as a result, one might, or might not, be introducing some degree of obfuscation into the process of trying to understand whether such words were actually present in the sample or one merely had discovered a way to come up with such words using the alphabetic fragments that were available in a given sample.

To claim that such words actually were present in the original sample -- but simply had degraded over a period of time -- is a problematic contention. After all, the foregoing two words (i.e., "hemagglutinin" and "neuraminidase") were not actually found intact in the sample one was studying but, rather, those words had to be constructed as possibilities based on what is known about the presence of various kinds of exemplars from an alphabet that were found in a given sample that contained both single instances of the alphabet along with various fragments of combined components of that alphabet from which the foregoing words might be constructed.

In any event, once again, just as was true in conjunction with the algorithmically constructed – and, therefore, entirely theoretical -- hemagglutinin gene sequence in which Dr. Reid and her fellow researchers were not able to identify anything in that sequence which might have enabled the proposed 1918 flu virus to be especially virulent, so too, the researchers came to the conclusion that their algorithmically constructed sequence – and, therefore, theoretical -- neuraminidase gene did not exhibit any properties that might suggest, or were known to be associated with, a capacity for enhanced virulence or lethality that was assumed to exist in the purely theoretical 1918 influenza virus.

For instance, there is a certain amount of alleged evidence to indicate that the loss of a glycosylation site in the neuraminidase gene at amino acid 146 might be associated with an increase of virulence in certain alleged, current influenza viruses. However, nothing of this kind was detected in the gene sequence of the theoretical neuraminidase surface protein from the 1918 tissue samples from Alaska, and, in passing, one also might note that correlating certain features in gene sequence with enhanced virulence is not the same thing as demonstrating that those gene sequence features are the cause behind observed increases in virulence ... in other words, correlation is not necessarily an indication of causality.

According to the theoretical phylogenetic analysis conducted by the aforementioned research group, the algorithmically generated neuraminidase gene sequence from, allegedly, the 1918 tissue sample was classified as being (in other words theorized as being) intermediate between mammals and birds. What exactly is entailed by the notion of "intermediacy" is not spelled out, but such considerations notwithstanding, the researchers contend that the alleged intermediary status of the theoretical neuraminidase viral protein indicates that the alleged virus was, most probably, introduced into human beings at some point just prior to the 1918 pandemic and that the source of the change in virulence is most likely rooted in an alleged avian source of some kind. Yet, the CDC article also goes on to note that the research group was not able to trace the precise nature of the pathway that, supposedly, led to increased virulence.

So, once again, one is talking about theories of virulence and theories of phylogenetic transitions that are bereft of the sort of concrete, detailed evidence which is necessary to be able to demonstrate that such theories possess credible empirical legs. Correlational possibilities and plausibilities are not the same thing as empirically demonstrated causalities.

The CDC article proceeds to mention further facets of the theoretical 1918 influenza research project that led to the appearance of articles focusing on, supposedly, six more of the theoretically proposed eight genes that are believed (and not known) to be present in the alleged 1918 virus. Thus, in 2001, a paper published in the *Proceedings of the National Academy of Sciences* was authored by

Christopher Basier and other individuals which provided a theoretical account of a nonstructural gene (NS) that was believed (but not known) to be present in the alleged 1918 influenza virus, and this was followed, in 2002, by a paper from an Ann Reid-led research group which appeared in the *Journal of Virology* and dealt with a hypothesized matrix gene that was alleged to be present in that same theoretical virus.

In 2004, a further study was published in the *Journal of Virology* that put forth an account of a theoretical nucleoprotein – NP gene – which is believed to have been present in the alleged 1918 influenza virus. Finally, a year later, Taubenberger -- et al. -- wrote an article that was published in *Nature* and focused on different hypothesized polymerase genes which also are considered (but not known) to have been a part of the alleged 1918 influenza virus.

All eight of the hypothesized genes that are believed (but not known) to make up the genome of the alleged 1918 influenza virus are theoretical constructs. None of those genes were actually discovered by examining the sequences of a genome that had been located within a virus that had been isolated from all other aspects of the tissues and cultures that served as the basis for the research that was being carried out by Basier, Reid, Taubenberger and their associates ... research that was being published as fact – rather than pure, computer-generated theory -- in a variety of prestigious scientific journals.

Following the publication of the foregoing papers, a program was set in motion that was intended to create a live version of the alleged 1918 virus. The first step in this process of going "live" involved the creation of plasmids, and this was done through the work of microbiologists Peter Palese and Adolfo Garcia-Sastre, both of whom worked at the Mount Sinai School of Medicine in New York City.

A plasmid consists of a tiny, circular strand of DNA. Such strands are capable of being amplified through means of laboratory controlled forms of replication.

The plasmids that were generated by Palese and Garcia-Sastre would be utilized in a process of reverse genetics that researchers hoped might enable them to study the possible relationships between theorized viral structure and hypothesized function. In turn, the foregoing sort of studies could, theoretically, help lay the basis for moving to the next phase of producing viable forms of alleged viruses which will be discussed shortly.

Once the foregoing plasmids had been created, they were shipped to the CDC. Because researchers at the CDC were going to use those plasmids during the process of generating allegedly live versions of the 1918 influenza virus, the CDC instituted what it considered to be rigorous protocols for ensuring that such research would take place within an environment that exhibited the necessary qualities of biosecurity and biosafety ... and these enhanced set of protocols turned out to constitute what is known as BSL-3, one level lower than the maximum conditions for biosecurity and biosafety that have been established in conjunction with BSL-4 labs.

Dr. Julie Gerberding -- who is now the executive vice-president for strategic communications, global public policy & population health, as well as the chief patent officer, for Merck & Co., Inc. but at the time of the proposed 1918 influenza reconstruction project was the Director of the CDC (and, therefore, is a very good example of the revolving door policy that links – in financially incestuous ways – the CDC and pharmaceutical companies) -- appointed a microbiologist, Terrence Tumpey, to be the individual who would be solely responsible for working within the BSL-3 containment facility in conjunction with the attempt to recreate, supposedly, a live viral version of the alleged cause of the so-called 1918 influenza pandemic. The foregoing proposal also had been approved by the National Institute of Allergy and Infectious Disease (NIAID) under the authority of Anthony Fauci.

The project actually got under way in the summer of 2005. The plasmids which had been sent to the CDC -- and, previously, had been constructed by Dr. Palese for each of the eight genes that were theorized to constitute the 1918 Influenza virus and -- were introduced into human kidney cells by Terrance Tumpey. Once inserted into the kidney cells, the plasmids induced those cells to generate what the members of the reconstruction project believed (but did not know) were a complete set of RNA sequences for the 1918 virus.

There is some question, however, as to whether, or not, the RNA sequences that are being alluded to in the foregoing claim actually captured the structural and functional properties that might have been present in the alleged agent of the 1918 pandemic. After all, Taubenberger and Reid -- together with their associate researchers who had been involved with the various studies that produced the hypothesized eight genes that, supposedly, made up the composition of the alleged 1918 influenza virus -- had acknowledged, as noted earlier, that they saw nothing in the theoretically generated genes that might be considered to be a possible causal source of the virulence that was thought to be present in the alleged 1918 influenza virus.

If the reconstructed edition of the theoretical1918 influenza virus had no obvious capacity for inducing infectious lethality in its hosts, then perhaps, something is missing from the reconstructed, alleged version of the 1918 influenza. Indeed, one should keep in mind that each of the eight genes that had been created by Taubenberger, Reid and others were, actually, all computer-generated constructs that were based on various kinds of software programs, algorithms, theoretical templates and the like in order to produce what was presumed -- on the basis of an array of hypothetical considerations, assumptions, and calculations – to be an accurate re-creation of the 1918 influenza virus. However, absent the presence of a causal mechanism for infectious lethality in such a model, then, perhaps, the researchers should have exercised some degree of scientific caution concerning precisely what it is that had been created and whether, or not, such a creation had anything to do with the agent that supposedly led to a pandemic in 1918.

An article, entitled: "Characterization of the Reconstructed 1918 Spanish Influenza Pandemic Virus" appeared in the October 7, 2005 edition of *Science*. Following the publication of the foregoing article, the researchers undertook a series of experiments which was conducted in order to assess – allegedly -- the pathogenicity of the reconstructed --but entirely theoretical -- entity.

In other words, the researchers wanted to evaluate the capacity of their creation to infect and disrupt the healthy functioning of organisms into which their reconstructed agent was going to be introduced. This process of evaluation involved conducting a number of experiments involving mice.

The CDC article proceeds to give an overview of the experimental procedures that were used and, in the process, indicates that one set of mice were infected with the reconstructed agent, while other sets of mice were exposed to various combinations of the eight genes that constituted the reconstructed agent that had been combined with various strains of influenza A viruses (H1N1) that affect human beings on a seasonal basis. These latter concoctions are referred to as "recombinant viruses."

There might, or might not, be problems surrounding the character of the foregoing experimental setup. For example, nothing is specifically mentioned in the CDC article about how the different sets of mice were infected or just what it was that constituted the vector that was being introduced into those mice.

To begin with, living organisms come into contact with potentially infectious agents by interacting with the surrounding environment. Therefore, unless the various experimental sets of mice were being exposed to a possible infectious agent via air, water, food, or through their physical interaction with the environment, then, one is using a mode of vector introduction into the test subjects which is of questionable scientific value.

Secondly, there are a number of questions that should be raised in conjunction with the nature of the precise contents of the potential infectious agent to which the test animals were being exposed. For instance, since the CDC reconstruction project supposedly had succeeded – at least theoretically -- in generating the RNA sequences for the complete genome of the purported 1918 virus, then shouldn't they have been able to produce completely isolated versions of the entities to which such RNA sequences give expression ... versions that would be uncontaminated or unadulterated by the presence of any other components such as would happen if one were to embed the reconstructed virus in some sort of culture which, supposedly contains said agents but, in addition, also often tend to contain a number of other components, as well, that are considered by researchers to be necessary to maintain a viable culture but which also might have pathogenic properties completely independently of the presence of any putative virus?

The term "viable" in the foregoing paragraph means something that might only serve the purposes of a group of researchers rather than something that necessarily reflects what is likely to happen outside of a laboratory. If the potentially infectious vector which is being introduced to experimental groups of mice consists of anything except a purified compilation of the reconstructed virus, or anything but a purified amalgamation of various kinds of recombinant viruses in control groups, then whatever other components are being mixed in with the reconstructed virus or mixed in with recombinant viruses that are being used as control groups might have the capacity to obfuscate the character of the biological dynamics that are taking place within organisms in conjunction with the possibly infectious agents to which they are being exposed?

According to the account provided by the CDC article concerning the foregoing experiments, there was a marked difference between the impact of the reconstructed version of the 1918 influenza virus on mice and the nature of the impact which the recombinant viruses had when they were introduced to various control groups of mice. For instance, mice that had been given the reconstructed version of the alleged 1918 influenza virus contained quantities of the replicated virus that were 39,000 times higher than were produced through one of the recombinant viruses.

One question that might be asked in conjunction with the aforementioned claim in the CDC article is the following possibility. Given the claim that mice which, somehow, had been exposed to the reconstructed version of the alleged 1918 influenza contained 39,000 times the amount of that reconstructed version of the alleged virus than did mice which were not exposed to the reconstructed version, then, how does one know that all the entities which are being claimed to be exemplars of the reconstructed version (some 39,000 times some given amount) are what they are said to be? In other words, have samples from the set of entities that arose in conjunction with the fully reconstructed edition of the alleged 1918 influenza virus been properly isolated, open up, and shown to contain intact RNA genomes that are the same as the reconstructed version from which the large quantity of replicated entities supposedly arose and which also can be shown (in accordance with the criteria set forth by Thomas Rivers), that the same kinds of patterns of replication are produced when materials are taken from allegedly infected mice and introduced to, yet, other mice?

According to the CDC report concerning the reconstruction project for the alleged 1918 influenza virus, another indicator of the claimed virulence of their reconstructed agent -- beside the degree of replication that is observed -- concerned the possible lethality of that agent. More specifically, the reconstructed edition of the alleged 1918 influenza virus was said to be 100 times more lethal than "one of the other recombinant viruses tested."

One wonders whether the foregoing claim means that the recombinant viruses were also lethal but 100 times less so than the fully reconstructed edition of the 1918 influenza virus, and, if this is the case, then why would such a recombinant virus have some degree of lethality? Furthermore, one might entertain various questions in relation to the extent of the lethality to which the article seems to be alluding in conjunction with the recombinant viruses which are not specified, as well as have questions about the nature of the mechanism of lethal pathogenicity that might be involved in those deaths.

In other words, if one accepts the premise that the fully reconstructed edition of the 1918 virus was 100 times more lethal than "one of the other recombinant viruses tested," then, just how lethal was the latter recombinant virus? How many mice in this group died, and what was the cause of death in those mice?

Moreover, there is a certain amount of ambiguity present in the CDC article with respect to experiments involving the reconstructed virus which indicate that the fully reconstructed version was 100 times more lethal than "one of the other recombinant viruses tested". In other words, does the foregoing claim in the CDC article mean that other versions of the recombinant viruses were associated with higher degrees of lethality than the one recombinant virus, in particular, that was tested and which, apparently is being referenced in the quoted statement. Or, alternatively, were the other recombinant viruses found to be more lethal than one of the recombinant viruses that was tested but were, to varying degrees, less lethal than the reconstructed edition of the alleged 1918 influenza virus, and, if the latter is the case, then, once again, what is the extent to which such recombinant viruses are associated with dead mice and why do such deaths occur at all?

The impression is given in the CDC article that it is the H1N1 virus which is killing the mice and that such a virus kills at a rate which is 100 times greater than the mice with recombinant genes. However, the precise nature of the cause of death for mice in the experimental group was not really made clear because, among other things, we don't actually know what is being introduced into the mice in the experimental group since the H1N1` genome has never been properly isolated/purified, sequenced, and proven to be infectious outside of computer models. That which is being given to the mice in the experimental group does not consist of just a purified pool of virus bodies and nothing else, but rather that concoction consists of many things that are a function of the culturing process through which experimenters claimed to have generated a virus "isolate" but, in fact, what is being called an "isolate" has not actually been shown to contain nothing but a properly isolated, purified amalgamation of something that has been proven to be the H1N1 virus and nothing else.

Conceivably, the concoction that was given to the mice in the experimental group might have been lethal. However, conceivably, such lethality could have been a function of the means through which such an "isolate" was delivered into the experimental mice, or such lethality might have been a function of what was in the "isolate" concoction as a result of the culturing process and not necessarily because there were any H1N1 virus bodies present in that "isolate".

For example, perhaps, on the one hand, the cytopathic event in the cell culture that led, supposedly, to the accumulation of an alleged "isolate" which, subsequently, was introduced into the experimental group of mice might have contained various kinds of toxic proteins that, say, either were being produced by bacterial and fungal microorganisms that had begun feeding off the decaying contents of the cytopathic event, or, possibly, on the other hand, the material from the culture that was introduced into the experimental group of mice contained decaying substances that, when given to the experimental group of mice, led to the awakening of bacteria or fungi in those mice and induced those microorganisms to generate toxins in certain stages of their pleiomorphic/pleomorphic cycle that caused the death of such mice. There are many forms of toxic substances that are capable of killing mice besides the presence of an allegedly lethal form of virus.

The CDC article does indicate that the theoretical HA or hemagglutinin gene from the fully reconstructed edition of the purported 1918 flu virus seems to play a critical role in rendering the virus to be lethal. The evidence for such a claim rests with an experiment in which the gene from the fully reconstructed edition of the alleged 1918 gene was removed, while the seven other genes from the reconstructed virus were combined with a seasonal influenza virus labeled as: "A/Texas/36/91" or in more abbreviated form: "Tx/91."

The latter, alleged recombinant virus did not result in the death of any mice. Furthermore, such mice did not undergo any sort of weight loss, whereas many mice exposed to the supposedly fully reconstructed rendition of the alleged 1918 virus not only died but, as well, some number of the latter group of mice lost up to 13% of body weight within two days of being exposed.

The foregoing experiment involving "TX/91" is described in a somewhat ambiguous manner in the CDC article. Presumably, the only difference between, on the one hand, the recombinant virus that combined seven genes from the fully reconstructed – but theoretical -- version of the alleged 1918 virus with the "Tx/91" control virus would have centered around the absence of the hypothesized HA gene. However, since nothing was said in the CDC article about the number or kinds of genes that might have been present in the "TX/91" to which the seven genes from the fully reconstructed version were being added, one is not really certain if the only difference between the allegedly fully reconstructed virus and the supposed recombinant "Tx/91" virus is the presence or absence of the hypothesized HA gene, or whether there were other differences in genomic structure as well.

Furthermore, the phrase: "lost up to 13% of body weight" which appears in the CDC article sounds like a lot of late-night television advertisements which indicate that if one buys a certain product, then, one can save up to "x" amount, or if one uses a certain product, then one's condition can improve by up to "x" amount, but, in reality, the amount which can be saved, or the benefit that actually accrues, turns out, in most instances, to be substantially less than whatever the indicated "x" amount might be, and, yet, the original statement would not constitute a lie because there were some cases in which "x" amount was saved or "x" benefit accrued. Consequently, to say that some mice "lost up to 13% of body weight" doesn't necessarily provide one with much information or provide any insight into what the nature of the dynamic was that might have caused such a loss in body weight.

One would like to know how many experimental mice exhibited the foregoing loss in body weight. One also would like to know how many mice in the experimental group exhibited little, if no, weight loss, as well as how many mice in the control group exhibited some degree of weight loss, even if not substantial.

Aside from the issue of numbers involving various kinds of weight loss, one might also like to know something about the causal issues underlying such weight loss. Why did some mice experience more weight loss than others, and what factors might have affected how much weight, if any, was lost?

Apparently, according to the CDC account of the reconstruction project, the presence or absence of the hypothesized HA gene had a marked effect on the symptoms that arise. However, exactly what role the hypothesized HA gene plays in the nature of the symptoms that arise, or do not arise, is not actually spelled out.

The CDC article describing the experiments involving the fully reconstructed gene version of the purported 1918 influenza virus also indicates that within four days of being exposed to the aforementioned reconstructed edition, mice displayed various forms of inflammation in their lungs that were reminiscent of, or similar to, the sorts of lung tissue inflammation that had been observed in conjunction with many human beings during the alleged 1918 pandemic. In other words, apparently, the lungs of the exposed mice filled up with fluids, or exhibited signs of pneumonia, or had some other kind of lung inflammation.

However, the term "similar" that appears in the CDC article is somewhat open-ended. As a result, one remains unsure as to the extent or degree of similarity between the sorts of lung complications that emerged in conjunction with the mice that were exposed to the fully reconstructed version of the purported 1918 virus and the kind of lung complications that were fairly common among the human beings who were said to be infected with the 1918 virus.

The CDC article also describes a set of experiments that were run using a human lung cell line referred to as "Calu-3 cells". More specifically, measurements were taken at 12 hours, 16 hours, and 24 hours following exposure of those cells to the alleged fully reconstructed edition of the 1918 virus, and, then, these measurements were compared with measurements that were made following the exposure of the human lung cell line to various forms of recombinant viruses involving different arrangements of certain genes from the fully reconstructed form and various kinds of seasonal flu viruses that supposedly affect human beings.

According to the CDC article, the reconstructed version replicated rapidly within the human lung cell line into which they had been introduced. In fact, the reconstructed virus produced "as much as 50 times" the amount of virus as various forms of the recombinant viruses did … but, once again, one needs to ask: What, exactly, is being counted as a virus and how does one know that what is being counted as a virus actually constitutes a virus?

Moreover,, the notion that one virus produces "as much as 50 times more" of that virus than does another kind of virus doesn't really explain how frequently this maximum of 50 times greater production actually occurred. Rather, the statement only indicates that there were some cases in which this sort of rate of multiplication was observed, but there also were other instances in which this kind of differential in production was not observed, but no details are given concerning the latter sorts of cases.

The CDC article goes on to state that one of the conclusions drawn from the aforementioned sorts of experiments is that the polymerase genes that were present in the artificially reconstructed viral form also appeared to play a significant role in the pathogenicity (i.e., virulence and capacity for infectivity) that was observed when human lung tissue was exposed to the fully reconstructed edition of the alleged 1918 virus. Nonetheless, what the nature of that enhanced role might be is not really spelled out, nor is it shown that the entities that, supposedly, were generated during such experiments were actually HINI viruses.

In addition, what takes place in a laboratory Petri dish is not necessarily an accurate reflection of what takes place in the much more complex environment of a living organism. Do the dynamics occurring within a laboratory dish point to certain possibilities in conjunction with life in the wild? Possibly ... however, there is a potential for many a slip twixt experimental cup and a living lip.

As noted earlier, Taubenberger and Reid were of the opinion that the 1918 influenza virus might have derived certain gain of function properties from an avian source ... properties that were theorized to have made a species jump at some point prior to the onset of the pandemic. The researchers had reached the foregoing point of view because they felt that the artificially reconstructed influenza virus had segments in its genetic sequence that seemed to be much closer to avian influenza A viruses (H1N1) than they were to various kinds of H1N1 mammalian influenza viruses, but what precisely was entailed by the notion of appearing to be "closer" to avian influenza A H1N1 viruses than to H1N1 mammalian editions of such viruses was not really specified or explained.

In order to test the foregoing thesis concerning the possible origins of the alleged 1918 influenza virus, 10-day old fertilized chicken eggs were exposed to the CDC reconstructed virus (or exposed to what was alleged to be such a virus) and, then, those results were compared with results from experiments that exposed the same kind of eggs to various editions of a modern human influenza A virus (or what were alleged to be such viral entities) that contained different combinations of the two, five, and seven gene recombinant viruses that had been created by Dr. Tumpey during earlier stages of the series of experiments that were being run through the CDC concerning the alleged 1918 influenza.

According to the CDC article, the fertilized chicken egg experiments indicted that the reconstructed version of what was assumed to be the virus at the heart of the 1918 pandemic had a much more lethal effect on the chicken egg embryos than did any of the recombinant versions of the human influenza virus (Why? What was causing this?). In fact, none of the recombinant viruses seemed to have the same degree of lethality in conjunction with the fertilized egg embryos as the fully reconstructed version did, but the CDC article is unclear about whether, or not, the presence of any of the recombinant viruses led to symptoms of one kind or another in the fertilized chicken embryos.

Furthermore, the pathogenicity of the fully reconstructed edition of the 1918 influenza virus in relation to fertilized chicken eggs was said to be "similar" to the kind of pathogenicity that was observed when fertilized chicken eggs were exposed to various kinds of current H1N1 editions of avian flu viruses (or what were claimed to have been such avian flu viruses). However, the nature of the alleged 'similarity' between, on the one hand, the fully reconstructed edition of the putative 1918 virus and, on the other hand, contemporary versions of avian flu viruses was not specified, nor was there any discussion in the CDC article concerning whether, or not, similar sorts of pathogenetic outcomes might have been produced in more than one way. Yet, if there were multiple possible paths to similar sorts of pathogenic effects in the chicken embryos, then, one couldn't necessarily conclude that the reason for such similar outcomes is necessarily due to the role that avian flu viruses (or what were claimed to have been avian flu viruses) might have played in the theorized gain of function that supposedly showed up in the alleged virus that supposedly caused the 1918 pandemic.

In addition, although the researchers believe that the foregoing experiments with chicken egg embryos showed – as the researchers also had concluded with respect to the human lung cell line experiments – that both the hypothesized HA, or hemagglutinin gene, as well as the hypothesized polymerase genes of the alleged reconstructed influenza virus played significant roles in enhancing the virulence of the putative 1918 influenza virus, once again there is an absence of details in the CDC article concerning just what the nature of those roles might have been, or how such capabilities actually came into being (rather than theoretically might have come into being according to inferences concerning computer algorithms), and why such features would have generated the kind of pathogenicity that had been observed in 1918.

Although much speculation within the CDC article, as well as elsewhere, has been focused on the possible mechanisms of pathogenicity to be found in conjunction with any given form of supposed influenza virus, one should keep in mind that not all mice died in the CDC experiments when they were exposed to such viruses, nor did all mice lose 13 % of their body weight within a couple of days following that exposure. Consequently, one must also take into consideration the characteristics of the organisms that are being exposed to an alleged virus in order to try to account for the differential outcomes that occurred in such experiments despite being exposed – supposedly -- to precisely the same reconstructed virus.

Death, like life, involves a dance between environment and organism. Why, despite being exposed to the same set of environmental features, some organisms die, while other organisms live, is an issue that cannot be reduced down to only questions of pathogenicity concerning an alleged virus, but, as well, one must take into consideration the degree of vulnerability, if any, that exists in various organisms and just what is entailed by such vulnerability. In short, one can't talk about the lethality of an alleged viral agent or entity without simultaneously exploring the susceptibility of an organism to certain kinds of difficulties that might arise when engaged in various ways by various elements within a given environment.

In fact, given the foregoing considerations, one might ask: Is the pathogenicity that is observed in such circumstances a function of the alleged virus or is it a function of the organism? Where is the locus of causality to be set?

If an organism is immune to the presence of a certain entity (say, some sort of alleged viral agent), then, in reality, the latter entity has absolutely no pathogenicity relative to such an organism. So, if another organism of the same kind displays various kinds of biological difficulties when exposed to the same sort of environmental agent, can one really say that it is the entity's pathogenicity that causes such difficulties or is the causal dynamic much more complex than assigning pathogenicity to a entity such as an alleged virus?

Perhaps, the reason why researchers have had such difficulty in delineating the causal process with respect to the 1918 pandemic is because their analysis should have been looking for something beyond the idea of an agent or entity that has some sort of capacity, all by itself, for generating pathogenicity in an organism. In other words, perhaps, they should have been looking into the complexities of how organisms interact with the environment and what both sides of the dynamic bring to the life, death, and well-being equation.

Finally, the research conducted by Taubenberger, Reid, Tumpey, and others that is, to a degree, delineated in the CDC article and which has been the focus of the present chapter, hasn't actually demonstrated that the reconstructed genome that arose through their efforts was the same as the viral agent that supposedly played such a devastating role in the events of 1918. Although they believe they have demonstrated that their reconstructed version is correlated with certain kinds of results in various sorts of experimental contexts, nonetheless, by their own admission, they acknowledge that their reconstructed genome does not seem to display any features which have been empirically demonstrated to be capable of generating the sort of virulence or pathogenicity that is believed to have been characteristic of whatever transpired in 1918.

They talk about a possible mechanism for entry into a cell (e.g., hemagglutinin – HA gene) as well as a possible means of being able to exit from cells (e.g., neuraminidase – NA gene). In addition, they allude to the possible role that various hypothesized polymerase genes in their reconstructed entity might have had in conjunction with the process of successful replication as well as possibly enhancing, in some way, the virulence of the alleged 1918 virus, but the capacity to enter, exit, and replicate do not necessarily give expression to a causal account of how such a virus generates its lethality within a human host

Consequently, the foregoing CDC account lacks causal concreteness. They cite experiments that were conducted at the CDC concerning the potential pathogenicity of their reconstructed creation, but none of those experiments demonstrate that their re-created entity is identical to what supposedly was at the heart of events in 1918, and, in fact, their experiments only indicate that in some fashion their reconstructed genome can be correlated with certain kinds of experimental results without being able to spell out what the precise causal dynamics were which underlay those experimental results.

Once can agree with the authors of the CDC article when she, he, or they conclude: "… that more work needs to be done." Whether the future work to which the CDC article is alluding will enable researchers to be able to causally prove that their computerized constructions constitute accurate recreations of the agent that, supposedly, was responsible for the public health crisis that occurred in 1918 remains to be seen.

Chapter 9: Seeking to Save Appearances

Virologists go through a sort of pseudo-methodological process in an effort to save the appearances of their viral theories. They claim that at the present time we do not have the necessary techniques or technological advancements to detect in the cells or tissues found in human beings the viruses which they believe are present in the cytopathic residue of a cultured cell, and, consequently, they have devised another technique which they believe provides evidence that the purported virus is present in a given ill individual.

The process to which the virologists are alluding is referred to as: "Unbiased De Novo (Anew) Next Generation Sequencing." I am indebted to the explanatory efforts of Dr. Andy Kaufman, Dr. Thomas Cowan, Dr. Stefan Lanka, Dr. Sam Bailey as well as her husband Dr. Mark Bailey, along with my medical friend who sought to help me long distance during a relatively recent bout of illness (a year and a half ago) and with whom I have had many long conversations, for quite a few years now, concerning all of the issues that are touched upon in this chapter.

Apparently, the meaning of the term "unbiased" in the foregoing phrase or term: "Unbiased De Novo (Anew) Next Generation Sequencing," is intended to convey the idea that the process is not being affected by the likes and dislikes of the investigator. However, as we shall see during the following discussion, the entire process seems to give expression to various biases and assumptions that virologists tend to carry and which also shape much of what takes place through the pseudo-methodology that is about to be described.

So, the question that needs to be asked is the following. How do virologists make the transition from: (1) a concoction consisting of human genetic material (in the form of a swab/sample taken from a ill or healthy individual), as well as consisting of materials from other kinds of genetic fragments arising from the Vero monkey kidney cells and fetal bovine serum that are used during the culturing process, in addition to, possibly, the genetic material that is present in whatever – if any – viral entities that are present (all of which would give rise to millions, if not billions, of genetic fragments from an array of: Human, bovine, Vero monkey kidney cells, and, possibly, viral sources) to: (2) some sort of credible claim that one can methodologically engage all such genetic materials and end up with only precisely those fragments that belong – allegedly – to, the hypothetical presence of a given virus?

Virologists begin to sort all of the different kinds of DNA and RNA that are present in a cell culture that has undergone a cytopathic event. Step one seems to involve the idea of removing all DNA fragments from the foregoing concoction.

The reason that tends to be given for undergoing the foregoing step has to do with the belief that, for example, SARS-CoV-2 is, supposedly, not a DNA virus (the discussion that occupies the following page focuses on SARS-CoV-2, but the ideas that are being explicated here actually apply to any and all hypothetical viral candidates). However, if one asks for the empirical basis that substantiates such a claim, virologists really have no independent way of justifying such a claim or step.

For example, if someone were to cite the particles being depicted in various Electron Micrographs as being non-DNA instances of SRS-CoV-2, then, the thinking becomes circular. This is because one starts out with certain assumptions about what is being depicted in such EMs, and, then, such assumptions bias the nature of the conclusions which one draws about what is, and is not, relevant to one's search for the presence of SARS-CoV-2.

Presuming that the SARS-CoV-2 exists, is it a DNA virus or is it a RNA virus? How does one demonstrate this independently of the allegedly "unbiased" Next Generation Sequencing process, because one would have to have such an independent confirmation of the nature of the genetic material in SARS-CoV-2 prior to the process of sequencing in order to justify eliminating all of the DNA fragments that one might find in the materials that are contained in the conglomeration of particles and fragments that are left behind in the cell culture that has undergone a cytopathic event.

The next step of the Unbiased De Novo Next Generation Sequencing process involves removing all of what are believed to be the RNA fragments that can be matched up with human or known microbial sequences. However, if one doesn't know what the actual sequence of SARS-CoV-2 is, then, one is no position to empirically establish whether any given RNA sequence comes from SARS-CoV-2, Vero monkey cells, human tissue, or fetal bovine serum since, among other possibilities, there could be various genetic sequences in the alleged SARS-CoV-2 virus that are held in common with RNA sequences from other organisms. What is the scientific principle that permits one to determine from where a given fragment of RNA might come?

Once again, a source of potential bias is being arbitrarily introduced into the De Novo Next Generation Sequencing process. Allowing such a bias to stand unchallenged has the capacity to affect the nature of the conclusions one might reach using such a method, and, as a result, the process is no longer unbiased and objective but is being shaped by certain kinds of assumptions that are being made but which cannot be scientifically justified.

After eliminating the DNA fragments and the RNA fragments that the virologists feel are irrelevant to, and even capable of obfuscating, their search for SARS-CoV-2, virologists will take the RNA fragments that remain and cut them up into fragments that are a certain number of base pairs-long. Purportedly, the purpose for proceeding in the foregoing fashion is so that, subsequently, researchers will be able to amplify different instances of those fragments by mixing in primer sequences that are capable of attaching to such fragments in the cultured materials that have broken down, and, then through the PCR process, the quantities of those fragments can be increased through various cycles of amplification.

At this point virologists add – not materially but algorithmically because the addition takes place through computer programs -- the entire set of genetic sequences that come from a previous corona virus so that it can be used as a comparison marker, of sorts, for detecting the degree of homology that might be in the viral genetic material (supposedly SARS-CoV-2) that could be somewhere in the ingredients that have undergone a culturing process and, then, a cytopathic event that causes the various biological ingredients in the culture contents to break down into a vast array of fragments, particles, and the like which the virologists are hoping will contain genetic material that will match up – to a degree – with some of the structural and sequential features of the previous corona virus   However, there are several problems inherent in the foregoing step.

First, aside from the questionable tenability of having removed various kinds of DNA and RNA from the culture without any real good scientific reason for having done so, one would like to know the etiology of how the entire set of genetic sequences that allegedly are from a previous corona virus came into being. Did someone discover or uncover an approximately 30,000 base-pair (A-T, G-C or G-U)) long sequence of actual molecules (in the form of adenine, guanine, thymine, or cytosine – in the case of DNA – and uracil instead of cytosine in the case of RNA, along with a certain kind of sugar molecule (different sugars for DNA and RNA) as well as a phosphoric acid molecule that is covalently linked to the rest of the components) that make up the nucleotides that form the backbone to which a genetic sequence is attached that supposedly give expression to the genome of such a corona virus?

The answer to the foregoing question is: No, someone did not find an actual entity -- that is, a molecular entity of some kind that exists in the world as opposed to being a series of 1s and 0s in a computer – which is approximately 30,000 base-pair long which matched the foregoing description. Every alleged viral sequence is entirely computational in nature in the sense that each of them has been generated through algorithmic program (such as "Muscle" and subsequent creations of a more sophisticated nature) that run through an array of interpolative, extrapolative and other sorts of possible interpretations of available data (in the form of molecules that are in the cultured conglomeration that has broken down following a cytopathic event, and in the process, such a computation supposedly produces a "best" estimate of what an alleged viral sequence might look like given related sequences that already have been worked out previously in similar sorts of algorithmically driven computations (e.g., an earlier edition of some other kind of a corona virus).

Libraries of the foregoing sorts of computations are maintained. The entries in those libraries are used for purposes of comparison with other on-going computations, and, as indicted in the present 'Unbiased De Novo Next Generation Sequencing' process', an entry from one of those libraries has been introduced into the computerized representation concerning the culture breakdown products (following the arbitrary removal of various kinds of DNA and RNA) which are to serve as something of a template for determining the extent of the complimentary matches that might arise.

In legal-court terms, I believe such a process would be referred to as leading the witness. The corona sequence from one, or another, library is actually framing the manner in which the computational-algorithmic process being used in the "Unbiased De Novo Next Generation Sequencing" goes about it processes of interpolating, extrapolating, and interpreting available fragments with respect to how they might have fit together prior to the cytopathic event that led to the cultured products breaking up into millions, if not billion, of molecular fragments, and, as such, the process is hardly "unbiased" since the presence of an "earlier" corona template is shaping the character of what transpires during the computations that currently are being conducted.

If the cultured conglomeration of cellular materials that is breaking down contains millions, if not, billions of fragments of RNA material, and if such fragments are further sliced up in accordance with the protocols of the "Unbiased De Novo Next Generation Sequencing" process, then, why wouldn't a "reasonable" person assume that one is highly likely – on just a random basis – to be able to produce a genetic sequence that has a fair degree of homology with the sequential nature of the corona template that has been introduced into the cultured products that are breaking down. This would be the case not necessarily because any such extended genetic sequence existed in the cultured conglomeration prior to the cytopathic event but because if one is only working with four genetic letters, then, the possible sequential combinations which might be assumed by those letters is likely to include the genetic sequence of the earlier template for an alleged corona virus that is being introduced into the culture. This is especially the case if the RNA fragments that are present in the cultured breakdown products are being helped to do so by the presence of a library template that tends to push the computational or algorithmic process in the sequential direction of such a template.

If one had introduced a different kind of priming template into the cultured conglomeration – say, polio, or measles, or small pox (all of which have been generated algorithmically and not biologically) – one would have produced different results during the "Unbiased De Novo

Next Generation Sequencing" process. However, a corona template was introduced into the cultured conglomeration precisely because the virologists were searching for – in the present example -- the presence of SARS-CoV-2, and, consequently, by so doing, their results were biased by the presence of that priming template which is being used to assess the degree of homology which might exist between the genetic residues that might be present in a given cytopathic culture and a template that has been drawn from an existing library of templates for other alleged types and subtypes of computer-generated, hypothetical viruses.

The parts of the computational process involving the cultured products breakdown that are homologous with an existing library template will be cited as proof that there is a close genetic connection between what had been drawn from the library and what is being computationally put together (constructed) during the process of so-called "Unbiased De Novo Next Generation Sequencing". The aspects of the two computations that do not match (one from the library and one from the algorithmic computational representation involving the current contents of a cultured conglomeration that has broken down following a cytopathic event) will be interpreted as constituting evidence supposedly demonstrating the presence of genomic aspects from a new edition of coronavirus. However, one needs to keep in mind that such "unique" aspects have been constructed through a computational, algorithmically driven process which, nonetheless, in time, will be entered into a computer-generated template library so it, at some point in the future, can be used in a similar way with some future cultured conglomeration that has broken down and is believed to contain some other edition of a coronavirus.

At no point during the "Unbiased De Novo Next Generation Sequencing" process is any 30,000 base pair corona virus actually found. Whatever is found is the result of a computational, algorithmic construction that is entirely theoretical in nature and which has been heavily influenced by the sequential structure of the corona library template that has been introduced by virologists into the process so that such "established" sequences can be compared with the alleged sequences that are found (via a computer program) in the breakdown products of the cultured conglomeration that has undergone a cytopathic event.

Are real genetic molecules present in the foregoing analysis? Yes, they are, but the sequence of those molecules is a reflection of the computational methodology being used and, therefore, does not necessarily constitute proof that such a sequence of genetic molecules had been present and intact in the cultured conglomeration prior to the cytopathic event that took place and is being analyzed by an algorithmically-driven computational process.

In fact, there is absolutely no evidence which establishes the existence of actual viruses independently of the foregoing sort of computational process. All claims concerning the existence of viruses are artifacts of a process of computational invention, and such claims are not based on any virologist having empirically uncovered an actual viral genome that can be sequenced independently of the computational/algorithmic processes being discussed above, and, therefore, such claims are entirely theoretical in nature.

Virology, for the most, is largely a theoretical system for arranging and interpreting the results of an array of computational/algorithmic forms of analyses that cannot be shown to be tied to any actual, instances of viral genomes that can be shown to have actual ontological status in the wild. As such, virology is about the theoretical entities that different virologists seek to project onto the world while simultaneously being devoid of any empirical proof that those projected theoretical entities actually exist independent of the theories of virologists.

Consequently, virologists tend to be the sorts of people who are not able to sway people with actual evidence. As a result, in accordance with the old adage that if one doesn't have evidence, then, one must resort to trying to dazzle people with bullshit ... and, in the present case, the BS is a complex of theoretical entities that are organized into libraries of arbitrarily invented sequences that are apropos of nothing real but which give expression to computational and algorithmic techniques that are so technically shiny that people are misled into believing that those techniques are capable of producing results that are substantive and credible but which are not actually either – that is, substantive or credible.

In a series of recent experiments, Stefan Lanka has been able to document important elements of the foregoing discussion. He used the same sorts of PRC priming techniques that is employed by virologists.

The PCR amplification process gives rise to an optical change (e.g., color or luminosity). This change enables an individual to see whether the sequence carried by a primer is present in the culture conglomeration that has broken down into fragments and, then, subsequently, sliced up a bit more so that the PCR protocol can be used.

One can't PCR the whole culture at once because the PCR process only works with sequences of a limited length, but one can use certain primers that are based – at least theoretically -- on short sequences in the corona template that virologists have taken from one of their existing libraries of sequences and fragments and which has been introduced – algorithmically, that is, as part of a computer program – into the analysis of the culture being investigated. Once the amplification process indicates there is a match between the sequence on a given primer and the some aspect of the contents of the cultured conglomeration being studied, then that match can be amplified and becomes visible through the PCR protocol.

In one experiment, Stefan Lanka ran through twelve cycles or amplifications of the primer sequences being sought (that is, twelve rounds of doubling the presence of such sequences) in a culture that contained the usual contents of a culture minus a tissue sample from a sick individual. He found 20% of the purported sequence of the SARS-CoV-2 genome (and, remember, the purported sequence of the SARS-CoV-2 genome is entirely theoretical in nature and has never actually been found independently of these sorts of computational analyses).

In the next experiment, Lanka increased the number of amplification or doubling cycles to 30. Nothing was added to the cultured conglomeration during this time of analysis.

He discovered that after 30 cycles of doubling, the primers matched up with 98% of the alleged SARS-CoV-2 genomic sequence. Once again, one must keep in mind that the foregoing genomic sequence is based on a computational-algorithmic methodology that has not been shown to have any independent connection with an actual – that is a material or substantive -- 30,000 base pair genome that has been found in nature.

One also should keep in mind that all of the foregoing activity took place without anything being added to the cultured conglomeration that had broken down. The only difference was the number of cycles of PCR amplification that were used.

Why did Lanka "find" only 20% of the alleged genomic sequence of SARS-CoV-2 at 12 cycles? Why did he "find" 98% of the alleged genomic sequence of SARS-CoV-2 after 30 cycles of amplifying cultured fragments?

As Kary Mullis has made clear on many occasions following his invention of the PCR protocol, the very nature of the PCR process is to be able to create a series of new sequences through that process. Given all the RNA fragments that were present in the cultured conglomeration being studied, if one runs the PCR process through enough cycles, one can reproduce almost any sort of sequence for which one might be searching based on the primers one is using.

None of the foregoing proves that SARS-CoV-2 was originally present – as a substantive, existential entity -- within the cultured conglomeration being investigated. Rather, Lanka's ability to reproduce 98% of the theoretical sequence of the SARS-CoV-2 genome was entirely an artifact of the PCR process when it is used in conjunction with certain primers (based on an earlier theoretical sequence concerning an alleged corona virus) that, in effect, biases the direction in which the PCR process goes.

Lanka goes on to indicate that 78% of the fragments and pieces that were "found" in his experiments were the result of the way the PCR process takes place. The PCR process is capable of rearranging sequences and fragments depending on an array of factors involving the sort of enzymes that are used, or the temperature at which things are run, as well as numerous other factors that are noted in the MIKE Guidelines that govern the techniques involved in so-called Quantitative PCR analysis (and I might add at this point that Kary Mullis, the inventor of the PCR methodology once indicated that the notion of "quantitative PCR" is an oxymoron).

One of the issues with which Quantitative PCR analysis is concerned (along with the MIKE guidelines that have been developed to govern such analysis) has to do with the tremendous differences in results that are possible due to the way in which the foregoing sorts of conditions under which any given PCR analysis is run can affect PCR analysis. As a result of those sorts of differences, researchers often encountered difficulties trying to have their own work verified or have had difficulty verifying the accuracy of the work of others precisely because those kinds of differences were not taken into account, and, as a result, analyses tended to vary and were not standardized in any fashion – as the MIKE guidelines try to do.

Lanka's experiments had been set up in a way that precluded the possibility that SARS-CoV-2 could have been present in the cultured system that he had established and which, then, underwent a cytopathic event. Nonetheless, he had been able to reproduce 98% of the alleged sequence – a theoretical sequence – as an artifact of the PCR process that was arbitrarily biased – via the primers that were used and which were based on a theoretical corona sequence that had been taken from a library – which would move the analysis in the direction set by the primers and not because SARS-CoV-2 had been present in that cultured system from the beginning.

The computational-algorithmic process that is used to piece together the different fragments through various modes of interpolation, extrapolation, and other forms of filling in the empirical gaps that are left by the limits and characteristics of the PCR process are stitching together – or inventing – a new sequence. However, that sequence cannot be shown to be capable of being independently tied to an actual particle of SARS-CoV-2 that has precisely the genomic sequence that virologists have theoretically claimed it has.

At no point has empirical reality been shown to meet up with the theoretical claims of virologists. This is the case both with respect to SRS-CoV-2 as well as any other alleged virus.

As noted previously, if one had used a different set of primers based on sequences in the theoretical libraries of virologists that had to do with measles, or polio, or some other alleged virus, then, despite the fact that there was no possibility that such entities had been in the original cultured conglomeration, nevertheless, after running the PCR process through 30 cycles, one would be able to generate sequences that were a 98% match with the alleged genomic sequences of such purported viruses from the library of genetic sequences. Once again, such results would be an artifact of the methodology being used, and the title of that methodology notwithstanding – namely, an "Unbiased De Novo Next Generation Sequencing" – the entire process is nothing but a series of biases that are being implemented, all of which undermine any claims concerning the reliability of the results that are have been, and are being published, by one virologist or another concerning the genomic sequences that they are supposedly discovering, and, thus, it turns out that such discoveries are only in their imaginations.

During an earlier portion of this book, I wrote several chapters concerning the alleged pandemic that took place in 1918. One of these chapters (Chapter 8 -- The Fraudulent Game of Virology) critically explored a CDC article whose title proclaimed: "The Deadliest Flu: The Complete Story of a Virus Influenza Pandemic," while the other chapter (Chapter 7) was entitled: "Jeffrey Taubenberger's 1998 PBS Interview Concerning the 1918 Influenza."

As far as Chapter 8 is concerned, at the time of writing that chapter I did not -- and do not now -- feel that the CDC account concerning the 1918 flu constituted a complete account of what transpired in 1918, The foregoing material examined some of the available data that tended to suggest there were many things that took place in 1918 which cannot be reconciled with the idea that what occurred back then was necessarily due to presence of an allegedly highly infectious virus.

One such point-counterpoint had to do with experiments that were run in both Boston and San Francisco during the year of the so-called pandemic. "Volunteers" – they were really individuals who were in trouble with either the military or the law or both and who had volunteered to participate in the experiments in exchange for certain considerations of leniency or forgiveness being made in their respective cases – were exposed to patients who were in various stages of whatever illness it was that they had (and was presumed to be some form of a virulent flu).

Materials were taken from ill patients (who might just have become sick, or who were in more advanced stages of their disease process, or who might be on the verge of death), and those materials were transferred to the volunteers. Sometimes the transfer took place through the patient coughing and breathing in the face of a volunteer who was just a foot, or so away, or ill patients might have sprayed spit or sputum on such individuals, or mucous discharges of the patient's would be put into various bodily openings of the volunteers (ears, noses, and so on).

Despite the foregoing experiments with – all told – probably 100 volunteers across an array of experiments in several studies in different parts of the United States -- none of the volunteers got sick. If the alleged 1918 influenza was so virulent and infectious, how does one account for what took place in the foregoing studies?

My essay: "Jeffrey Taubenberger's 1998 PBS Interview ..." critically examined Taubenberger's account of his efforts to reconstruct the H1N1 virus that he believed was as the heart of the 1918 Influenza pandemic. According to Taubenberger, the H1N1 influenza genome that he believes was active in 1918 consisted of eight genes.

An important piece of data to keep in mind with respect to the foregoing is that no one has ever been able to discover – either in the tissues of ill people or via various cultured scenarios – the actual molecular genome of the alleged H1N1 virus. Both the H1N1 genome and its alleged eight genes are theoretical constructs concerning how virologists believe that alleged virus is structured and operates.

No one has witnessed that those eight genes actually perform in living organism in the manner that theory claims takes place in conjunction with such genes. During the 1998 PBS interview, Taubenberger indicates that his research group took a look at five genes in order to try to get a sense of what the overall genetic properties of the alleged virus might look like, but the genes at which they took a look had not been found as genetic, molecular structures in nature but, instead, had been constructed through various kinds of computational-algorithmic programs of the kind that have been critically examined by Lanka and others.

For instance, during the 1998 PBS interview, Taubenberger indicates that his research group had been able to piece together the 1800 base-long components of the hemagglutinin gene (the H in H1N1) and which supposedly codes for one of the proteins which is said to be present on the surface of the alleged H1N1 virus. However, what Taubenberger means by the idea of piecing together is that his research group came up with a theoretical computer model for constructing such a gene.

Similarly, the foregoing sort of thinking also extends to the neuraminidase gene that – according to theory -- codes for another surface protein that appears on the surface of the purported virus. Neuraminidase is the N in the H1N1 configuration.

However, since no one has ever isolated and purified an actual ontological instance of the H1N1 virus and, thereby, been able to demonstrate the actual nature, character, and sequence of such an alleged entity, then, Taubenberger and his research associates have not actually proven that their theoretical computer model of either the five aforementioned genes or the overall genomic sequence they were trying to work out for H1N1 was reflective of anything more than a theory. Both the hemagglutinin and neuraminidase genes (and resulting proteins) are nothing more than theoretical constructs that have been put together through various kinds of computer modeling.

According to theory, the hemagglutinin gene produces a protein that enables the alleged H1N1 virus to gain access to the cells and tissues of living organisms. The neuraminidase gene, on the other hand, produces a protein that supposedly enables a virus to exit cells once the virus has – presumably through its other six theoretical genes – been able to take over the replication machinery of a cell and generate as many copies of the virus as are deemed necessary (and one wonders about how the alleged H1N1 virus determines that the necessary number of viral replications has taken place).

Yet, none of the foregoing dynamics have ever been empirically demonstrated to actually take place. Obviously, one must clearly delineate between what the H1N1 theory of viral action claims takes place and what actually has been empirically demonstrated in this respect – which is really nothing at all.

According to the 1998 PBS interview, Taubenberger claims that there are 14 different subtypes – or variations on a theme – of the hemagglutinin gene, to go along with nine different subtypes of the neuraminidase gene. Taubenberger maintains that the H1N1 subtype combination played a key role in the 1918 flu crisis, and, yet, all of Taubenberger's claims are predicated on the various facets of the computer model that he and his colleagues put together when, literally, they invented or constructed the alleged H1N1 virus.

All of the foregoing considerations concerning Taubenberger are consistent with what has been said throughout the earlier analysis of how virologists go about making claims that they have discovered and sequenced SARS-CoV-2 (which is why I consider what Taubenberger said in the PBS interview to be "strangely familiar" when considered in the context of claims that have been made in conjunction with SARS-CoV-2). In both cases, virologists are confusing – in what seems to be a very delusional manner -- the process of producing computer models and theories with the process of actually being able to generate hard-core empirical proof that such theories and computer models are capable of accurately reflecting the character of concrete, molecular, and genetic reality. Lacking real empirical proof for their theories, they treat the concepts that give expression to their theories as if they possessed the same ontological status as such empirical proofs would be able to establish, and, as a result, theory is projected onto reality like some sort of palimpsest arrangement and, and, as a result, reality becomes obfuscated and covered over by a purely theoretical narrative.

Chapter 10: Debunking Some Modern Research

During my earlier book: *Observations Concerning My Encounter With COVID-19 (?),* I provided an overview of the work of Canada's Christine Massey and her New Zealand colleague –- work which established that evidence indicating that the SARS-CoV-2 virus actually exists is so overwhelming that more than 130 medical establishments, universities, research labs, government health ministries, and an array of other scientific-medical organizations and institutions are unable to cite even one study that is capable of lending credence to claims that such a virus exists. However, while Christine Massey accumulated a considerable number of official affidavits indicating that a variety of health, scientific, health, research and government agencies admitted that they did not possess or know of any documentation that was capable of demonstrating the existence of SARS-CoV-2, nevertheless, the absence of documentation capable of supporting the SARS-CoV-2 hypothesis does not necessarily mean that her findings constitute incontrovertible evidence that SARS-CoV-2 does not exist., Instead, the extensive survey conducted by Christine and her research partner only indicates that none of the organizations and individuals which had been contacted were aware, apparently, of any paper, article, or document that gave expression to evidence indicating that some individual or research team had been able to properly isolate and determine the genomic sequence of such a properly isolated SARS-CoV-2 particle.

In order to definitively address the latter issue, one must take a much more direct and active approach. More specifically, one needs to show how and why the methods of virologists are incapable of demonstrating that the SARS-CoV-2 virus exists.

There are variations in methodologies which permit certain degrees of freedom to be exercised in developing protocols for culturing an alleged virus and generating what virologists refer to as an "isolate." Nonetheless, all of those variations work off an underlying set of methodological procedures which has not really changed since the mid-1950s when John Enders began to do such work, and this underlying set of methodological procedures needs to be explored.

The normal format for a professional research paper consists of a number of sections. These include sections involving material covering: an abstract; introduction; methodology; results; discussion, and, finally, a conclusion.

While each of the foregoing sections has a role to play, one of the most important features of such a research paper lies within the section on methodology because the methods that are used will have a pervasive impact on the structure and character of all of the other sections of the paper. To get a sense of an article or paper, many people will read its abstract, but the real measure and value of such articles tends to be found within the section on methodology because that is the section of the article that actually informs a reader how any given experiment is run.

Let's consider some research that was conducted in late 2019, or early 2020, and was led by N. Zhu, (et. al.). For example, the title of one paper (Reference #1) is: "A Novel Coronavirus from Patients with Pneumonia in China," and it was published in the *New England Journal of Medicine* (382), pages 727-733, 2020. The title of a second paper (Reference #2) that was authored by L.L Ren and others) is: "Identification of a Novel Coronavirus Causing Severe Pneumonia in Humans: A Descriptive Study," This latter study was published in the *Chinese Medical Journal* (English), pages 1015 -1024, 2020).

The title of the first paper – (Reference #1) -- indicates that a Novel Coronavirus was discovered in conjunction with some patients who had pneumonia in China. The title of the second paper – Reference #2 – claims (more forcefully) that a novel form of coronavirus has been discovered that is capable of causing severe pneumonia in human beings (rather than being just something that correlates with the presence of pneumonia).

The Discussion section of Reference #1 states that the researchers have discovered a species of coronavirus that is "likely" to have been the cause of severe pneumonia in the patients that were being studied in Wuhan, China. The Discussion section goes on to assert that:

"Although our study does not fulfill Koch's postulates, our analysis provides evidence implicating 2019-nCoV in the Wuhan outbreak."

If one has not fulfilled the requirements of Koch's postulates (and, more accurately, if one has not satisfied the requirements of Rivers' updating of the Koch postulates for use with possible viral materials), then, one has not shown the following – namely, that researchers have successfully isolated and purified a given entity which supposedly emerged after having been cultured in conjunction with some sort of swab from a patient suffering from a severe form of pneumonia. Moreover, one has not shown that a properly purified edition of such an entity is capable of inducing other people to whom such an isolate is transmitted to also exhibit the same sort of severe pneumonia.

So, one can't help but wonder just why anyone should suppose that whatever it is that a group of researchers believe they have discovered to be present in the specimen swab taken from a patient ill with severe pneumonia is "likely" to be the cause of the observed severe pneumonia. In addition, one can't help but wonder what the nature of the alleged evidence is that supposedly some given "isolate" is the cause of such pneumonia despite the absence of any evidence that is capable of satisfying any of the Koch-Rivers conditions for determining causality with respect to the etiology of a given form of severe pneumonia.

According to Rivers' reformulation and extension of Koch's postulates, a virus must be capable of being shown to be present in every instance of the disease for which it is purported to be a cause. If the disease occurs without the presence of that putative virus, or if the alleged virus is present, but the disease is not actively being manifested, then, one has a prima facie case indicating that the relationship, if any, between an alleged virus and a given disease is problematic if not questionable.

Rivers also maintained that one needed to be able to completely isolate a putative viral entity from a person's body and from all other products associated with a given disease process in order to be able to ascertain that it is the virus which is causing a disease and not some other artifact that might be part of the disease process. Rivers goes on to stipulate that the alleged virus must be grown in a pure culture, and, as we will soon see, this really isn't something that virologists are able to accomplish in any sort of convincing manner.

Finally, one must be able to demonstrate that an isolated/purified virus is capable of producing the same disease as the one which is associated with the swab that has been taken from an ill person. If one were to purify an alleged virus, and then, expose, say, animals to that putative virus, and, yet, those animals did not exhibit any of the sorts of severe pneumonia that had been observed in the patient from whom a swab had been taken for purposes of culturing, then, once again, one has reason to question the nature of the relationship, if any, between an alleged virus and a given form of pathology, such as severe pneumonia.

In the discussion section of Reference #2, one finds the following words:

"These findings primarily indicate that the novel CoV is associated with the presence of severe pneumonia. However, it remains to be determined whether this novel CoV is capable of causing similar diseases in experimental animals."

Yet the title of the paper in which the foregoing quote appears is: "Identification of a Novel Coronavirus Causing Severe Pneumonia in Humans."

There is a considerable disconnect between what the title of the article asserts and what actually is being confessed with respect to the absence of any Koch-Rivers confirmation concerning the capacity of a given form of CoV to be able to cause severe forms of pneumonia in humans during the Discussion section of that same paper. Unfortunately, many academics, researchers and medical doctors who are often pressed for time might tend to look only at the title of a paper, and, perhaps, its abstract before moving on to other things. Anyone who had limited themselves to doing things in the foregoing curtailed manner -- and, therefore, had failed to actually read the paper in its entirety -- would be under the impression that some researchers in China had proven that CoV caused severe pneumonia when by the admission of the authors themselves in the paper's Discussion section, nothing of the sort had been demonstrated.

Let's consider – in more detail – another paper entitled: "The Pathogenicity of SARS-CoV-2 in hACE2 Transgenic Mice." The paper involved research by Bao and others. It appeared in *Nature*, Volume 583, in the July 30, 2020 edition of that journal.

The title of the paper makes a claim. It states that the pathogenicity of SARS-CoV-2 can be shown to be actively present in hACE2 transgenic mice.

Mice do not usually express ACE2 receptors (and this presupposes that such receptors actually exist). Consequently, one has to breed transgenic versions of those mice that are capable of expressing ACE2 receptors (Considerations indicating that such receptors might not actually exist will be presented in a later chapter of the present book).

Such transgenic processes tend to lead to alterations in other aspects of the physiology of mice that extend beyond a capacity to manifest alleged ACE2 receptors. Therefore, due to the presence of such alterations, the nature of whatever parallels are believed to exist between transgenic mice and human beings is uncertain.

There were two control groups in the Bao study. One group consisted of mice that had not been bred through a transgenic process and, therefore, were without a gene that, supposedly, was capable of being expressed in the form of ACE2 receptors.

Another alleged control group was referred to as being mock-infected. The mice in this group were also transgenic, but they were not given the concoction that supposedly contained whatever was causing the sort of illness that was observed in the individual from whom a swab of some sort had been drawn originally, and, instead, they were administered a phosphate buffered solution.

However, the foregoing mock-infected test subjects do not really constitute a true control group. To qualify as such a control, the transgender mice in this group should have been given bodily fluids of some kind that came from a healthy organism rather than a phosphate buffered solution.

The study indicates that the non-control group of transgenic mice was "given" the alleged virus. However, this actually obfuscates what is taking place.

Materials were taken from an ill organism and transferred to the transgenic group of mice. There was no evidence that what was transferred contained the alleged virus, nor was there any evidence that even if present, such a virus was responsible for whatever illness was being observed.

Other materials were added to whatever was taken from an ill patient. Among other things, the resulting concoction contained Vero kidney monkey cells.

Vero kidney cells are a line of cells that were developed in 1962 in conjunction with African Green Monkeys. They are used in the culturing process because of the high degree of homology between the genetic contents of monkey cells and human genomes, and, as such, they are believed to be able to serve as a sort of credible stand in for what might take place in human cells.

In addition to the Vero kidney cells, the process of culturing a virus also contains a number of other ingredients. Among these extra materials are: DMEM (Dulbecco's Modified Eagle Medium, a growth medium); fetal bovine serum; streptomycin, penicillin, or other antibiotics such as gentamicin and, sometimes, anti-fungal agents (e.g., amphotericin B) – all of which can be quite poisonous to Vero kidney cells.

Thus, when one considers the process of culturing an alleged virus, one should understand that whatever swab of material comes from an ill organism (and quite independently of the issue as to whether such a swab does, or does not, contain viral material of some kind), that swab is co-joined with an array of other materials. These other materials have properties that are capable of obfuscating and confusing a person's understanding about whether, or not, viral particles actually exist in such a concoction.

A more rigorous way of trying to determine whether alleged viral particles exist in the original swab that is taken from an ill organism would be to institute something akin to the following protocol. First one would need to filter the lung fluid in the original sample in order to remove cell-sized objects since the objects for which one is searching are, supposedly, far smaller than a cell.

Next, one would want to run the filtered material that was derived in step one through a density gradient centrifuge process. This will result in particles that have the same density being bound together in tight bands that permit one to distinguish such bands from other chemicals and particles that possess different density properties.

Third, one would need to identify the kind of density band in which one felt that alleged viral particles of a certain kind were most likely to be found. Then, one would use a pipette or syringe to gather together whatever was in the density gradient band in which one was interested.

If one believed that a certain density gradient band contained the alleged virus in which one was interested, then, the final step would be to take the identified band which had been removed via a pipette or syringe and, then, transfer the material, through one method or another, to the transgenic mice in the experimental group. Once that material has been transferred, one would wait to see whether, or not, any form of pathology or illness emerged and whether, or not, the nature of that illness or pathology was similar to whatever the nature of the disease process that had been present in the ill individual from whom test swabs had been taken originally.

Clinical manifestations were recorded in conjunction with the three groups of mice during the Bao experiment that currently is being explored. The symptoms that were observed by the researchers consisted of various degrees of weight loss and instances of slightly bristled fur, and, moreover, less than half of the mice in the study developed any symptoms at all.

Presumably, weight loss and, especially, slightly bristled fur are not typical symptoms associated with COVID-19 – at least in humans. None of the mice in the study exhibited coughs or had any sort of respiratory problems, and, yet, experimenters had been claiming that what took place in the mice was evidence capable of demonstrating – as the title of their paper stipulated – "The Pathogenicity of SARS-CoV-2 in hACE2 Transgenic Mice."

On June 8, 2020, the *Lancet* published an article that provided some details about autopsies that had been performed in conjunction with 38 patients who had tested positive for COVID-19. Given what already has been stated concerning the lack of credibility that surrounds the whole process of PCR testing, let's put aside that aspect of the *Lancet* and focus on some of the results of those autopsies.

Among other things the autopsies revealed that many of the bodies of the examined patients exhibited diffuse damage in conjunction with the system of alveoli sacs in the lungs (where oxygen and carbon dioxide are exchanged). In addition, there was considerable interstitial edema (congestion of fluids); necrosis of pneumocytes (these consist of several types of surface epithelial cells of the alveoli); metaplasia (involves a transformation of normal adult cells into abnormal forms of those cells); hyaline membranes (a form of lung injury that involves a deficiency in a surfactant – consisting of six lipids and four proteins – that is responsible for helping to maintain surface tension and providing stability for the alveoli), as well as an array of blood clots in small arterial vessels within the lungs.

Now, irrespective of whether, or not, the foregoing set of problems noted during the autopsies was due to SARS-Co-V-2 is a separate issue. Nonetheless, many people were labeling such a list of effects as indicators of the presence of COVID-19 (primarily because such individuals had been misled by the presence of a positive PCR test that had been assigned to such deaths ... tests that were actually meaningless as indicators of the presence of disease).

Yet, even if we were to suppose that the foregoing findings of the 38 autopsies that were performed in Italy were due to the presence of SARS-CoV-2, what has any of that got to do with the Bao paper that is being discussed and which, on the one hand, had a title claiming that it was presenting evidence which demonstrated the pathogenicity of SARS-CoV-2, and, yet, on the other hand, all the results which were reported in that paper merely indicated that some of the mice (in all three groups) exhibited some degree of weight loss, while others showed signs of bristled fur, and less than half of any of the mice developed any symptoms at all?

Anyone who merely read the title of the paper in question might believe that here was another piece of evidence in which not only had SARS-CoV-2 had been proven to exist, but, in addition, SARS-CoV-2 had been shown to be a virus that had a certain kind of profile of pathogenicity to which that alleged virus gave expression. Unfortunately, the paper by Bao, (et. al.,) was devoid of any such proof or evidence.

Autopsies of the mice in the Bao study were done. Unlike the 38 autopsies of humans performed in Italy, no edema of any kind was detected in any of the mice. There were no hyaline membranes found in the mice. There had been no indications that metaplasia occurred within any of the mice. There was no evidence of blood clots of any kind within the mice.

If one looks at the alleged culturing process of any given virus, one comes into contact with a standard methodological protocol template that has been used by virologists and microbiologists since the time of John Enders in the mid 1950s. The general character of this set of methodological protocols for such a culturing process has already been touched upon in the previously discussed Bao experiment.

One takes a sample or swab from a diseased organism and introduces that swab/sample into a culturing process. The latter process consists of: Taking a Vero kidney monkey cell; adding some sort of growth medium; mixing in a soupçon of fetal bovine serum; throwing in a few antibiotics that often are poisonous to the Vero kidney monkey cells, and, finally, putting the whole conglomeration in a minimal nutritional state.

What occurs next is a cytopathic event. In other words, one observes the death of the Vero cell, and for decades virologists and microbiologist have attempted to claim that such an event is proof that the swab/sample from the ill person contained a virus that was introduced into the culturing process and, necessarily, is responsible for the death of that cell. This end product of the culturing process constitutes the alleged "isolate" through which, supposedly, the putative virus has been induced to assert its lethal presence.

Stefan Lanka has done something relatively recently that most virologists and microbiologists have never done. He decided to run a controlled experiment in which everything would be exactly as it had been during the standard culturing experiment in virology (i.e., Vero kidney cell, growth medium, fetal bovine serum, various antibiotics would all be present, and the whole mixture would be subjected to a condition of nutritional starvation), but instead of introducing a swab/sample from an ill person, he added a swab/sample from a healthy individual.

The same cytopathic event took place in conjunction with the swab from a healthy person. In other words, the cell being cultured died.

However, because there was no swab/sample from an ill person that had been introduced into the culturing process, one couldn't blame the death of the cell on the presence of an alleged virus that had been hypothesized to be present in the swab/sample from an ill person. The reason that the cell died in both instances was because the components that made up the culturing process were responsible for the death of the cell and not because there had been any kind of exogenous organism or viral body that had been introduced into the culturing process.

Back in the mid-1950s, John Enders actually had run the same sort of controlled experiment as Stefan Lanka did relatively recently. Enders too had discovered that the reason why the cells died in the two culturing processes (one involving material from an ill person, and one involving material from a health person) had nothing to do with the presence of an alleged virus but was due, instead, to the cytopathic nature of the culturing process in and of itself independent of the presence of possible viral agents.

Unfortunately, subsequently, virologists only seemed to want to remember the part of the Enders experiment that involved taking samples/swabs from an ill person, culturing that material, and, then, observing that there was a cytopathic effect which – enabled (although problematically) virologists to conclude that the manifestation of such an effect (i.e., the death of the Vero monkey kidney cell) proves that there was some sort of putative virus present which was responsible for that cytopathic event. Yet, simultaneously, they also seemed inclined to want to forget or ignore (probably because to remember that John Enders also demonstrated that the same cytopathic effect occurred when added swabs from healthy people into the culturing process undermined their narrative concerning the idea of viruses) that if one performed the same process of culturing with material from a healthy person as has been done with a swab/sample from an ill person, and, thereby, established a control group for the first part of the experiment involving a swab/sample from an unhealthy person, then, the result of running the control group gives rise to the same cytopathic effect – that is, kidney cell dies, lyses, and releases all of its biological contents into the culture due to the toxic nature of the culturing process and not because of the presence of an alleged virus.

The foregoing process of ignoring what happened in the control group within the Enders experiment is really a case of willful blindness. Such people are only willing to see what they want to see and the significance of what occurred with the control group in the original Enders experiment (which has been confirmed by Stefan Lanka) be damned.

When the cytopathic effect takes place in the Vero monkey kidney cell and the cell lyses, the contents of that cell are emptied into the cultured conglomeration. In addition, one also has additional sources of biological content coming from the fetal bovine serum that was part of the culturing process, plus whatever cellular and biological material came from the swab/sample that was taken from either a healthy or ill individual.

As noted earlier in the present book, electron micrographs are often recorded in conjunction with certain products or objects or entities that come forth during the process of lyses that takes place during cell death. Small particles often can be observed in these electron micrographs, and after a research person highlights some of those particles or draws arrows to draw attention to their presence in the EM imagery, the claim is often made that such objects constitute the virus (e.g., SARS-CoV-2, or chicken pox, or polio, or measles, or whatever other virus one believes to be present) and, yet, the very same objects/entities could be seen if one were to go through the same culturing process and a Vero kidney cell dies in conjunction with a healthy swab/sample (rather than from an unhealthy source) because it has been added to a culturing process that is inherently toxic and constitutes the actual reason why the Vero monkey cell dies irrespective of whether the swab/sample that is added is from an healthy or unhealthy individual or organism.

The many particles that can be imaged following the aforementioned cytopathic event in the cultured sample are believed by virologists to be the result of a viral replication process that is enabled by the presence of the culturing medium. According to theory, a virus needs either the living tissue of a host (say in the area of the lungs) or a culturing environment in order to be able to replicate itself, and the particles that are depicted in various Electron Micrographs are said to give expression to the end result of the viral replication process.

Nonetheless, there is no data in the EM which demonstrates how the particles being depicted actually arose. There is no experimental evidence (but there are lots of theories) which purportedly demonstrates how a virus supposedly gains entrance to cells (whether in living tissue or a cultured medium). There is no experimental evidence (but, again, there are plenty of theories concerning this issue) which shows how a virus takes over a cell's capacity to replicate, and, then, proceeds to replicate until sufficient numbers of viral particles have been produced to lyse the cells in living tissue or lyse the Vero monkey kidney cell, nor is there any actual experimental evidence (although there are considerable theories concerning such an issue) to show how a virus actually goes about the process of cell lyses.

Specialized genes have been proposed for all of the foregoing functions (e.g., the ability to gain access to a cell's interior; the ability to take over a cell's machinery of replication; the ability to engage in the process of cell lyses in order to be able to exit from one cell and move on to other cells within a given instance of living tissue). Yet, unless one can demonstrate that such genes are actually contained within however many base pairs make up the alleged genome of a putative virus, then, all of the foregoing is nothing more than a theoretical account of how things might work.

Electron Micrographs are static images. If virologists had something more than such static images -- that is, if they had been able to capture dynamic images of the genes of a virus accessing, entering, taking over replication, and, then, exiting a cell (whether being cultured or in actual tissue) -- those virologists wouldn't just be showing people EMs and, then, trying to interpret what is being depicted in that static image.

The sort of evidence – i.e., EM – that is being presented by virologists actually reveals the weakness of their perspective. If they had the sorts of dynamic imagery that are being alluded to above, (which would constitute a form of rigorous evidence that strongly supported claims concerning the presence of a virus in living tissue or a cultured cell, as well as documented proof concerning the actual nature of their activity with respect to cells in living tissues or in conjunction with the culturing process), virologists wouldn't have to restrict themselves to presenting static EMs and, then, trying to convince viewers that the particles seen in those images are actually virus particles despite the absence of any independently derived evidence capable of confirming that such particles actually were viral in nature.

Circling, or pointing toward, or highlighting particles in an EM does not, in and of itself, actually prove anything about the actual nature or identity of the particles that are being singled out. One needs to examine those objects through whatever methods are available in order to try to determine what the nature of their internal composition might be.

Do those particles harbor some given number of base pairs that are capable of uniquely identifying such particles as instances of one kind of virus rather than another? Or, is the internal compositional nature of those particles indicative of some other kind of particle -- such as endosomes (tiny – viral sized -- intracellular organelles that might play a role in storing and/or transporting and/or cleaning up various materials within a cell) or exosomes (tiny – viral sized – organelles that tend to be membrane bound and could have arrived from the extra-cellular environment surrounding a cell and is either in the process of being absorbed by a given cell, or such a particle could be in the process of being released by a cell to serve purposes beyond the membrane of the cell to which the exosome is temporarily bound).

If the particles or objects in the Electron Micrographs to which virologists are pointing were, say, SARS-CoV-2, then, one should be able to discover that, yes, the particles under consideration all consist of 30,000 base pairs of genetic material (this is the theoretical estimate concerning the alleged size of the SARS-CoV-2 virus). Furthermore, one also should be able to sequence such a genome and identify those aspects of the sequence that are unique to SARS-CoV-2 and, thereby, which differentiate it from all other species of virus.

Surely, virologists have succeeded in doing all of the foregoing. Surely, they have shown that when one examines the particles depicted in the EM, then, one discovers an approximately 30,000 base pair genome that can be sequenced to show that, say, SARS-CoV-2 has a unique structure that in some way differentiates that virus from all other viruses (and this unique feature would be the very thing that any credible test for the presence of SARS-CoV2 would have to be able to detect and which the Drosten PCR test cannot demonstrate can be satisfied in any credible manner and which is why the PCR test is completely useless and meaningless).

Some researchers have claimed that they have sequenced the whole genome of SARS-CoV-2. Recently, Stefan Lanka ran a series of tests – and is running further entries in that series – to determine whether such a claim is defensible.

Lanka took a cell culture to which no materials from an ill or healthy person had been added, and therefore, there was no possibility that any virus was present in the culture. The culture contained the usual materials consisting of a Vero monkey kidney cell, fetal bovine serum, a growth medium and antibiotics of one kind or another. In addition, according to standard procedure, the culture was placed in a minimal nutritional condition (i.e., it was starved).

The culture underwent a cytopathic event and, as a result, broke down and released its contents. In one of the experiments conducted by Lanka, he added mRNA to the foregoing concoction.

The mRNA was from an easily accessible form of commercial yeast. There was no virus present in the yeast.

The concoction to which the mRNA was added contained various fragments of the broken-down Vero cell that were the result of the cytopathic event that had taken place in the Vero cell. In addition, the concoction contained fetal bovine serum, antibiotics or antifungal agents of one kind or another, as well as some limited or minimal level of nutrients.

Lanka next examined the contents of the foregoing concoction of materials, in order to try to detect the presence of an assembly (presumably via the activity of the mRNA that came from the yeast) of 30,000 base pairs (the letters of the genetic code) that gives expression to the SARS-CoV-2 genome. He did not find such a genome, nor did he discover any sort of set of 30,000 base pairs that had a sequence which could be shown to be uniquely specific to the alleged SARS-CoV-2 virus.

In fact, nowhere in the entire history of virology has anyone ever been able to take a cell culture similar to the one with which Lanka was working and demonstrate -- after it undergoes a cytopathic event -- that one can find in such a culture the base pairs for a viral genome that can be sequenced to show that such a sequence is unique to a given virus and, thereby, differentiates it from all other forms of viral material. Moreover, if one looks at any of the experiments that were reported early on in China, Canada, Australia and elsewhere concerning claims that they had located and sequenced the SARS-CoV-2 virus, one will not find any evidence in those experiments which shows that some 30,000 base pair genome had been discovered in their cultures and, then, showed that the researchers had been able to properly sequence those base pairs and, also were further able to demonstrate that the foregoing genomic sequence was both infectious and lethal.

Those papers (like the Zhu, Ren, and Bao papers examined earlier in this chapter) are all smoke and mirrors. In each case, paper or article titles are presented that claim one thing, but when one actually examines the sections covering methodology, results, and discussion, there often is a game of bait and switch taking place, and, presumably, the authors of such papers/articles are counting on the laziness of readers and/or counting on the time constraints under which, many researchers operate to obfuscate the fact that claims in the title or the abstract section have not been substantiated with actual evidence in other sections of the paper/article.

Chapter 11: There Is No Immune System

The last four chapters have contained a considerable amount of information indicating that viruses in the modern sense of the term do not exist. In other words, if one considers viruses to be nano-sized entities that contain a set of internal sequences consisting of either DNA or RNA (but not both) which are encapsulated within some sort of glycoprotein packaging, and that such entities are capable of: (1) entering cells, (2) taking over part of the genetic machinery of those cells in order to use it to generate copies of themselves, and, then, (3) exiting such cells in a manner that causes the deaths of the cells from which such entities are departing before (4) finding their way to new cells to enter (i.e., infect), then, the discussions which have taken place in each of the last four chapters provide evidence to substantially demonstrate – despite claims to the contrary by most virologists, microbiologists, and medical practitioners -- that such entities have never been proven to exist.

Toward the beginning of Chapter Three in the present book, I indicated that **if** the existence of viruses cannot be proven, then, allopathic medicine is confronted with a substantial set of problems. More specifically, in the aforementioned chapter a series of illnesses was cited which, supposedly, are caused by viruses – namely:

"Mumps; Hepatitis A, B, and C; HIV/AIDS; colds (some of which, supposedly, are due to various forms of coronaviruses); influenza (e.g., swine flu, bird flu); small pox; measles; polio; chicken pox; HPV (human papillomavirus); rabies; certain forms of meningitis; viral pneumonia; SARS 1 and 2; Epstein-Barr; mononucleosis; RSV (respiratory syncytial virus); an array of hemorrhagic fevers including Ebola, Lassa Fever, and Marsburg; hantavirus; yellow fever; dengue fever; some researchers believe that 15% of cancers are due to viruses of one kind or another; West Nile Virus; Zika; Western Equine Encephalitis; Herpes Simplex Virus I and II; shingles; roseola, as well as monkeypox."

Additional viral candidates could have been included in the foregoing list of illnesses that, allegedly, are caused by viral entities.

However, if viruses -- as the last four chapters have tried to indicate -- do not exist, then, the medical establishment really has no clue as to what the nature of the illnesses are to which the foregoing names are alluding nor do they have any idea about what might cause those illnesses, and, therefore, at best, clinicians are merely treating symptoms independently of any context of causality.

In the next chapter, the idea of vaccines will be engaged in a critically reflective manner. After all, if many – if not most -- vaccines are supposedly directed toward providing recipients of those injections with supposed immunity against this or that virus, then, the possibility that the very viruses against which such vaccines allegedly are providing some sort of immunity might not actually exist becomes something of a deeply disturbing embarrassment if not medical crisis. This is because vaccine ingredients are being introduced into the bodies of individuals (often children) through such injections, and as will be pointed out in the following chapter, many of those ingredients are toxic.

Therefore, such injections have no business being introduced into the bodies of human beings because those jabs have no provable capacity to immunize someone against non-existent viruses and, in fact, those injections often carry some sort of demonstrable toxic effect with respect to the human body. Indeed, if viruses do not exist, then, whatever statistical data is put forth in an effort to demonstrate that such vaccines work constitutes a complete distortion concerning the alleged significance of that data because there would be nothing in the contents of the injection which could be shown to have anything to do with a non-existent virus ... unless, of course, one wishes to argue that whatever data that exists serves as evidence that injections which do not contain viral material of any kind for purposes of defending against non-existent viruses is nothing more than a placebo of some kind which people have been tricked into believing helps prevent certain kinds of diseases.

However, before moving on to the issue of vaccines in the next chapter there is another related idea that requires attention because it tends to frame the issue of vaccines in a biased manner, and this related idea is the focus of the current chapter. More specifically, just as it makes no sense to inject people with anti-viral vaccines if viruses do not exist, so too, it makes no sense to talk about vaccines as enhancing the immune system if the latter sort of system does not actually exist. One even might argue – and I will -- that, perhaps, the primary reason for the existence of the term "immune system" might be because that phrase serves to lend credence to the idea of vaccines which supposedly lend support to, and allegedly enhance such, a theoretical system.

While the human body does possess a variety of defense mechanisms that play essential roles in helping to maintain the health of the biological terrain of an individual, none of these defensive activities are necessarily rooted in a dynamic which confers some sort of immunity on a person's body. Instead, the discussion in this chapter will be geared toward trying to show that the defense system of human beings seems to entail processes that either seek to maintain some sort of biological stability or involve various modes of detoxification rather than give expression to processes of immunity.

If the foregoing claim is true, then, because vaccines often introduce a variety of toxic substances into the human body, vaccines actually serve to undermine the body's primary means of defense against environmental toxins and poisons – that is, the body's tendencies to stabilize and or detoxify its biological terrain. Instead of helping the body to detoxify, vaccines actually increase the problem of toxicity and biological instability with which the body must deal by virtue of the nature of the ingredients that tend to be present within those vaccines.

Although what follows will not be a definitive account of the detoxification-stabilization defense system that exists in our bodies, hopefully, there will be enough information which will be presented during the ensuing overview process that could, at the very least, induce a reader to re-consider the whole issue concerning the idea of an immune system and ask whether that term might be something of a misnomer and ask, as well, whether that phrase might serve as a beneficial smokescreen for the vaccine industry due to the problematic manner in which the term frames the issue of how the body actually works and given the latter dynamic whether vaccines actually serve any useful purpose as far as the issue of immunity is concerned. Of course, since the notion of the immune system is so deeply entrenched in most of our minds and ways of thinking, then, objectively entertaining the possibility that such a system might not actually exist becomes a rather daunting task, but let's proceed with that challenge and see where it might lead us.

The alleged immune system is often described as consisting of two major components: Namely, an innate system and an adaptive system. One of the alleged primary differences between these two defensive components is that the innate system tends to have no memory of its interaction with potential challenges to the well-being of the biological terrain, whereas, the so-called adaptive system supposedly remembers – in some sense and to varying degrees – its interactions with previous encounters involving challenges to the well-being of an organism, and that sort of adaptive memory is at the heart of the notion of immunity.

For example, consider one dimension of the body's innate system of defense: The skin. Approximately one millimeter below the surface of the skin one finds the basal layer of cells which consists of modified stem cells that generate new skin cells on a constant basis, and, as these new skin cells come into existence, they begin their journey to the surface during which they will push previously generated skin cells outward, toward the exterior of the body, where, eventually, such cells will die and be sloughed off.

As a result of the aforementioned pushing process, there are roughly 50 layers of dead cells between the basal layer and the surface of the body. These layers of dead cells serve as a barrier that helps protect against various kinds of pathogens – whether in the form of agents like toxins or poisons or some sort of microbiological entity from gaining entry to the interior of the body.

The foregoing barrier arrangement does not confer any sort of immunity, nor does it necessarily form an impenetrable barrier. Toxins and poisons that the barrier of dead cells might have kept from entering the body at one point in time might find channel-ways through that barrier at some other point in time.

In both instances, the dead cells have no memory of having previously encountered those agents. The barrier operates as a physical impediment to penetration and does not operate as some sort of immunological dynamic involving a process of adaptive memory.

As skin cells mature, they develop longish spikes which form an interlocking network with other cells that, collectively, establish a wall-like structure, of sorts, that helps prevent toxins, poisons and various kinds of microbiological entities from entering the body. Skin cells also are capable of releasing substances such as the protein keratin.

Keratin not only helps make the nails in the tips of our fingers and toes hard, but, also helps provide the skin with a certain element of toughness or hardness. Therefore, keratin not only helps fortify the aforementioned interlocking network of skin cells but, as well, helps to fill in some of the gaps that might be present in such a network.

Skin cells also contain what are known as lamellar bodies that release fats filled with substances called defensins. Like keratin, the fats which are released by the lamellar bodies offer, yet, another layer of protection that can resist penetration by poisons, toxins, and other possible protagonists, while, on the other hand, the defensins molecules that are present in that fat help to establish a resistant and/or inhospitable environment for various kinds of substances or agents that, under certain circumstances, might have a potential for creating health difficulties for human beings.

Defensins are described as constituting several subclasses of molecular-assemblages that have the capacity to poke holes in various entities that it encounters. Apparently, if enough defensins gang together, they are capable of poking enough holes into an entity to reduce the latter into some sort of dysfunctional state.

Defensins, supposedly, are very particular about what they choose to attack. What enables them to be so specific with respect to how they are able to identify which objects or entities are to be targeted and which objects or entities are to be left alone is not entirely understood.

While their existence might give expression to a defensive response of the body, that response is not necessarily immunological in character. In other words, it is possible that the presence of defensins does not confer a form of immunity so much as it part of an arsenal of tools that can be activated as needed in order to try to maintain a stable form of dynamics within a given dimension of the biological terrain

For example, the wall of interlocking skin cells plus keratin, and lamellar body-created fats and defensins could be understood to be establishing a wall-like, fortified structure that helps establish a set of ecological conditions, along with the aforementioned layers of dead skin cells, that are conducive to maintaining a certain level of stability within some facet of a given biological terrain (in this case, the skin).

If the foregoing wall-like structure which makes up the composition of the skin should be penetrated in some way from without, then that structure loses some of its capacity to protect the body rather than loses some sort of capacity to render the body to be, or become, immune to potential pathogens (and pathogens can be toxins and poisons as well as some manner of microorganism). Furthermore, one also should keep in mind that if there various forms of dynamics within a human being that interfere with the body's ability to generate new skin cells, or to be able to produce appropriate amounts of keratin, or to possess fully functioning lamellar bodies, then, this undermines the body's capacity to create effective ecological barriers to intrusion from without rather than undermines some sort of immune process.

A dike – even though it has protective value -- doesn't serve to immunize the land against which the sea is impinging when it pounds against the dike. Each wave must be engaged on its own, as well as, be dealt with collectively as a series of such encounters.

Similarly, the complex barrier being described here does not immunize the body against whatever might be seeking entry into the interior of the body. Nonetheless, that set of interlocking barriers, like the dike system, does have protective, stabilizing value.

As indicated previously, the skin does not seem to have any sort of memory concerning its past encounters with potential threats that entail possible ways in which the barrier system that has been erected by the skin cells might be breeched. All instances of a potential for breeching that system of barriers tend to be treated as being independent of one another -- and let's put the issue of allergies aside for the time being because the presence of allergies seems to indicate an absence of sort of immunity rather than its presence.

The poisons or toxins that land on the surface of the skin on one occasion are met with the same sort of layered barrier system of protection as existed during earlier encounters with such poisons and toxins, and, therefore, one such encounter does not confer any sort of immunity with respect to ensuing encounters involving those same toxins and poisons.

Conceivably, the foregoing set of interlocking defenses could be shaped, in part, by a process of learning in which the way the genome expresses itself at any given point in time is altered by a set of dynamics that are epigenetic in character. More will be said about the issue of epigenetics in a subsequent chapter, but at the present time, all I wish to note is that to whatever extent epigenetic processes assist the biological terrain to better deal with potential threats to well-being, those sorts of processes do not necessarily give expression to some form of immunological adaptation but, instead, might be directed toward helping the body to better defend itself ... much like a boxer who is paying attention to her or his opponent learns to vary tactics in order to enhance his or her defensive and/or offensive perimeter and, yet, none of these improvements necessarily confers any sort of immunity with respect to either preventing being effectively attacked again in ways that are similar to previous encounters, nor do such improvements necessarily guarantee a successful outcome with respect to those kinds of encounters.

Like a boxer, the biological terrain might learn, through epigenetic processes, how to get hit less frequently or not get hit as directly or as forcefully as in previous rounds or fights. Or, like a fighter, the biological terrain might learn, through epigenetic transitions, how to better pace itself and, thereby, be able to fight for a more extended period of time. Or, like a fighter, the biological terrain might learn, through epigenetic modifications, how to vary certain detoxification and stabilization tactics from round to round or fight to fight, and so on.

However, none of the foregoing sorts of adaptive forms of learning necessarily enable the biological terrain to avoid the fight or provide that terrain with any sort of immunity that allows the terrain to idly sit in the corner while a designated stand-in goes out and KO's an opponent. In fact, removing a particular opponent from the ring will not necessarily return the biological terrain to a condition of symbiotic stability or return a given microorganism to a condition of pleiomorphic/pleomorphic stability.

Moreover, the dynamics of immunity should not be confused with the dynamics of detoxification. Countering the presence of a non-symbiotic form of a given microorganism through the process of removal that is entailed by the dynamics of detoxification is not at all the same as the process of removal that is entailed by the dynamics of immunization.

In detoxification there is no memory of whether something is toxic or poisonous. There is only the capacity of toxins and poisons to destabilize the biological terrain and, in the process, induce microorganisms to transition away from their normally symbiotic relationship with that terrain, and it is the presence of the condition of destabilization and accompanying undermining of effective functioning in the biological terrain that leads to processes of detoxification beginning to kick in,

Since there is no proof that viruses exist, there would appear to be no need for an immunological system capable of remembering previous encounters with an inexhaustible set of non-existent entities. Furthermore, in the case of diseases such as diphtheria, tetanus, and cholera the use of injections can be understood as a means of helping to detoxify the poisons or toxins that are released by bacteria when the latter are induced to transition out of a harmless condition into a non-symbiotic state.

Interestingly enough, in the case of tetanus and cholera, not all instances of the bacteria carry the toxin or poison that has the capacity to cause illness. These bacteria must go through what is known as a lysogenic cycle in which under normal conditions they are harmless, but if they attacked by a "virus or phage" which introduces the DNA into the bacteria that is capable of making the problematic toxin or poison, then such bacteria become potential threats to health.

Yet, previously, I stated that there are no viruses. So, if there are no viruses, then, what are phages?

One possibility is that bacteria which manifest a phage of one kind or another are merely giving expression to one of the pleiomorphic forms of those sorts of bacteria. In other words, bacteria are harmless when in certain stages of their pleiomorphic/pleomorphic cycle. Yet, when induced by the surrounding terrain to enter into a non-symbiotic mode of functioning, then they have the capacity to become toxic by, among other things, altering their morphological and functional character through, among other things, the appearance of a phage structure on the bacteria.

Under certain conditions of the biological terrain, the gene or genes for the phage structure are not activated. When those conditions change – perhaps through some sort of epigenetic transition process – the genes might become activated.

Leaving such considerations aside, let's return to the issue of adaptive learning that was being discussed earlier and which might come through epigenetic changes of some kind. Such changes could be considered to be adaptive in the sense that they help enhance the body's capacity to establish greater ecological stability in conjunction with some facet of the biological terrain. Alternatively, whatever learning is taking place within the biological terrain might be adaptive due to the manner in which it helps the process of detoxification to work more effectively.

However, none of the aforementioned sorts of adaptations confer immunity of any sort. The body merely learns how to put up a better fight with respect to potential threats that will happen again and again ... threats that cannot be short-circuited by some sort of immunological response. There are all manner of modalities of adaptive learning which are not immunological in nature – that is, such learning does not automatically prevent certain kinds of problems from arising but, instead, merely provides the individual with a better chance to survive in order to be in a position of the sort of adequate well-being that might enable the individual to take on similar fights in the future.

To alter the metaphor somewhat, a baseball batter who is able to figure out what the pitch sequence is that a given catcher is calling for or a given pitcher is seeking might have a higher probability of getting on base during that at-bat than if he would if he were unable to correctly surmise what pitch or pitches might be coming, but this does not enable the batter to become immune to striking out or getting out in the future – even with the same pitcher. So too with the defense systems of the body ... each encounter with pathology tends to be independent of other encounters even if it should be the case that as with baseball hitters certain kinds of adaptive learning occur – perhaps epigenetically -- along the way which enhance the chances of the body responding more effectively on some – but not necessarily all – occasions in the future.

Given – in the light of the information presented in the previous four chapters – that there does not seem to be any proof that viruses actually exist – I am going to remove such entities from the following discussion. Consequently, the ensuring conversation concerning potential threats to well-being will be restricted to pathogens in the form of toxins, poisons, and microbiological entities such as bacteria and fungi. However, one should keep in mind that Béchamp, Enderlein, Rife, and Naessens – along with a variety of other researchers -- all indicated that the pleiomorphic/pleomorphic nature of microorganisms tended to be activated as a result of changes in the biological terrain which served as part of the ecological environment within which such entities existed.

Thus, if – let us say as a result of some form of intense stress that were being experienced by a human being – the biological terrain that is shaped by the dynamics of skin cell processes becomes disrupted in some way or is undermined to varying degrees, then, such changes might induce various pathogens that are present on the surface of the skin – or, perhaps, that are nestled in some way among the interlocking skin cells -- to enter into other phases of their pleiomorphic/pleomorphic cycle. Moreover, if one will recall, in Chapter Four, mention was made in passing about Naessens contention that under normal, healthy conditions of functioning, the somatid cycle was limited to only three of its possible 16 or 17 cycle stages, but if some given aspect of the biological terrain became destabilized, then, other stages of the pleiomorphic/pleomorphic cycle of a given somatid might become manifest as various forms of bacteria or fungi that are capable of releasing toxins and/or poisons as part and parcel of their normal mode of metabolic functioning and that are capable of adversely affecting the biological terrain in which they are released.

Such toxins and poisons could have the capacity to create various sorts of micro-lesions in the barrier that has been erected by the dynamics of skin cells. Such areas of toxicity might become focal points of various facets of the body's defense system to bring about processes of inflammation that give expression to the way in which different dimensions of the body's defense system are marshaled to counter whatever toxicity might have arisen in the biological terrain of the skin at that location.

Once again, however, none of the foregoing dynamics constitutes something which might be called an immune response. Whatever the body is doing is directed toward countering the toxicity that exists, and should such toxicity arise again in the future, the body will not be immune to its presence but will, once again, have to mount a similar sort of defense that is intended to detoxify the presence of such poisons and, thereby, help return the biological terrain – in this case, the skin – to stable forms of functioning in which (if Naessens is correct) only the first three stages of a given somatid's pleiomorphic/pleomorphic cycle are operational.

When a given aspect of the biological terrain was considered to be healthy, Béchamp, Enderlein, Rife, and Naessens all tended to indicate that whatever microorganisms might be present in that terrain tended to have a symbiotic relationship with one another from which both microorganisms and the terrain derived benefit. When that condition of health became destabilized due to some sort of dysfunctional dynamic within a given aspect of the biological terrain, then only at that point might some of the microorganisms which were present be induced to depart from their normal symbiotic relationship with the surrounding terrain and begin to enter into other non-symbiotic stages of their pleiomorphic/pleomorphic cycles that had the potential to present challenges of one kind or another for the surrounding terrain and, as a result, would require different facets of the body's defense system to become active and intervene.

In a sense, from the perspective of people such as Béchamp, Enderlein, Rife, and Naessens, the whole point of medicine is to assist the body to go through whatever processes are necessary to be able to help return the microzymas, endobionts, or somatids that exist in the body to be in a condition of symbiotic functioning within the dynamics of the biological terrain (and all of the those individuals considered the foregoing entities to be more basic than cells, while also being central to, the proper functioning, of the cell). As such, one of the best defenses against ill-health was to finds ways to stabilize the state of symbiosis which tied normal functioning in the biological terrain, and this was accomplished primarily through working to maintain only certain, limited stages of the pleiomorphic/pleomorphic cycle of the microorganisms which inhabit that terrain.

In other words, the preeminent threat to the well-being of any given organism's biological terrain was not invasion by infectious germs from without. Rather, the primary threat was – for whatever reason (e.g., poor nutrition, exposure to toxicity, environmental poisoning of one kind or another) – the deterioration of, or transitioning of, some part of the terrain to a less effective form of functioning which would, in turn, run the risk of inducing some sort of pleiomorphic/pleomorphic change in one, or more, of the microorganisms that are present and, in the process, de-stabilize the terrain and complicate its way of functioning by altering the nature of relationship between microorganisms and the terrain from being symbiotic to that of being non-symbiotic.

Maintaining a condition of symbiosis is best achieved through (a) processes that lend support to the ecological stabilization of the biological terrain of an organism and, when necessary, (b) the dynamics of detoxification involving that same ecology rather than through the dynamics of immunity. No process of immunity could prevent microorganisms, microzymas, endobionts, or somatids from entering into problematic stages of their pleiomorphic/pleomorphic cycles, but, instead, what is necessary is to find ways of stabilizing healthy forms of symbiotic relationships between such entities and the surrounding biological terrain, and this was best accomplished by helping that terrain to perform within stable parameters of operation that were unlikely to induce whatever microorganisms that might be present within the terrain to change their morphology or mode of functioning and, thereby, become pushed into or pulled into problematic, non-symbiotic stages of their pleiomorphic/pleomorphic cycles.

For example, under the right set of conditions, people sweat. Sweat brings salt to the surface of the body.

Some people maintain that the presence of that salt tends to repel certain kinds of microorganisms. In addition such individuals indicate that there are antibiotic-like substances present in the skin that have the capacity to kill certain kinds of microbes.

Whether such alleged antibiotic-like substances come from the previously mentioned lamellar bodies within skin cells or they arise from some other source, there is another way of looking at the situation being described. Rather, than having antibiotic-like properties there might be substances – such as the previously mentioned defensins -- that are excreted by, say, the skin cells which are intended to help stabilize the biological terrain and render it less likely to be able to induce the microorganisms, microzymas, endobionts, or somatids that are present to enter into non-symbiotic stages of their pleiomorphic/pleomorphic cycles.

After all, we are told that defensins are very particular concerning the nature of their targets although how targets are selected and why they are selected or when they are selected is, apparently, not, yet, known. Given the degrees of uncertainty concerning the functioning of such entities, then, the aforementioned substances which are present in the salt that are brought forth by sweating or which are released from the lamellar bodies in skin cells are not necessarily antibiotic-like but might have functions that are other than being responsible for killing entities that reside on, or in, the skin and, instead, might be intended to help to stabilize conditions in a given aspect of the biological terrain – in this case, the skin … a process of stabilization which is directed toward maintaining conditions of symbiosis between whatever microorganisms are present within the surrounding terrain.

There is a multiplicity of microorganisms on, and in, the skin of the human body. There is no need to kill those entities with antibiotic-like substances if those microorganisms can be coaxed into continuing on with their symbiotic relationship with the surrounding biological terrain through the presence of substances (perhaps, for example, that are present in sweat and secreted by, say, lamellar bodies within skin cells) which lend stabilizing support to the continuation of those symbiotic relationships.

Even if such substances did have antibiotic-like properties of some kind, the purpose of their presence might not be to kill microorganisms in general but, rather, to help resist the emergence of various forms of bacteria that might arise if certain microorganisms were induced to enter into a stage of their pleiomorphic/pleomorphic cycle that was non-symbiotic in character. Microorganisms will always be present on, and within, the skin because there are billions of them and, therefore, they cannot all be exterminated – irrespective of what they body does or does not do – and, furthermore, not all microorganisms that inhabit the biological terrain should be eliminated because of the ways in which they contribute to the health of the body, and, consequently, to suppose that whatever is present in sweat or is secreted by lamellar bodies in skin cells must have an antibiotic-like function seems to make little sense, and, instead, it might make more sense to suppose that such substances serve the task of helping to lend stability to the symbiotic interaction between the pleiomorphic/pleomorphic cycles of the microorganisms which are present and the surrounding biological terrain.

Similar sorts of considerations might be entertained in conjunction with the issue of pH. Some individuals believe that because the skin tends to have a low pH value -- and, therefore, is somewhat acidic – then that this condition serves to rebuff many kinds of microorganisms from taking up residency on, or in, the skin.

There is another way of looking at the foregoing situation. Instead of allegedly serving to rebuff microorganisms in general from taking up residence in a given aspect of the biological terrain, perhaps, the relatively low pH value of the skin might be what is most conducive to maintaining a stable relationship between whatever microorganisms are present and the surrounding biological terrain (i.e., the skin), and part of the nature of that process of stabilization involves the way in which the relatively low pH value might help to resist the emergence of certain forms of the pleiomorphic/pleomorphic life cycle of a given entity from entering into non-symbiotic modalities of expression with the surrounding biological terrain or, alternatively, to help maintain a given microorganism in a symbiotic aspect of its pleiomorphic/pleomorphic cycle.

The same might be true with respect to determining what will constitute optimum pH values in different parts of the biological terrain. In other words, an optimum pH value for any given aspect of the biological terrain that is under consideration will be a function of what sorts of conditions are necessary to help maintain the most stable form of symbiotic relationship between whatever microorganisms are present and the surrounding biological terrain. Furthermore, part of what makes certain kinds of pH value optimum in different facets of the biological terrain is the extent to which certain kinds of pH values help to prevent, or establish a certain resistance with respect to, microorganisms that are present being easily able to enter into non-symbiotic modalities of functioning.

As Béchamp, Enderlein, Rife, and Naessens were able to demonstrate – but contrary to the claims of Pasteur – the blood is not sterile. All manner of microorganisms are present within the blood.

The pH of blood is not necessarily intended to establish the sort of hostile environment that will rebuff the presence of microorganisms. Rather, the pH of blood has optimum value when, on the one hand, it lends support to helping to maintain a stable symbiotic dynamic between the biological terrain (in this case, the blood) and whatever microorganisms might be present within that terrain, while, on the other hand, simultaneously serving as a countervailing force to the possible emergence of stages in the pleiomorphic/pleomorphic cycles of whatever entities are present that could be induced to enter into non-symbiotic stages of those cycles should the condition of the surrounding terrain change in certain ways.

The defense dynamic of the human body does not make decisions about which microorganisms will be permitted to settle into a given aspect of its biological terrain. Rather, the defense dynamic of the human body operates to try to create conditions which are optimum because they are most conducive to (a) stabilizing the symbiotic relationships between the presence of various kinds of microzymas, endobionts, or somatids within different dimensions of the biological terrain that constitutes the human body, and (b) serving as ecological buffers or sources of resistance to the emergence of certain modalities of the life cycles of pleiomorphic/pleomorphic organisms that are non-symbiotic in nature in the context of a given aspect of the biological terrain.

The human body responds to the presence of toxins, poisons, de-stabilization of the biological terrain, and microorganisms that are induced to enter into non-symbiotic stages of their pleiomorphic/pleomorphic cycles. None of this response is necessarily oriented in an immunological manner but tends to operate according to the nuances of each case as it arises and, with the exception of some relatively minor considerations, each case develops largely independently of whatever has taken place previously. The same, or similar, sorts of problems often show up again and again until the underlying problems with the biological terrain as well as various non-symbiotic stages of the pleiomorphic/pleomorphic cycle of various microorganisms that have arisen in conjunction with the foregoing sorts of problems are properly addressed.

If one runs down through the list of components that often are considered to constitute part of the immune system, I believe it is possible to re-frame the issue as a function of the dynamics of stabilization and detoxification rather than immunity. For instance, macrophages are frequently described as being the largest sort of cell that exists within the immune system -- indeed, the size of a macrophage cell relative to an average human cell is a number of orders of magnitude greater than the size of the latter.

Purportedly, macrophages have a variety of abilities. They are said to: (a) be able to mend wounds in various ways; (b) have the capacity to engulf or eat entities – both dead and alive; (c) breakdown the materials that are consumed to their basic constituents, which can, then, be recycled, and also (d) help coordinate bodily defenses to different degrees.

One should note before moving on that approximately one million cells are estimated to die every second in the human body. Somehow, such cells know that they have come to the end of their life-cycle, and as they prepare to self-destruct through a process known as apoptosis, they release a signal to the rest of the body which indicates what is taking place, and, as a result, macrophages have the capacity to find their way to such self-terminated entities, consume them, and, then, salvage whatever components might be salvageable.

None of the foregoing abilities or activities is necessarily inherently immunological in character. All of those processes could be understood as giving expression to the dynamics of stabilization (e.g., recycling materials, helping to heal wounds co-ordinate defenses) and detoxification (i.e., engulfing, eating, processing, and removing various materials, whether dead, dying, or compromised) from a given location – whether inflamed or just the site of cellular apoptosis.

Much of immunological data is theoretically parsed. Different theories will lead to different modalities of interpreting the data and, as a result, tend to lead to different kinds of conclusions concerning the precise nature of the dynamic that a given theoretician believes might be taking place.

If, on the one hand, Pasteur and his subsequent acolytes are wrong about the monomorphic nature of germ theory – and there seems to be considerable evidence (some of which has been presented already in earlier chapters) to suggest that this notion of germ theory is essentially incorrect, while, on the other hand, if Béchamp and his scientific heirs are correct about the pleiomorphic/pleomorphic nature of microorganisms including the principle that germs do not attack us from without but are induced to enter into non-symbiotic stages of their pleiomorphic/pleomorphic cycles by the condition of the surrounding biological terrain in which they reside, and if, finally, viruses do not exist (and I believe the evidence is overwhelming in this regard), then, just what immunological functions are being performed by macrophages? Macrophages are not eliminating all microorganisms from the body so that one never has to – supposedly -- fight or resist the latter again, but, instead, macrophages appear to be directing their activities against whatever entities (whether in the form of dead dying, compromised, or molecular detritus) which are present that are undermining the stability of the aspect of the biological terrain that has become destabilized/inflamed and using the dynamics of detoxification (i.e., engulfing/eating and removing) to assist the destabilized facets of the biological terrain to work its way back toward stability and healthy functioning.

If the organism should return to a state of health, the activities of the macrophages do not appear, in any way, to have helped to confer a condition of immunity on the organism. Should a similar sort of destabilization events take place in the future and, as a result, the biological terrain becomes compromised in some fashion, and this, in turn, leads to microorganisms which normally have a symbiotic relationship with the terrain being induced to enter non-symbiotic stages of their pleiomorphic/pleomorphic cycle and, as a result, release toxins and poisons that adversely affect the functioning of the surrounding terrain to some further degree, then, the organism will not exhibit properties of immunity with respect to the unfolding events but, instead, will have to fight the earlier battle all over again – although, as indicated previously, the body's capacity to do battle again might have been enhanced in certain ways as a result of, say, epigenetic forms of adaptive learning that might have taken place in the meantime.

Similar sorts of things could be said in conjunction with the activities of neutrophils. Neutrophils are short-lived modalities of bodily defense that die within a few days of coming into existence.

Like macrophages, neutrophils are capable of engulfing certain kinds of cellular detritus and removing that material from the biological terrain. Because of this capacity to consume cellular debris, macrophages and neutrophils are both classified as phagocytes.

Neutrophils are believed to be far more prevalent in the body than are macrophages. Moreover, estimates indicate that there could be as many as one hundred billion of these kinds of cells that come into existence, as well as die, every day (apparently, the body produces one billion neutrophils for every kilogram of body weight).

Since we are working on the assumption – based on considerable evidence – that viruses don't exist, and since there is a great deal of evidence to support the notion of pleiomorphism/pleomorphism which runs counter to the monomorphic theory of Pasteur which, among other things, holds that human beings are constantly under attack by invading hordes of bacteria, one might wonder what all of the neutrophils are doing in our bodies.

Like the National Guard, they are on stand-by in case of different kinds of emergencies – that might run from minor to extensive in severity. To begin with, even if nothing of a pathological nature were happening in the human body, there is still the task of dealing with the one million cells that are undergoing apoptosis each second.

However, lived life is filled with all manner of incidents that either destabilize certain aspects of the biological terrain or threaten to do so if not properly attended to. Macrophages and neutrophils both cruise the byways of the human body looking for signs of potential or actual problems, and, as such, they are both agents of maintaining or helping to maintain, conditions of stability, and, when necessary, to undertake processes of detoxification.

Somehow, neutrophils are capable of picking up on whatever biological chatter is occurring within the terrain, and, if necessary, they will find their way to the area of inflammation or destabilization, and, among other things, either consume detritus from the area of inflammation or have the capacity, on occasion, to erupt and cast a net of chemicals that help to seal off and begin to detoxify the area of inflammation or destabilization.

Some individuals speak about the capacity of neutrophils to, under certain circumstances, to generate what is referred to as a NET or Neutrophil Extracellular Trap. When this occurs, the nucleus of the neutrophil begins to dissolve and release its DNA into the surrounding cellular cytoplasm, and as this occurs, different kinds of proteins (both enzymatic and structural) become attached to the released DNA. Eventually, the whole developing complex is shot out into the extracellular medium surrounding the former neutrophil and forms a matrix-like formation that traps dead, dying, compromised, and molecular detritus within the chemical net.

According to some immunologists and virologists, the aforementioned sort of netting phenomenon traps whatever pathogens -- such as viruses and bacteria – that might be present and, as a result, prevents those entities from escaping their date with termination. Alternatively, one might also argue that since viruses have not been proven to exist and since whatever bacteria are present might be dead, dying, or compromised in some fashion, the so-called net is not really a trap as much as it is a way of cordoning off an area that is designated for a complete process of detoxification and re-stabilization, and, as such, is not really immunological in nature as much as it is reparative in scope.

Given that neutrophils are believed to have a potential for generating a lot of collateral damage under certain circumstances, the whole process of generating a matrix-like network that seals off a given area of the biological terrain might be a form of apoptosis. If so, the NET mechanism constitutes something of a fail-safe mechanism which is built into the neutrophil and enables it to contribute to the process of re-stabilization even as it removes itself from further activity.

Platelets –- which are not cells but fragments of cells known as megakaryocytes, and the platelets break-off from the squid-like appendages that grow outward from their home in the bone marrow and, eventually, connect to different blood vessels) -- also find their way to the site of inflammation. Such platelets, together with whatever red blood cells happen to be caught in the chemical net that has been cast by certain neutrophils will collectively work to seal up whatever sort of breach might have occurred in the skin or tissue and, thereby, prevent loss of important bodily fluids, such as blood.

Platelets – because of their fragmented nature -- also seem to have the capacity to slice and dice various forms of dying, dead, compromised, and molecular structures that might be found within the zone that is being sealed off. This helps with the process of detoxification but has no immunological properties

Once again, as indicated above, none of the foregoing dynamics involves any sort of immunity dynamics. If a similar crisis arose in the future, then, similar sorts of dynamics will unfold and the organism will have to cycle through its litany of defenses yet, once again, because it has not been made immune to anything.

Eating once does not render one immune from having to eat again. Sleeping once does not confer some sort of immunity on an individual and thereby, enable the person to forgo the need to sleep again. Recovering from a cut or a broken bone does not make one immune to any future need to attend to cuts or broken bones. Being exposed to an environmental toxin or a poison does not immunological relieve one of the task of having to deal with the ramifications of such exposures during subsequent incidents.

Since the pathological potential of the microorganisms that live on and within us is a function of the condition of the biological terrain that surrounds those microorganisms, then dealing with a given instance of destabilization in the biological terrain that induces one, or more, microorganisms to transition away from a normal state of symbiosis and, thereby, presents an individual with the problem of trying to find ways of returning the destabilized biological terrain to a condition of well-being or health once again does not protect that individual from having to go through the foregoing process yet again on some future occasion should the biological terrain become destabilized in a similar manner. Through all of the foregoing, there is no immunological activity taking place, but, rather, there is just a constant process of trying to maintain stability or re-establish stabilization through an array of detoxification processes that must be repeated as needed.

The presence of inflammation within one, or more, facets of the biological terrain is not necessarily a signal for some alleged immune system to kick into operation. Instead, inflammation might just be the first sign that destabilization of some kind is affecting one, or more, areas of the biological terrain, and, as a result, the organism is beginning to experience a form of stress that falls beyond what is necessary for normal modalities of functioning ... a form of stress that is problematic, if not destructive, and, consequently, serves no useful purpose as it does in conjunction with such activities as curiosity, creativity, learning, exercise, motivation, sexuality, and other modalities of social interaction.

The five indicators of inflammation are said to involve the presence of: Pain, redness, swelling, heat and some degree of dysfunctional activity. However, the only reason the foregoing phenomena occur is because there has been some kind of destabilization within the biological terrain, and, therefore, it is the destabilization that leads to the emergence of the aforementioned five symptoms.

The foregoing 5 symptoms, or whatever combination of them manifest themselves, are all indications that some form of inflammation exists which has summoned or activated the set of dynamics that have brought about such symptoms. Nonetheless, those symptoms are not the inflammation but are the body's response to the presence of inflammation.

In the foregoing context, some individuals mention Mast cells as entities that contain the sorts of molecules that, when released, are capable of causing inflammation. Once again, however, one should distinguish between, on the one hand, the actual cause of inflammation – that is, whatever is responsible for the destabilization of some facet of the biological terrain to which, say, a human being gives expression – and, on the other hand, the response of different components within the body to try to find ways of helping to re-stabilizing and detoxifying the part or parts of the biological terrain that has or have become destabilized.

Similarly, there are individuals who claim that one of the tasks of the macrophages and neutrophils is to help maintain a condition of inflammation. Such a perspective is somewhat oxymoronic in character because macrophages and neutrophils are only found at the scene of some given inflammatory event which has summoned such entities to the site of initial breakdown in the biological terrain that constitutes the actual ground zero of inflammation.

Therefore, at best, macrophages and neutrophils should be added to the previously noted 5 signs concerning the presence of inflammation. They are like the little cards at a crime scene indicating that somewhere amidst those symptom (crime) cards there is a condition of inflammation or destabilization that has led to the appearance of such markers being stuck in the biological terrain at this location.

One of the issues that is both intriguing and mysterious at the same time in all of the foregoing is the following. What is the nature of the signal that the initial conditions of destabilization-inflammation send out which draws different bodily resources to themselves and how, as well as in what way, do different components of the body's indigenous medical team understand those signals?

At this juncture, the term cytokines is often mentioned. Cytokines is the collective term that is used to refer to a group of proteins (numbering in the hundreds) that are believed to be bearers of information. There are several classes of cytokines: One version of this molecule goes according to the rubric of: chemokines, and these are largely responsible for helping to guide different elements to places of inflammation, while the other kind of protein are known as cytokines and are considered to be responsible for the transmitting of an array of other kinds of information.

Most immunologists today believe that the cytokine system constitutes an integral part of an alleged immune system. Nonetheless, one might be willing to concede that cytokines have the capacity to transmit information within the biological terrain without necessarily supposing that the information being transmitted is immunological in character.

Every time some modality of inflammation or destabilization of the biological terrain occurs and the body responds to that destabilization with any of the previously noted 5 symptoms that are commonly interpreted as constituting signs indicating the presence of inflammation – signs that have emerged as a result of information that has been conveyed (we will assume) to appropriate cells by one or another cytokine protein – there is nothing necessarily of an immunological dynamic which is taking place. The body is being prepared to undertake a set of re-stabilization and/or detoxification processes, and it is not being prepared to by-pass such an undertaking as one might expect in the case of some sort of immunological phenomenon.

If macrophages, neutrophils, Mast cells, platelets, salt, various kinds of proteins, plasma, intercellular fluids, and the like are being signaled by an array of cytokines to show up at a given location of inflammation, how is any of this immunological in character? Every time inflammation occurs, the same set of functions have to be set in motion, and there is no general, immunological form of protection that will guarantee that either simple inflammation will occur or that simple inflammation -- despite the assistance which is being directed to the indicated area of the terrain -- will not descend into chronic inflammation.

Even if the destabilization that gave rise to some form of inflammation had been sufficient to induce microorganisms living in the affected area of the biological terrain to enter into some non-symbiotic stage of their pleiomorphic/pleomorphic cycle and, as a result, lead to further modalities of inflammation, there is nothing necessarily of an immunological nature that can prevent the foregoing sequence of events from happening. The cytokine system of communication might help guide the body to initiate and coordinate a set of responses that are intended to assist the biological terrain to regain its normal stability or integrity by properly addressing whatever caused the existing condition of inflammation, but nothing in the defensive arsenal of the human body can stop the original cause of inflammation from happening and, therefore, perhaps there is no immunological response to inflammation.

Sometimes, for unknown reasons, the cytokine system becomes inflamed – that is, the portions of the biological terrain within which and through which cytokine proteins convey their information becomes destabilized and dysfunctional. As a result, the body is unable to mount any sort of systemic response to that kind of inflammation because the very system of protein informants that is needed to direct and coordinate an appropriate response is out of commission and unreliable, but this does not necessarily constitute a breakdown of the immune system but, rather, it could be a breakdown in the system that is believed to play a key role – via information processing -- in helping the body to return to its original condition of stability and well-being.

If the foregoing is the case, then, disease is not being prevented in the way in which the immunological model holds. Rather, health – if possible -- is being re-established.

Inflammation might be followed by infection, and infection might exacerbate the degree of inflammation that is taking place. Nonetheless, the two are not synonymous with one another.

Infection – whenever it might occur -- always follows from some form of initial destabilization or ground-zero mode of inflammation within the biological terrain. Infection appears to be a more advanced or complicated form of the foregoing ground-zero incident of inflammation that initially destabilized the biological terrain in some manner.

In a sense, infection is a condition in which the dynamics of re-stabilization that were set in motion in conjunction with the original, ground-zero cause of destabilization within a person's biological terrain are unable to resolve the underlying problem that helped to give rise to some sort of destabilizing form of inflammation, and, as a result, the portion of the biological terrain that has become destabilized becomes caught up in a struggle of stabilization due to an on-going, and incomplete struggle to detoxify the dead, dying, compromised, and molecular detritus that have been accumulating in the destabilized area, as well as unresolved problems with respect to whatever microorganisms within the microbiome have been induced to transition away from symbiotic behavior and, as a result, have complicated attempts of the body to re-stabilize and detoxify the biological terrain.

Microorganisms that have been induced to transition away from their previously symbiotic relationship with the biological terrain do not infect that terrain. Rather, the problem which such microorganisms tend to pose arises in conjunction with the toxins that such entities release either as a result of normal metabolic activities or due to some sort of self-defense dynamic.

These poisons usually come in the guise of proteins of one kind or another that are toxic to the biological terrain of human beings. The microorganisms that are associated with pathologies such as botulism, tetanus, cholera, diphtheria, anthrax, meningitis, pneumonia, and so on tend to do their damage through the release of toxins and not as a result of some process of cellular infection.

Such toxins do interfere with or undermine various aspects of cellular metabolism. However, just as cyanide cannot be said to infect human beings, so too, the toxins released by microorganisms do not infect human beings but, instead, disrupt normal cellular functioning.

It is interesting that while macrophages and dendritic cells were, supposedly, clever or lucky enough to develop a system of receptor sentinels capable of recognizing and, according to theory, organizing a coordinated attack against the microorganisms that, under some circumstances (i.e., when induced to transition away from symbiotic modes of behavior) and, therefore, only actually represent a potential threat (that is, they are safe until they transition away from symbiosis) but never seem to have been clever or lucky enough to develop the capacity to detect the presence of, and coordinate an attack against, the toxins which are released by such bacteria and are the actual threat represented by those microorganisms. One also wonders how macrophages and dendritic cells came to "understand" that the reason such microorganisms had a potential to help bring about some form of pathology had to do with toxins that were released rather than anything to do with the microorganism in and of itself.

The foregoing sorts of microorganisms might proliferate within the biological terrain, but that sort of proliferation just enhances the extent to which toxicity of some kind is being released. The formation of such colonies within the biological terrain does not so much constitute a condition of infection as it sets in motion the release of a set of toxic forces that can only exacerbate as well as complicate whatever event or set of events first led to the de-stabilization of the biological terrain of a given individual.

Septicemia, sometimes referred to as blood poisoning, is often described as what takes place when bacteria find their way into the blood stream. However, as Béchamp, Enderlein, Rife, Naessens, and other students of pleiomorphic/pleomorphic dynamics have all pointed out, the blood stream is not the sterile environment that Pasteur claimed it to be.

Microorganisms inhabit the blood stream of even healthy individuals. What is critically determinate in the possible onset of septicemia is whether, or not, such microorganisms are induced to transition away from their normal symbiotic relationship with the surrounding biological terrain (the blood) in which they reside.

The same seems to be true in with respect to the pathologies known as necrotizing fasciitis and toxic shock syndrome. There are a variety of microorganisms that – if induced to transition to a non-symbiotic state as a result of the de-stabilized condition of the surrounding biological terrain – are capable of releasing toxins that are capable of leading to the death of different kinds of soft tissue in the case of necrotizing fasciitis as well as lead to multiple organ failures in the case of toxic shock syndrome.

When inflammation becomes chronic, then, some organ, tissue, cellular activity, or metabolic process within the biological terrain has become destabilized in a continuous or semi-continuous manner. The plasma (the liquid dimension of blood), intercellular fluids, salt, and proteins that have been drawn to the destabilized area of the terrain help to underwrite the occurrence of the five symptoms that were noted previously that are associated with the presence of inflammation and, as such, are, as previously intimated, symptoms that have been created by the body's unrequited response to whatever the nature of the initial source of inflammation might have been.

Idiopathic chronic inflammation can have deadly consequences. In fact, 50% of the people who die each day is due to some underlying condition of chronic inflammation which has never been properly resolved – often because such pathologies have never been properly diagnosed and/or properly treated since the cause of this sort of inflammation or destabilization of the biological terrain has, to varying degrees, eluded the understanding of the attending medical practitioners.

There is a reason why, during each past decade, millions of people have died at the hands of well-intended doctors (this is based on actual research and not hyperbole), and that reason has to do with the ignorance which governs the understanding or lack thereof, concerning an array of pathological conditions which such doctors treat. There is a reason why -- with each, new ensuing decade -- millions of people will continue to die at the hands of presumably well-intentioned doctors, and this reason seems to have to do with the unwillingness of all too many doctors to acknowledge their ignorance or to acknowledge even the possibility of their ignorance concerning so many known unknowns within medicine. And, as the body count mounts into the tens of millions of human beings, one can't help but question whether such individuals are so well-intentioned after all.

Since the 1949 release of: *The Production of Antibodies*, by MacFarlane Burnet and Frank Fenner, the world of immunology has been deeply influenced by the idea that, somehow, an organism and each of its subset of organs, tissues, and cellular systems are able to tell the difference between self and non-self. Naturally, the question arises as to what the nature of this "somehow" is that enables such distinctions to be made.

One of the primary attempts to account for the foregoing sort of capacity to be able to differentiate between self and non-self involves a process that is referred to as 'microbial pattern recognition'. More specifically, there are proteins which have been discovered that are referred to as "Toll-like receptors" which generally are found on macrophages and dendritic cells which have surveillance roles that, among other things, parse the biological terrain on a fairly continuous basis as they scan for signs of danger – actual or potential -- and, then – if necessary -- pass this information along to other facets of the stabilization-detoxification system so that the latter processes can try to help the terrain regain its biological integrity or health.

Dendritic cells are not to be confused with the similarly sounding dendrites that are associated with neurons in the brain. The former dendritic cells bear the name they do because of the tree-like structures to which they often give expression.

Their etiological origins are situated in the bone marrow, but their roots also can be traced to leucocytes that are generated by the lymph system. Theory maintains that there are sentinel-like receptors on both macrophages and dendritic cells that have developed the capacity to recognize a menagerie of bits and pieces from an array of microorganisms that, supposedly, have the capacity to do the body harm and, consequently, when such bits and pieces are detected as being present in the biological terrain, macrophages and dendritic cells begin to transmit the information to the rest of the body so that appropriate steps might be taken (e.g., such as the schooling and activation of T-cells) which will enable the biological terrain to deal with such entities.

Let's leave aside questions concerning how macrophages and dendritic cells supposedly were able to acquire, over time, the sort of adaptive learning skills that enabled them to develop an ability to be able to recognize, as well as, understand the significance of what was being encountered by means of different receptors or proteins. Furthermore, let's shelve questions concerning how other dimensions of the biological terrain acquired the capacity to understand the nature and significance of the communications that were being passed on to them by macrophages and dendritic cells. Even given – for purposes of argument -- both of the foregoing concessions, there are still a variety of important questions that remain.

When I was an undergraduate, I took a course in philosophy with Morton White who later went on to spend time at the Institute for Advanced Study that is associated with, but independent of, Princeton University and which has served as a sort of theoretical research womb for the development of so many interesting, talented, and creative thinkers. One of the themes for the aforementioned course concerned the issue of causality.

Can one say, without the need for any sort of amending addendum, that the reason that a match lit was because someone struck it against the right kind of surface? The answer is: "No, one cannot."

If there is not enough oxygen in the space where one tries to light the match, it will not light. If the ratio of chemicals in the match head does not have the right set of chemical components or those components are not in the right ratios, the match is not likely to light. If the matchstick has an insufficient amount of tensile strength, then, the match head might not be able to ignite. If the force that is used to draw the match head across a given surface is not sufficiently strong, the match might not light. If there is a wind blowing in the area where one is trying to light the match, one might not be able to induce the match head to light. If the match head is damp or if the conditions are sufficiently humid, one might not be able to light the match.

What is the nature of the biological epistemology which enables part of an individual's terrain (say, in the form of macrophages or dendritic cells) to be able to grasp what the "cause" of the destabilization of the body might be in any given instance? As the foregoing example from a past course in philosophy indicates, determining causality is not an easy issue to resolve in philosophy, and the same set of problematic considerations extend into law, science, medicine, theology, history, as well as everyday life and, yet, (with tongue firmly planted in cheek) somehow, organisms are purported to have the capacity to develop a whole science involving patterns of recognition which enables them to differentiate between microbial friend and foe merely on the basis of protein receptor shapes

Allegedly, there are trillions of microorganisms within the human body. According to some individuals, there are far more microorganisms than there are human cells, while others believe that such a claim is more of a myth than a reality.

Whether one is talking about billions of microorganisms or trillions of microorganisms that give expression to the human microbiome, where do all the receptors go on a macrophage or a dendritic cell that allows these two entities to differentiate between not only microorganism and human cells but, also, given that such cells come in many different sizes, shapes and modalities, how do macrophages and dendritic cells differentiate between one human cell and another? If there were just one kind of receptor which was able to distinguish between human cells and microorganisms and, thereby, relieve the biological terrain of the burden of having to use different protein receptors to differentiate between various human cells and the microorganisms that make up the microbiome which inhabits that biological terrain, then what is the identity of that protein because, too date, no one has been able to provide a plausible answer?

What enables macrophages and dendritic cells to differentiate between symbiotic microorganisms and non-symbiotic organisms? What if the critical difference between symbiotic and non-symbiotic microorganisms is not a matter of morphology but shows up with functionality as a given microorganism transitions from symbiotic to non-symbiotic behavior and there very few, if any, commonalities which link functionality with morphology?

If this were the case, then the problem which confronts macrophages and dendritic cells is somewhat like that which faces a colonial power that is caught up in a modality of guerilla warfare in which the former soldiers cannot tell the difference between friend and foe among the local inhabitants on the basis of external considerations and will only be able to learn after the fact – that is, through functionality – whether some resident of the country being invaded is friendly or not. If this is the case, then coming up with some kind of receptor system to sort out such problems would seem to be a rather tricky and very complicated affair – although, I suppose, one might hypothesize that macrophages and dendritic might somehow have developed a capacity to generate sets of algorithms which, on the basis of the behavioral patterns of individuals, might be able to provide some degree of intimation concerning which entities were most likely to attack one in the near-future, but, if this were the case, one has difficulty understanding how that kind of algorithmically driven system would operate off of some set of receptors on the macrophages and dendritic cells or how such protein-receptors would come to stand for one kind of behavioral pattern (e.g., a non-symbiotic one) rather than some other kind of behavioral pattern (e.g., a symbiotic one).

Recall from the discussion in Chapter 5 how Gaston Naessens indicated that only three of the 16-17 stages of the somatid pleiomorphic/pleomorphic cycle were part of a healthy functioning, and, therefore, when the biological terrain becomes destabilized, the somatid cycle departs from what is normal and healthy and transitions to stages that have different morphological and functional properties, not all of which are necessarily symbiotic in character? Further recall that Naessens indicated how cells with different functional requirements were populated by somatids that are different in some way from the somatids that populate other cell or tissue types, and, therefore, there is a likelihood that different organs and tissues will have pleiomorphic/pleomorphic cycles that are unique to them, and, as a result, once again, questions arise as to how macrophages and dendritic cells develop the sort of specialized knowledge that would enable them to differentiate between symbiotic and non-symbiotic stages of any given pleiomorphic/pleomorphic cycle?

Conceivably, macrophages, dendritic cells, and other components of the re-stabilization-detoxification dynamic do not bother with self non-self distinctions nor become preoccupied with being able to identify particular microorganisms as the alleged "cause" of some sort of departure from well-being. Instead, the entire set of processes that are entailed by the dynamics of re-stabilization-detoxification come into play as needed or indicated (for example, by macrophages, neutrophils, dendritic cells, and/or cytokines) according to the nature of the destabilization which has occurred to one or more aspects of the biological terrain.

Whatever communication that is taking place within the body might be entirely about what steps are to be taken in order to return the biological terrain to its original condition of integrity during which it had nothing but symbiotic relationships with the surrounding members of the microbiome that inhabits the body. If this is the case, then the aforementioned sorts of communication are about re-establishing health or stability or symbiotic relationships and not about preventing disease through being able to differentiate between self and non-self.

Perhaps, the body operates in accordance with a set of 'emergency medical service' protocols or a set of battlefield protocols that are narrowly directed toward trying to re-stabilize the aspects of functioning in the biological terrain that, for whatever reason, have become destabilized. This would be a set of protocols that do not require 'the cause' to be identified in order for re-stabilization dynamics to be released.

This process of re-stabilization could be done in a way that will, in a period of hours, days, or a few weeks, help resolve the issue of destabilization, or the dynamics of re-stabilization are designed to help keep the individual alive until help of some kind (family, doctors, hospitals) can take over and provide the compromised individual with that person's body can't do for itself or can't do without assistance. In either case, the body's EMS protocols operate much like doctors do in a clinical setting when they are dealing with some sort of idiopathic problem – that is, different protocols are pursued (some which work and others which do not) in order to stabilize a patient and, thereby, buy extra time to determine what might be the underlying problem for what is transpiring.

Macfarlane Burnet's first foray into the issue of the alleged self and non-self distinction involved the process of digestion. He believed that any organism which exists by virtue of being able to digest other organisms must have the capacity to distinguish between 'self' and 'non-self.'

The foregoing belief seems to take a rather problematic manner of engaging the way in which organisms – say, human beings -- operate. The digestive process has its own characteristics, and one of those characteristics is that under normal circumstances, the system does not digest itself.

If food is digested, this is because it is digestible through the means that are available. Consequently, while food is being digested, the body is structured in such a way that the process of digestion only affects the food and not the processes that are responsible for such digestion, and, therefore, there is no need to distinguish between self and non-self because things unfold according to the inherent properties of that which is being digested and that which does the digestion.

In short, the digestive system is structured in such a way that it does not have features that have the property of being susceptible to digestion. This has to do with the way in which something is made and, therefore, appears to have nothing to do with any sort of self and not-self distinction.

A metal stove does not melt itself because its inherent structural nature removes such a possibility from consideration and not because the stove has developed a system for distinguishing between what is self and what is not-self. That which is placed within the stove and is vulnerable to the heat generated by a metal stove will burn while the container within which such temperatures rage has been built from materials that are capable of withstanding the heat that is being generated and, therefore, will not burn ... irrespective of considerations of self and not-self.

Another building block for Burnet's idea of the self and non-self distinction in biological life was rooted in his work involving the issue of lysogeny. Lysogeny is said to be the process in which the nucleic acid of a bacteriophage (supposedly some sort of virus) becomes merged with the genome of an associated bacterium such that whatever information is contained in the transfer and fusing of nucleic acid from a bacteriophage to the bacterium becomes capable of being passed on to that bacterium's progeny. In addition, Burnet felt that lysogeny involved properties that differentiated it from classical forms of bacteriophage which he felt were either independent parasites or were entities that, somehow, had been separated from bacteria) and among these differences were certain kinds of functional principles.

Without going too deeply into the foregoing perspective, one might note the following. Burnet considered bacteria and viruses to be separate kinds or classes of entities, and, as well, he believed that the process of lysis which took place in conjunction with bacteriophages was different from the process of lysogeny which occurred in bacteria.

Conceivably, Burnet could not see the forest through the trees. The trees were all of the phenomena that he considered to be separate from one another, and the forest was the pleiomorphic/pleomorphic approach to microorganisms that was capable of tying together all of the aforementioned phenomena which Burnet considered to be separate from one another.

More specifically, if viruses do not exist – and there is good evidence to support such a hypothesis – then, it is possible that bacteriophages are not viruses but are different morphological expressions of the pleiomorphic/pleomorphic cycle of some given somatid or microzyma or endobiont or microorganism. Moreover, if the foregoing is true, then, perhaps, the phenomena of lysis and lysogeny to which reference is being made are merely different functional properties of one and the same microorganism or microzyma or somatid or endobiont during different stages of its pleiomorphic/pleomorphic cycle.

For Burnet, lysogeny gave expression to a fusion of selves in which the alleged viral character of a given bacteriophage became one with the self of the bacteria to which the aforementioned bacteriophage had been attached. Nevertheless, when considered from the foregoing pleiomorphic/pleomorphic perspective, there is no dissolving of one kind of self (i.e., a virus) with another kind of self (i.e., the associated bacterium), but, rather one is merely talking about different stages of the pleiomorphic/pleomorphic cycle of one and the same entity.

There are other reasons for questioning Burnet's approach to the foregoing issues. For example, he published about 98 papers on the topic of viral influenzas during a nearly 25-year period of time between 1935 and 1958.

The papers being alluded to above provide, among other things, an account of the research that he had completed concerning the development of various methods for cultivating viruses. Unfortunately, there are a bevy of red-flags concerning the viability of such research because of the problems that have been pointed out in previous chapters in the present book which strongly suggest, if not demonstrate, that the issue of whether, or not, viruses actually exist or have been properly isolated in any of the cultures that have been prepared has not, yet, been resolved in a way that is capable of proving that virology is not an empty science.

Yet, on two separate occasions Burnet was nominated for the Nobel Prize in conjunction with his work on cultivating viruses and turning his techniques of cultivation into analytical methods that allegedly measured the extent to which viruses were present, virulent, infectious, and so on. Apparently, not only had Burnet become deeply invested in Pasteur's monomorphic theory of germs, and he also was invested in the modern notion of virus as entities capable of infecting human beings and causing various kinds of pathology, but, as well, the individuals that were nominating people like Burnet for the Nobel Prize in conjunction with that sort of research were also deeply invested in, and biased by, such a perspective.

Burnet, himself, felt that his most important contribution to science involved a theory in which he introduced the notion of antibody production being rooted in a process of clonal selection. More specifically, he argued that whenever a new antigen was encountered by the body, then one of the individual's antibody-producing cells would generate two lines of antibody clones, one of which supposedly was directed toward the immediate task of defending against the intruding invader or antigen, and a second lineage which was dedicated to being prepared to be ready to rally against future encounters with that same antigen.

Subsequently, experimental evidence was forthcoming that was believed, at least by some, to lend support to Burnet's clonal selection theory of antibody production. On the other hand, in passing, one might raise the following question: If Burnet's theory of clonal selection of antibody production is true, then why do allergies tend to persist?

While I will hold off, for the most part, critically reflecting on the notion of so-called evidence and what such evidence might, or might not, signify in any given instance, I would like to offer a caveat concerning the claim that empirical evidence has accrued which is consistent with, or lends support to, the foregoing theory. That caveat is as follows: What is believed to constitute evidence is often a matter of how the data which gives expression to that "evidence" has been processed, understood, and shaped by a variety of assumptions that are used to frame a viewer's engagement of that data (including the view of the person who is providing such "evidence") so that data is seen as 'evidence' rather than being seen as merely amorphous, unrelated information.

At this juncture, the foregoing caveat is given advisedly and, as is said the law courts, without prejudice. Consequently, the foregoing is not intended to serve as any sort of definitive declaration concerning Burnet's theory but, rather, it is merely offered for critical reflection and consideration.

How does the body know that something is an antigen? If the pleiomorphic/pleomorphic theory is correct, and the default state of the human body involves a symbiotic relationship between, on the one hand, the general health of the biological terrain and, on the other hand, the microbiome that inhabits that terrain on a continuous basis, and if there are no such things as viruses, then, what is an antigen?

From the pleiomorphic/pleomorphic perspective, the offending antigen is not necessarily some microorganism. Instead, perhaps what induces microorganisms to depart from their condition of symbiosis with the surrounding terrain have to do with changes to the condition of the terrain itself.

Conceivably, human beings are not made vulnerable through the attacks of external pathogens or antigens, but, rather, the human body has the capacity to render itself susceptible to a process in which microorganisms that inhabit our biological terrain transition out of their normal state of symbiosis and enter into non-symbiotic states that may induce our bodies to generate various kinds of health issues and symptoms in response to the transitions undergone by various microorganisms in our microbiome. Given the foregoing possibility, then, there is a sense in which the biological terrain that has become destabilized within this or that individual is the primary antigen in any disease since as a result of unknown processes (at least initially they might be unknown), something (not a microorganism) has destabilized the condition of the terrain and induced one, or more, morphological and/or functional transitions to take place with one or more microorganisms within an individual's microbiome, and, as a result, the process of transitioning away from a condition of symbiosis is a symptom of, not the cause of, the underlying problem.

The underlying cause of the initial destabilization that preceded microorganisms in the microbiome transitioning away from a state of symbiosis could be due to any combination of the following factors: Diet, stress, lack of exercise, a person's emotional/psychological state, poverty, as well as exposure to thousands of environmental toxins and poisons such as pesticides, industrial chemicals, manufacturing contaminants, vaccines, or non-ionizing radio waves and other forms of electromagnetic impulses that constitute the woof and warp of the modern world. Some people maintain that if one understands the properties and functionality of different stages of a given pleiomorphic/pleomorphic cycle, then, the morphological and functional changes that manifest themselves in microorganisms during the aforementioned sorts of periods of transition can, actually, be used as a guide to help the individual or a clinician to work her or his way back to a condition of symbiosis and health with those very same entities.

Given the foregoing perspective, the task of the body is not necessarily to identify or designate (or to develop a capacity to identify or designate) this or that microorganism as being the antigen which causes disease. The task of the body might be to undertake whatever processes are required and are feasible under a given set of conditions which could help return the biological terrain to its original state of symbiosis with the microorganisms that have been induced to transition away from the symbiotic manner in which those microorganisms tend to function during times of health – an induction process that is due to a dynamic of destabilization which is not initially due to the action of a given microorganism.

The so-called "complement system" consists of more than 30 different kinds of proteins. Their size is on the low end of the nanometer scale and, therefore, smaller than the size of purported viruses.

Supposedly, the all-protein complement system serves a number of different functions. For example, some of them have the capacity to not only induce certain elements within the re-stabilizing-detoxifying dynamic to become active but, as well, to also be able to help shape or guide the functioning of those activated components.

In addition, other members of the complement system supposedly have the capacity to either incapacitate or kill certain entities. Now, in light of the fact that some individuals have estimated, give or take a few proteins here or there, that there are at least some 15 quintillion complement proteins (this amounts to either a 1 followed by 18 zeros or if one is British, a one follower by 30 zeros) that are being pushed and pulled throughout the biological terrain of our bodies at any given point in time, and given that there are billions, perhaps trillions of, microorganisms within the microbiome that occupies virtually every part of the body, and given that those billions – perhaps trillions – of microorganisms are not being ripped to shreds or maimed at every turn by the 15 quintillion members of the complement system that are elbowing their way through – among other places – the microbiome, then, perhaps one might wish to re-conceptualize their inherent nature.

For instance, a masked individual comes into a room and begins to handle an array of sharp, destructive instruments. Is the individual Dr. Mengele, the infamous 'Angel of Death', or is the individual someone by the name of Dr. Khan, a famous thoracic surgeon, who has operating privileges at the local hospital?

An alternative scenario might be as follows: A hooded individual walks into a room carrying a box of tools, many of which have the potential for maiming or, perhaps, killing someone. Is the person a young carpenter who has just come inside from a cold and snowy day outside and is ready to go to work, or is the individual someone who is preparing to torture prisoners and wishes to keep her or his identity concealed?

If one approaches the complement system from the perspective of Pasteur's monomorphic germ theory, then, the complement system exists for no other reason than to engage in search and destroy missions that target germs which have breached various perimeter defenses. If one approaches the complement system from the perspective of Béchamp's pleomorphic/pleomorphic position in which microorganisms are capable of being induced to transition into non-symbiotic stages of their life cycle, then, the instrumentation which is represented by the various members of the complement system constitute tools that might have a role to play with respect to helping an individual's body to re-stabilize and detoxify.

Do surgeons sometimes have to cut away problematic tissue in order to address whatever difficulties beset a given individual? Yes, they do, but the cutting is primarily a constructive process rather than being, primarily, a destructive dynamic.

Do carpenters sometimes have to use their tools to tear down certain elements within a house that is being remodeled? Yes, they do, but the tearing down is really a prelude to building something that is more desirable and/or more stable.

Similarly, the different components within the complement system might have the capacity for cutting, tearing, and even destroying certain elements within a destabilized portion of the biological terrain. However, the foregoing sorts of actions have not necessarily been undertaken in order to maim, kill, or place the lives of microorganisms under a constant state of attack, but, instead, they might have been undertaken as part of a process that helps to re-stabilize and detoxify some facet of the biological terrain which has become destabilized.

Notwithstanding the foregoing considerations, one should note that irrespective of whether one adopts a monomorphic or pleiomorphic/pleomorphic point of view concerning the body, none of what the complement system is doing seems to have anything to do with giving expression to an immunological function. Whether the complement system is preoccupied with hunt and destroy missions involving various microbial intruders or the complement system is focused on activities that, in some way, assist the biological terrain to return to a condition of health, there doesn't appear to be anything taking place which will relieve the human being from having to go through such a process again should some sort of health crisis arise in the future.

Somewhat ironically, microbiologists tend to reject pleiomorphism/pleomorphism because of its claim that the life cycle of microorganisms enables the latter entities to change their morphology and mode of functioning under different circumstances. Yet, at the heart of the complement system is the principle that all complement proteins have two different morphological structures and that when such morphology changes, then, so too, does functionality.

In one state of morphology, a complement protein is inactive. When that modality of morphology is induced to change, then so too does it becomes active and becomes able to express functionality.

Pleiomorphic/pleomorphic organisms are both similar to, but more complex than, complement proteins. In one morphological shape, those microorganisms interact with the biological terrain in a symbiotic matter, but when those same microorganisms are induced to transition away from that state and, thereby, assume a different modality of morphology, then, they also often display different kinds of functionality, some of which might be non-symbiotic in character.

Immunologists who claim that notwithstanding the capacity of the complement system to be able to kill, maim, and cause trouble for microbial intruders, the different members of the complement system the complement system is even more effective against viruses. Since any, and all, viruses have never been successfully isolated in a manner which demonstrates that they actually exist, then the foregoing claim concerning the alleged capacity of the complement system to dominate viruses and remove them from our systems is nothing more than creative fiction, and since there is no concrete evidence indicating that the complement system actually can or does remove said viruses from the biological terrain, there is no real-world immunological function that is being performed ... the theory is nothing more than a narrative.

The notion of "self-enforcing cascades" plays a central role in the perspective of immunologists. The foundational precept of the foregoing notion is that within the human body there is a process in which one complement protein has the capacity to activate other complement proteins and, within a short period of time, many members of the complement system supposedly can be activated to form structures and processes that are capable of engendering a considerable amount of biological destructiveness.

For instance, supposedly, the most important facet of the self-enforcing cascade dynamic begins with the complement protein known as C3. According to immunological theory, C3 can be induced to change its morphology or shape, and once this happens, it separates into two further components, one of which is known as C3b.

If C3b cannot find something on which to latch in less than a second's time, it will be deactivated. If it does find something on which to latch within the small window of opportunity of activity that it has available to it, then, it will change its conformation, and this new morphology has the capacity to not only corral other complement components and, in the process merge with the new component and, together, the new arrangement begins to attract other complement members and starts to form a structure capable of recruiting still other C3 components.

None of the foregoing dynamics have actually been seen taking place in real time. It is all a theoretical construct which might, or might not, have a real-world counterpart, and even if such a real-world counterpart actually exists, one can only speculate about what its actual function is, or functions are, and whether, or not, those functional properties are consistent with a monomorphic theory of germs or a pleiomorphic/pleomorphic approach to microbiology.

According to immunological theory, the foregoing process of self-enforcing cascade generates an amplification effect that enables bacteria to become completely covered with components from the complement system. From the perspective of many immunologists, the foregoing cascade creates a living hell for the bacteria that are being entombed.

However, until one knows what is actually going on between such complement components and the bacteria to which they are attached, perhaps, one should consider the possibility that the bacteria are not necessarily being entombed and prepared for death but, instead, could be being placed within some sort of surgical or healing chamber in which different constructive tasks can be performed. To be sure, one possible task for such a cascade might be to eliminate an entity that is dead, dying, compromised, or which has transitioned to a non-symbiotic stage of being, but, perhaps, just as easily, the encompassed microorganism could be undergoing an event that is somewhat like that of a caterpillar which is wrapped up within a cocoon so that it might be able to undergo a transformation or transition to some other morphological form ... in other words, maybe the engulfment process involving complement proteins is prelude to a process of transitioning back to a more symbiotic stage of its pleiomorphic/pleomorphic cycle of life.

In either case, the effect of the self-enforcing cascade is not necessarily immunological in character. According to one scenario, a microorganism that is dead, dying, compromised, or which has transitioned to some non-symbiotic form of microorganism is being removed from a destabilized aspect of the biological terrain, whereas in the other scenario, a microorganism is being rehabilitated, but in both cases the process seems more like an attempt to re-stabilize and detoxify the biological terrain rather than an attempt to confer some sort of Immunological properties on the biological terrain such that if a similar set of circumstances were to occur in the future, the same type of dynamic would be required to re-surface in its entirety once again.

To be sure, the biological terrain has a way to counter different modalities of pathology which might arise within the body. However, there is no automatic form of protection or immunity which is present.

Each case of inflammation or destabilization must be engaged anew, or from scratch, on every such occasion.

The term used by some immunologists to capture the foregoing dynamic of engulfment by complement proteins is opsonization. The word's etymology is derived from a Greek word that refers to the idea of some sort of side dish that is considered to be delicious.

Apparently, one is supposed to believe that macrophages, neutrophils, dendritic cells, and the like find such encapsulated microorganisms delicious. Macrophages and other components of the so-called immune system might, or might not, find the foregoing supposition to be the case, but one would have a very difficult time proving what the phenomenology of a macrophage or neutrophil might be if they were devouring such cocooned complexes.

Earlier in the chapter, the phrase "dendritic cells" was introduced. According to immunological theory, dendritic cells are distributed throughout the biological terrain and are constantly engaged in a process of scanning the terrain for signs of trouble. If viruses don't exist – and four chapters of the present book have indicated that there is no substantial evidence that they do – and if the normal, default position for microorganisms that inhabit the biological terrain is one of symbiosis, then, for what, exactly are dendritic cells searching.

One possible answer might be that they are looking for bacterial or fungal parasites of one kind or another. How does a dendritic cell learn to detect the presence of a parasite?

Presumably, the parasite has to do something that, somehow, catches the attention of the dendritic cell in a way that enables the dendritic cell to understand or grasp the problematic significance of what is taking place. Also, presumably, the parasite only becomes a problem if it is able to destabilize the biological terrain of the host in some manner.

Let's leave aside the issue of whether all biological terrains are equally vulnerable to the presence of any given parasite and, therefore, eschew questions having to do with whether diet, or stress, or poverty, or exposure to different kinds of chemical pollutants might render some biological terrains more susceptible to the presence of a given parasite than might be the case if someone who had a healthy terrain were exposed to the same kind of parasite. In other words, let's assume that all biological terrains are equally susceptible to the presence of parasites.

Let us assume that some given parasite engages in its parasitic ways and, in the process, one, or more, aspects of the host's biological terrain becomes destabilized or dysfunctional. How does a dendritic cell come to know that it is a parasite rather than any number of other genetic, epigenetic, metabolic, energy related, and/or cellular activities that is responsible for such destabilization? How does a dendritic cell solve the problem of causality and, as a result, becomes able to zero in on a given parasitic species as the cause of a given form of destabilization?

According to immunological theory, there are numerous occasions within any given twenty-four period during which dendritic cells consume and, then, vomit out what has been consumed. The total amount which is consumed and, then, released in the foregoing manner comes to a multiple value of the dendritic cell's volume.

Apparently, when dendritic cells go through the aforementioned process, they are engaging in a sampling dynamic of some kind. What, exactly, is it that they sampling, and how do they know what the significance might be of those samples?

Why not simplify the issue. What if we were to suppose that the dendritic cells were not scouring the biological terrain in order to detect the presence of viruses, bacteria, or parasites, but, instead, what if one were to suppose that the dendritic cells were searching for signs of destabilization within different facets of the biological terrain.

Perhaps the reason why dendritic cells are so omnipresent throughout that terrain is not necessarily because of any sort of presumed need to be able to detect the presence of on-going threats concerning the possibility of being invaded by infectious agents from without. Instead, maybe, the presence of dendritic cells throughout the biological terrain only has to do with a need to be able to detect signs of destabilization in that terrain (and such a process of detection might key in on just a few elements), and, then, to transmit that information to different facets of the body's re-stabilization-detoxification system (such as the lymphatic system) in order to activate certain dynamics that -- barring any further complications – might be capable of successfully addressing such an issue and, thereby, return the biological terrain to a condition of detoxified stability?

To make a much longer story considerably shorter – but, hopefully, not in a manner that distorts actual biological dynamics -- dendritic cells must be able to transmit the information which they have picked up through their sampling process and which, potentially, concerns the condition of health in the biological terrain to something that is capable of correctly parsing that information. For instance, the major histocompatibility class II complex refers to receptor proteins which are found on all nucleated cells of the body (thus, this leaves blood cells which are not nucleated as the only cells that do not have these receptors) and which, supposedly, have the task of presenting samples that, in one way or another, have been transmitted by dendritic cells to T-cells.

T-cells are leucocytes or white blood cells that emerge from certain kinds of modified-stem cells in the bone marrow. T-cells are alleged to have T-shaped receptors along their membranes.

The shape of the foregoing receptors is not the reason why they are called T-cells. Their name actually comes from the thymus gland to which they eventually migrate for purposes of some kind of maturation process. The thymus is part of the lymphatic system.

T-cells are said to entail several different modalities of expression. One species is regulatory; another edition has cytotoxic properties, while a third version of the T-cell lends assistance in various ways – such as determining when it is appropriate to activate said T-cells -- and, consequently, are known as Helper T -cells.

All three of the foregoing kinds of T-cells can be understood as having regulatory capabilities rather than necessarily giving expression to functionality that is immunological in character. More specifically, if one were to adopt the pleiomorphic/pleomorphic perspective, then, what is foundational to health is maintaining a condition of detoxified stability in which there is a symbiotic relationship between the biological terrain and the microbiome that occupies that terrain.

T-cells could be engaged in maintaining an on-going condition of detoxified stability (and in this respect T-cells could play an active role in processes of detoxification that help a stable biological terrain to remain stable). Alternatively, T-cells might have responsibility for helping to organize events within the biological terrain in a way that will lead to the removal of dead, dying, and compromised cells.

T-cells might also be engaged in processes that are directed toward the removal or rehabilitation of microorganisms that have departed from a symbiotic relationship with the biological terrain, or whether T-cells have changed their morphology and/or functionality in order to ensure that conditions warrant the activation of T-cells/ In this respect, T-cells might serve as something akin to a fail-safe system which helps to maintain detoxified stability in the biological terrain.

All of the foregoing possible modalities of functioning of the T-cell could be understood to be serving what might be considered to be the prime directive of the biological terrain – namely, to maintain a condition of detoxified stability. If so, then, T-cells need not be framed in terms of a narrative that is cast in hues of immunological activities.

The scouting reports which are being delivered by dendritic cells to the major histocompatibility complex II receptors on, say, the membrane of the thymus could all be about whether, or not, detoxified stability is present in different segments within the kingdom of the biological terrain. The information which is being transmitted to T-cells via major histocompatibility complex II receptors also could be about how to deal with such information in a way that either might help to maintain a condition of detoxified stability or that might help to initiate the activation of T-cells in certain ways that could be needed to help re-stabilize the aspect of the biological terrain that has become destabilized.

If the foregoing perspective were true, then, as intimated previously, the activity of T-cells need not be about the process of generating and finding the right molecular receptor connection to some given antigen that has been, and, currently, is being detected in the biological terrain. Instead, everything might be geared toward just one set of tasks: Maintaining or regaining the status of detoxified stability in the biological terrain.

The reason why there is a system of verification in conjunction with Helper T-cells in conjunctions with T-cell activation which requires independent sources for determining whether T-cells are to be activated in a given set of circumstances and, if activated, whether that activation is to assume one form of functioning rather than another, is because not all forms of T-cell activation are necessarily appropriate for a given set of circumstances that currently exist. The biological terrain and the surrounding environment are constantly changing, and, therefore, adjustments, of one kind or another, might have to be made in the way in which a given T-cell is configured so that it will be best prepared to deal with whatever might be transpiring within the biological terrain.

Moreover, conceivably, in certain biological contexts, some modalities of T-cells could have a greater cytotoxic impact on the terrain than is the case with respect to other modalities of T-cell expression, and as a result, the kind of cytotoxicity that is being introduced into a given facet of the biological terrain could exacerbate the condition of destabilization that already exists in the biological terrain. The poisons that exist in venoms (from certain snakes, spiders, etc.) and which also are released by different kinds of microbial pathology (e.g., botulism, anthrax, cholera, etc) tend to be proteins, and, therefore, conceivably the body might exercise a certain abundance of caution in order to ensure that none of the proteins that are affixed to the membranes of T-cells will generate cytotoxic effects on healthy cells or tissues rather than on entities that are dying or compromised in some way.

Helper T-cells are also described as being able to offer different modalities of assistance other than the aforementioned activation issue. For example, Helper T-cells have the capacity to release various kinds of cytokines which co-ordinate the activities of different facets of the on-going dynamics that take place in conjunction with areas of inflammation that might exist within the biological terrain.

Apparently, Helper T-cells also have the capacity to extend the life span of macrophages. Normally speaking, macrophages are pre-programmed to undergo apoptosis after a certain period of time has passed, but Helper T-cells actually appear to have the capacity to intervene and re-set that time of termination ... as many times as might be required according to whatever conditions might prevail at a given location of inflammation or destabilization.

Helper T-cells also have the capacity to end their life cycle. When the time is right – and how they determine what time is right is anybody's guess – they will undergo the process of apoptosis.

According to immunological theory, there are some Helper T-cells which are alleged to have the capacity to transition into what are known as 'memory helper T-cells'. Supposedly, these cells are able to remember – in some sense of this word – the properties of a specific enemy antigen.

Such a memory is said to provide one with immunity with respect to certain diseases. Purportedly, this is because by virtue of such memory cells one is said to be able to quickly recognize the existence of such a threat through a process of detection concerning an antigen of some kind which supposedly signifies the presence of that threat.

Before accepting the foregoing idea, there appear to be a few things that need to be known before what is a theoretical concept can make the transition to biological fact. For instance, once again, one would like to know how such a cell is able to figure out what is causing a given instance of destabilization or inflammation in some aspect of the biological terrain, and one also might like to know how such a cell comes to 'grasp' that a given antigen signifies that some given form of microorganism constitutes being a threat when, in actuality, it is the toxins that are released by such microorganisms that tend to be the actual troublemakers.

One can understand the narrative that is being spun by immunological theorists. The problem arises when one tries to understand the dynamic details that supposedly underwrite how the establishment of such a reliable system of 'memory' or signification actually comes about or how it actually functions.

None of the foregoing necessarily serves any sort of immunological function in which the job of the dendritic cells is to identify known biological felons and call in defensive measures through T- cells that have been pre-programmed to deal with just such known felons. Conceivably, what a memory helper T-cell actually might be able to do is to improve the speed with which the stabilization-detoxification system implements certain facets of the set of protocols that are used to either help maintain or re-establish detoxified stability.

In other words, the epigenetics of the ecological conditions within and outside of life might have changed. As a result, it is possible that certain aspects of the genome might become re-programmed to help speed up response times to the presence of inflammation or destabilization in the biological terrain. However, some individuals (e.g., immunologists) have interpreted the foregoing sort of epigenetic sort of adaptive learning as being an immunological function of activity within the 'memory helper T-cells' when such learning actually might be a function of epigenetic dynamics that are shaping the behavior of the cells which are being referred to as 'memory helper T-cells', and, as such, whatever kind of memory exists is a function of certain kinds of epigenetic changes that have taken place in the thymus or in the major histocompatibility complex II receptors, or in the way certain T-cells function and, therefore, such changes are not necessarily inherent in the so-called 'memory helper T-cells per se'.

The task of returning a given biological terrain to a condition of detoxified stability is not necessarily at all the same kind of phenomenon as developing a system for detecting, identifying and, then, arranging for the disappearance of different species of biological terrorists. Speeding up response time with respect to certain facets of the process of maintaining or re-establishing detoxified stability need not have anything to do with remembering specific antigens that supposedly represent or signify the presence of certain kinds of pathogens.

The Lymph system to which dendritic cells transmit information concerning the status of the biological terrain has a variety of functions. One of those tasks is to serve as a drainage system in which extracellular fluid that, to varying degrees, has accumulated in the interstitial spaces between cells and which, in one way or another, has managed to escape from the flow of plasma through the capillary by-ways of the blood system is slowly returned to the latter system.

Just as blood cells actually are carried along by the plasma that flows through the blood system, so too, various elements are carried along by the fluids of the lymph system and, surprisingly enough, that fluid is known as lymph. That fluid or lymph can have different colors depending on what is being transported within it.

Consequently, the lymph system not only serves as a drainage system which prevents the body from swelling up and, possibly, bursting, by slowly reintegrating the accumulation of such extracellular liquids back into the blood system from which they originally came but, as well, the lymph system also serves as something of a sewer system. A great deal of biological detritus gets picked up by lymph as that fluid winds its way through miles of lymph-related vessels that run throughout the body.

Such detritus tends to consist of, on the one hand, dead, dying, and compromised cells of one kind or another (some of which might be microbial in nature), or, on the other hand, such detritus also consists of the molecular wreckage that tends to come into existence as a result of various kinds of biological transactions and metabolic processes (whether anabolic or catabolic in nature). However, some of what is picked up by the lymph fluid might have to do with signs of destabilization or stress in different parts of the biological terrain.

There are some 600 lymph nodes located throughout the body. When indications of destabilization in some aspect of the biological terrain are picked up by the lymph, then, that information might, presumably, be processed, relatively quickly, by the nearest lymph node – although if such indices of destabilization are permitted to remain in the lymph (rather than be removed) additional analysis might take place at some subsequent lymph node way-station. Such lymph nodes might have the responsibility of differentiating between the usual, on-going detritus of biological life and signs of destabilization within the biological terrain, and different lymph nodes might be looking for different kinds of signs of destabilization.

The foregoing task need not involve any kind of process of trying to identify or classify microorganisms per se or involve any attempt to definitively establish issues of causality. Instead, lymph nodes might be processing the fluid lymph merely for the presence of more generic and less complicated signs of destabilization or potential danger and, then, proceed with activating a set of protocols that, hopefully, will assist the biological terrain to return to a condition of detoxified stability.

As noted previously in conjunction with an earlier discussion that mentioned dendritic cells in passing, there is nothing in the lymph system that necessarily involves some sort of immunological functioning. Rather, one of the primary functions of that system, and one of the reasons why there are some 600 lymph nodes distributed throughout the human body might have to do with providing a wealth of venues for detecting the presence of signs of stress within the biological terrain which indicate that some facet of that terrain is in a condition of being destabilized and, therefore, in need of assistance.

There is the old adage that to a hammer, everything looks like a nail. Similarly, to immunological theorists everything is interpreted through the lenses of a framing process that casts many biological dynamics as serving an immunological function when, possibly, the reality is much, much simpler than, and quite different from, such a scenario.

Let's turn to one last facet of immunological theory – namely, the issue of "antibodies". The notion of antibodies seems to go to the very heart of the idea that the body has an adaptive immune system which is capable of learning how, in a supposedly unique fashion, to pair up or match the receptors on an antibody with receptors on some kind of an antigen that is connected, in some way, to a pathogen (such as a bacteria or virus) and by accomplishing this task not only prepare the body to be able to resist such pathogens in the present, but, as well, be able to resist such pathogens in the future ... that is to have acquired a stable memory of some modality of pathogenicity that enables an organism – such as a human being – to become pre-programmed to dispense such threats in an automatic fashion much like a bouncer might prevent a potential troublemaker from ever entering a given establishment beyond some established perimeter.

One of the problems with the foregoing scenario is no one has been able to prove that "antibodies" actually exist. In other words, no one has been able to demonstrate that within the body there exists a molecular configuration – believed to be protein in nature – that has a specific affinity for one, and only one, kind of antigen (something capable of inducing antibodies to emerge), and, in the process can be shown to be capable of nullifying or destroying that antigen and its associated pathogen.

In order to flesh out what is being alluded to in the foregoing paragraph, perhaps the best way to begin is to provide an overview of how most immunologist have come to parse the concept of antibodies. However, as one is going through the following presentation, one should keep in mind that while there might be a great deal of data that touches on the notion of antibodies, and while there might be a great many theories that use such data to construct models that purport to "inform" us about what antibodies supposedly are, and what they might look like, and what their function or functions might be, and how that function might be served, and/or how antibodies might be produced, nonetheless, there is actually nothing in the way of empirical data that can be pointed to as establishing a reliable basis to indicate that any given theory or model concerning antibodies (and there have been many) can be reliably and repeatedly tied to concrete evidence capable of showing that the entity or molecular configuration which underlies all such theories – namely, an "antibody" -- actually exists.

To borrow a phrase from a song by Jon Mitchell, it is all "sandcastles in the air". In this respect, immunology, like virology, is nothing more than a fictional narrative ... sets of memes that have captured and regulated the thoughts, behaviors, and careers of thousands of biologists, scientists, researchers, medical practitioners, media representatives, and entrepreneurs – all of whom have made a great deal of real world money, and were showered with accolades of one kind or another due to a mere fictional narrative, just as a lot of people often make real money and might even have collected accolades of one kind or another as a result of turning some Stephen King story (short or long) – which are all nothing more than fictional narratives -- into a movie that has concrete, frequently lucrative ramifications for the lives of, at least, some people associated with the process. So, with the foregoing caveat having been stated, let's take a look at some of how 'sandcastles in the air' get to be built

Emil von Behring introduced the idea of an antibody in 1890. It was a notion that was intended to help make sense of, among, other things, how human beings seemed to be able to ward off certain kinds of diseases, as well as, perhaps, to provide an account for how and why vaccines might operate.

The term wasn't introduced because antibodies had been isolated, purified, and, then, physically characterized. The term was purely theoretical and introduced as a heuristic device – that is, as a concept which might be able to push research and understanding in a fruitful and constructive direction.

In 1923, for example, Michael Heidelberger, an American chemist who is considered by many individuals to be the father of immunology, published a paper, along with Oswald Avery, that supposedly demonstrated that the polysaccharides in the membranes of pneumococcus III microorganisms were capable of serving as antigens. However, given that the notion of an antigen stipulates that in order for something to be able to qualify as an antigen, then that something must be a foreign agent or toxin of some kind which is able to induce an immune response, and given that when Heidelberger injected the aforementioned polysaccharide into test animals no immune response was generated, then, it would appear that Heidelberger had not actually demonstrated what he – and others on his behalf -- claimed to be the case.

Later, in 1929, Heidelberger, along with a doctoral student Forrest Kendall, released a paper which indicated that antibodies were proteins. In general terms, the two researchers made an assumption that the protein content of the immune precipitates which were being studied could be determined by measuring the nitrogen content of that precipitate using something called the Kjeldahl procedure.

Whether Heidelberger and his co-investigator were, or were not, correct in relation to the foregoing assumption concerning the significance of whatever nitrogen content that might have been detected through the foregoing methodology – I.e., that it signified the presence of proteins – is, in a sense irrelevant. The really important assumptions that were being made by Heidelberger and his partner – but which had not been stated explicitly – and which, therefore, need to be pursued more critically are: (a) that the precipitate being studied is actually residue from an immune response rather than from some other kind of biological dynamic, and (b) that if the precipitate being studied does contain proteins, then it is the detected proteins that play a role of some kind in order for the immune process to occur.

The 1929 paper did not actively demonstrate in the body of document's contents or passively demonstrate in the form of references that the precipitate being studied was, indeed, the precipitates of an immune reaction. To prove that the precipitate was from something called an "immune response" one would have to be able to present – in an empirically compelling manner -- the whole back story concerning the dynamics of immunity and how it worked, and this would require one to be able to show that the precipitate's contents could be caused by only such an immune dynamic, and, then, one would have to be able to show that such a dynamic actually took place in the human body.

Furthermore, even if one were to concede that such a precipitate was generated from an immune response, and even if one were to concede that measuring the nitrogen content in that precipitate constituted a reliable way of determining the presence of proteins, one still would have to be able to demonstrate that the detected proteins played some sort of key role in the immune response rather than merely being present because they were part of some sort of metabolic process that might, in some fashion, be associated with the dynamics of immunity but were not necessarily part of the immune dynamic.

In 1942, Merrill Chase proposed that the idea of "immunity" should be bifurcated into kinds of processes – namely, a cellular or innate component and an adaptive component in which antibodies played a central role. The foregoing proposal was not based on the sorts of facts that showed or proved how, indeed, there were two kinds of immunological dynamics taking place in the biological terrain of, for example, human beings, but, instead, the Chase proposal was an attempt to organize and make sense of available data, and, as such, it was an interpretation of what Chase believed the available data indicated.

Chase's 1947 idea of a bi-furcated immune system in which there is an adaptive component based on antibody functioning is consistent with Emil von Behring's 1890 notion of an antibody as well as consistent with Heidelberger's 1929 idea that antibodies consist of proteins. However, while the foregoing set of ideas do give expression to an intelligible narrative, nonetheless, that narrative is entirely theoretical in character because no one has actually shown that an immunological system is actually present in the human body that does all the things that an immunological system is supposed to be able to do or that there is an adaptive system of protein modification within certain immunological processes that take place in the body which are capable of carrying out immunological functions and, therefore, satisfies the conditions that are considered necessary to call something an "antibody."

In 1972 Rodney Porter and Gerald Edelman were awarded a Nobel Prize for research which, supposedly, uncovered the structural nature of antibodies. The prize was given in recognition of a body of work that had been conducted in the early 1960s, some 30 years after the work of Heidelberger and others concluded that the molecular nature of antibodies was protein in nature.

In the Porter and Edelman research, samples of proteins were taken which were assumed to have some sort of immune function, and, as a result, were referred to as being immunoglobulins. To lend credence to such an assumption, one would have to be able to isolate and purify those proteins and, then, proceed to show that they, indeed, did play a certain kind of role in an immune dynamic which also could be demonstrated to be present in human beings.

Porter and Edelman didn't establish any of the foregoing. They took molecules that were considered to have the functionality of immunoglobulins and proceeded to break those molecules down through the use of enzymes and different chemical methods.

Once the proteins were broken down into a variety of fragments, the two researchers began to analyze whatever biological and physiological properties seemed to be present in those fragments. On the basis of their analysis of the fragments, they began to develop ideas or hypotheses about how those fragments might be re-assembled to produce a functional protein that had immunological properties.

They decided that the best way to put the fragments together involved a glycoprotein configuration which contained four polypeptide chains, Two of those chains were – relatively speaking -- heavy as well as being identical to one another, while the other two chains were – relatively speaking – light. Based on his analysis of, and thoughts concerning, the disulfide bonds which Edelman believed were present in the heavy chains of the finished protein, apparently, he maintained that the overall structure of the four peptide chains was in the shape of a 'Y.'

Porter and Edelman did with the aforementioned fragments what modern virologists do when, allegedly, they set about allegedly sequencing some given virus whose existence has never been proven. That is, they created a molecular structure that was not based on something which had been observed in nature, but, rather, what they did was based on a set of assumptions, hypotheses, and theories concerning how certain proteins – which were believed to be immunoglobulins -- might be structured.

No one has isolated and purified a 'Y'-shaped protein which had been shown to carry out immunological functions in the human body. In fact, none of the fragments that were used to construct the 'Y'-shaped end product had any of the reactivity of the proteins with which their research began.

One might also note that whatever 'reactivity' the starting proteins might have had, one cannot necessarily conclude that such reactivity was a sign of an immunological process. One would have to be able to study such proteins in a natural setting and show that their role in that setting was immunological in nature rather than reflecting some other kind of biological functionality.

Edelman and Porter were merely carrying on the tradition that had been initiated by Emil von Behring some 90 years previously when he conjured up the idea of an antibody as a way of providing a possible explanation for what might be happening in cases of vaccination and what might be happening in human beings quite independent of vaccinations. In addition, Edelman and Porter were following the path trodden by Michael Heidelberger in which questionable assumptions were made about what the character of antigens were and whether whatever proteins that might be associated with a given antigen – assuming it was one -- were necessarily immunological in character.

The ideas of Emil von Behring, Michael Heidelberger, Rodney Porter, and Gerald Edelman did not demonstrate that antibodies exist, consisted of proteins, or that they have a certain kind of structure and shape. They all contributed to the creation of a variety of hypothesis that became part of a theoretical structure or paradigm or framing process which was little more than a narrative that stood in need of real world proof that antibodies – in the form of 'Y'-shaped protein structures – actually existed and that those molecules were part of an immunological system in which the body protected the human being inhabiting that body by means of a process that was capable of the sort of adaptive learning that established immunity in relation to certain kinds of pathogens and, thereby, automatically prevented such pathogens to give rise to pathologies in a given biological terrain more than once, or, allegedly, as in the case of vaccines, ever taking root at all.

Such proof has never been forthcoming because 'Y'-shaped proteins having immunological functions of a certain kind have never been isolated and purified from any sort of sample that is derived from a human being. Macrophages, neutrophils, dendritic cells, T-cells, B-cells, the complement system, cytokines and so on might all exist, but their existence has not been, and, perhaps, cannot be, exclusively tied to a set of immunological functions except through various kinds of assumptions, hypotheses, and theories.

All of the foregoing components might have roles to play in helping the biological terrain to maintain or try to re-establish a condition of detoxified stability in which pleiomorphic/pleomorphic microorganisms engage in symbiotic relationships with the dynamics that take place in the biological terrain. However, there is nothing -- as the rest of this chapter has sought to point out -- which requires that those roles must be immunological in character.

Just as T-cells derive their name from the Thymus gland where they are believed to mature in various ways, B-cells derive their moniker from the bone marrow which is – and this is also true for T-cells -- their place of birth, but unlike T-cells, B-cells do not leave the bone marrow. Supposedly, like T-cells, B-cells have a specificity to them which enables them to recognize – and, therefore, engage -- one, and only one, antigen, and antigens are components that, allegedly, can bind to only one facet of the immune system.

However, one might note in passing that researchers have known for quite some time (at least for a few decades) that entities which are believed to be, or are being identified (on the basis of various assumptions and modes of interpreting data) as being, polyclonal or monoclonal antibodies both have been shown to be able to cross-react with a variety of elements within any given aspect of the biological terrain. Consequently, the alleged specificity that theoretically connects T-cells and B-cells with that terrain is not necessarily always present, and, as a result, one cannot necessarily be sure what a given entity – which is presumed to be an antibody – is doing or why it is present at a given location because the theorized specificity that is supposed to be a characteristic feature of antibodies is often absent.

For example, Clifford Saper, who was editor-in-chief for the *Journal of Comparative Neurology* between 1994 and 2011, wrote a couple of open letters to readers of the journal concerning the idea that monoclonal antibodies supposedly (at least according to theory), bind to one and only receptor, and he stated unequivocally that such an idea entailed a great many problems. Among other things, Saper noted that those entities which are being called monoclonal antibodies will, in fact, bind with any protein that has either the right kind of complementary sort of peptide structure as the alleged antibody or will bind with a peptide sequence that has a complementary structure that is very similar to the more precise, complementary structure being alluded to above.

Molecules that are referred to as monoclonal antibodies are sold commercially as reagents for laboratory research in such areas as neurology. The foregoing molecules are used to serve as indicators that certain kind of molecule – say a given neurotransmitter -- is present in the brain at a given location because it is believed that such a monoclonal molecule – said to be an antibody – has a very specific shape that will only bind to a specific kind of target ... in the present case a neurotransmitter of some kind, and, thus, is believed to serve as something of a stain or marker that identifies the presence of a unique kind of structure.

However, when what are known as 'knockout mice' was introduced, difficulties began to be encountered. Knockout mice are mice that have been genetically modified so that they do not express a particular gene – say, one for a given neurotransmitter.

If the theory of antibodies were correct (and this would require that one can show that the property of specificity is present in phenomena that are being described in terms of the alleged dynamics of antibodies), then, knockout mice should produce results that are very different from regular, non-genetically modified mice when one uses proteins that, supposedly, are monoclonal antibodies, as a means of determining if one can detect the presence of a given neurotransmitter that supposedly uniquely binds with the monoclonal antibody being used as a reagent. Unfortunately, data indicated that knockout mice (i.e., in this case, mice missing the gent that leads to the expression of a given neurotransmitter) showed the same staining characteristics as non-genetically modified mice (that is, mice that possessed the gene for expression of that neurotransmitter), and, therefore, one could only conclude that the entities being referred to as monoclonal antibodies were able to cross-react with other substances and, therefore, were not necessarily uniquely specific in their binding proclivities.

As a result of the foregoing considerations, the reliability of many research papers in neurology was brought into question. Moreover, because of the capacity of so-called monoclonal antibodies to cross-react with a variety of candidates, researchers also experienced considerable difficulty trying to replicate previous experiments because the use of such alleged monoclonal antibodies led to inconsistent results in different laboratories.

Saper tried to establish a few rules or principles for diminishing the foregoing sorts of problems. However, there were different kinds of problems entailed by each of his guidelines and, as a result, while the degrees of possible error might have been lessened if such guidelines were to be followed, nevertheless, one could never be quite certain that a given result really showed what was claimed for it because of the many factors that permeated the reactivity of so-called monoclonal antibodies, and, therefore, had the capacity to skew or undermine whatever conclusions might have been reached on the basis of using such monoclonal molecules as markers capable of specifically identifying the presence of this or that molecule..

Unfortunately, so many questions, problems, and uncertainties arose in the research community as a result of the rules that Saper had set in place to help improve research by rendering it more reliable and capable of being replicated, many researchers simply avoided sending their research to the *Journal of Comparative Neurology* to be peer reviewed. Instead, they sent their articles to journals where the criteria for publishing a paper were not so stringent, and, as a result, a lot of work got published that wasn't necessarily reliable if the underlying research relied on the use of so-called monoclonal antibodies as reagents that could specifically isolate the presence of certain kinds of molecules in their laboratory work.

One should keep in mind that none of the foregoing problems were about immunology per se. The commercial materials being sold and which were being referred to as monoclonal antibodies were being used as reagents in a staining process that was intended to identify whether, or not, a certain kind of molecule might be present in a given sample.

Consequently, quite independently of whether, or not, such commercially sold materials can be shown to have immunological properties and, therefore, actually deserve to be described as antibodies (that is, agents which are capable of arising in response to the presence of certain antigens and also be able to neutralize or destroy the latter as well as any pathogens associated with those antigens), the notion that antibodies are necessarily uniquely specific to particular elements within the biological terrain has been shown to be false even if one could prove that such reagents actually had some sort of immunological properties.

In addition to the foregoing set of considerations, one might note that there are people who might test positive for some given antigen and, yet, remain asymptomatic and in addition, do not show any evidence of having produced antibodies that are considered to be evidence that a person has, in some way, been exposed to whatever microorganism is believed to be associated with the antigen that has been positively detected in such a person's system. There also are people who recover from what has been diagnosed as a given microbial sort of disease who do not necessarily show any evidence of the sort of antibodies that one might expect – based on theory – to be present in a person who has recovered from such a disease,

So, when data is generated – say through a test of some kind -- which, allegedly, indicates that something which is being called an antibody shows up in someone's system, can one conclude that the presence of such entities constitutes evidence that antibodies necessarily have an immunological function? The entities in a given sample that are being referred to or classified as antibodies might well be proteins. Moreover, the proteins that are present might well have some role to play in helping someone re-establish a condition of detoxified stability, but none of those roles need be fundamentally, or even peripherally, phenomenological in character.

In addition, one might keep in mind that some 80-100,000 different kinds of proteins have been discovered within the human biological terrain despite the fact that the genome has a coding capacity for only somewhere between 15,000 and 20,000 proteins. The thousands of proteins that are **not** ensconced within the established genome might very likely be products or expressions of epigenetic dynamics of one kind or another and that realm will be explored a little more deeply in a subsequent chapter. For now, perhaps what can be said is that the biological terrain seems to have the epigenetic capacity to produce tens of thousands of proteins that might be involved in processes contributing to either maintaining, or working toward re-establishing a condition of detoxified stability that have nothing to do with immunological functioning of any kind.

By using current immunological theory to serve as the lens that is to be used to frame what we "see" and, therefore, shape or frame how we might parse data concerning the sort of epigenetic processes that are being alluded to in the previous paragraph, we tend to shut ourselves off from possibilities that, conceivably, could have the capacity to reflect the dynamics of the biological terrain much more accurately than the current theory of immunology does. This is similar to what has happened and continues to happen when various biological scientists tend to frame everything they do in terms of what can be viewed through certain kinds of light microscopes or electron micrographs, while excluding the work of those who have specialized in darkfield microscopy or who use quartz lenses rather than regular glass lenses (the latter lenses cannot access, as quartz lenses can, objects that are visible in ultraviolet light ... objects that tend to appear to be "invisible" in regular light, and, therefore, are presumed to be non-existent), or those individuals who actually were able to learn by having access to, and using before the cabal of allopathic medicine rendered them dysfunctional or "disappeared" them, the paradigm-shattering tools of microscopy that had been invented by Royal Rife or Gaston Naessens.

Before moving on, I would like to note, in passing, one more facet within the modern theory of immunology. This has to do with the notion of Plasma cells.

Eventually, B-cells transform into what are known as Plasma cells. Plasma cells are said to be responsible for the production and release of antibodies.

Estimates have been made that as many as 2,000 antibodies/per second can be generated by a Plasma cell. Given that no one has actually isolated and purified proteins in a way that can be shown to have immunological functions and which also can be shown to be the way the body actually operates, one has difficulty knowing what to make of a process that supposedly is able to produce 2,000 units per second of something that has never been shown to actually exist.

In light of the discussion that has taken place over the past ten pages, or so, what does it mean to claim that B-cells, just like T-cells, need to go through a rigorous process which checks, and, then, re-checks things in order to make sure that the antibody binding connections that are made will be unique to antigens of one sort or another and, therefore, will not bind, in problematical ways, to substances that are crucial for life within the biological terrain? After all, if, for example, antibodies – as the previously noted research of Saper has indicated -- are able to cross-react with a variety of candidates, then, how can one be sure that those entities won't cross react with elements that play important roles in the metabolism of different kinds of cells, tissues, and organs?

Macrophages, neutrophils, dendritic cells, cytokines, the complement system, the major histocompatibility II receptor complex, T-cells, B-cells, Plasma cells, and antibodies might all be ensconced in a system of communication with one another. However, what are the topical themes that define the nature of that communication process?

Immunologists would say that the aforementioned system has to do with a set of principles that are directed toward establishing a system for generating immunity within certain kinds of organisms – such as a human being. Yet, the present chapter has focused on pointing toward another kind of possibility.

If 'antibodies' in the sense in which immunologists use the term actually existed, then, one might suppose that all one would have to do is collect those antibodies together which are associated with a given antigen and transfer them to another person, and the latter individuals should be protected against whatever the disease is with which such an antigen is supposedly associated. The makers of vaccines don't do this.

Instead, they put together something akin to a Rube Goldberg machine in which one arranges a very intricate and overly complex set of dynamics to bring about, in a very indirect way, some result that might be produced in much simpler and more direct ways (such issues will be discussed in the next chapter on vaccines). The more simple and direct method would be – as indicated above -- to collect the antibodies in a given human being (assuming that one could find them and that they actually had immunological properties) that, supposedly, are specific to the antigens associated with a given disease and inject them into another individual without having to add anything – such as adjuvants – to help enhance antibody production.

Vaccine makers cannot pursue the foregoing simpler, more direct method because they have not discovered a means that allows them to isolate and purify antibodies in a manner that would show that what has been collected is capable of neutralizing or killing the pathogens that are associated with the antigens that supposedly are capable of inducing such antibodies to come into being with shapes that uniquely bind to such antigens/pathogens. Instead, vaccine makers concoct induction machines (i.e., vaccines) that, supposedly, are capable of generating what the vaccine makers are incapable of accomplishing independently of such devices.

How does one know that such a Rube Goldberg-like process will lead to the emergence of antibodies that are specific to a given antigen that is associated in some way, with some pathogen? Evidence already has been put forth that materials which are being referred to as 'antibodies' are not necessarily uniquely specific to antigens.

If antibodies have not been isolated and purified, then, how does one know that whatever is being induced to surface in the biological terrain of a recipient by means of a vaccine actually has some sort of immunological function? What is the standard against which such entities are to be measured which identifies them as being antibodies that have immunological functions rather than some other kind of function?

The seroconversion tests that are used to serve as indicators for whether, say, elevated levels of antibodies might be present in a given blood sample, are all indirect, surrogate markers that tend to be based on certain assumptions about the nature, properties and characteristics of antibodies ... assumptions, properties, and characteristics that are all based on theories about what antibodies are, how they are made, and what they do. None of the seroconversion tests can be independently verified and, therefore, shown to be based on evidence that comes from direct observation of antibodies which have been isolated and purified and also demonstrated to have immunological properties.

A considerable amount of information has been put forth in four earlier chapters of the present book indicating that viruses do not seem to exist. If they do not exist, and a serological test is administered to a person which indicates that, for example, elevated levels of HIV are present, then, clearly, there appear to be methodological ways that enable one to generate positive results for the existence of something which considerable evidence can be bought forward (as was done in four earlier chapters in the present book) that entities – such as viruses -- do not seem to exist and, yet, there are tests which can be run which, supposedly, are capable of detecting the presence of such non-existent entities.

Suppose one were to assume that what is showing up and being called an antibody is actually present in order to try to attend to the damage that might be being introduced into the biological terrain by means of, say, a vaccine. Perhaps, the more those kinds of antibodies show up as a result of a given vaccine, then, perhaps, this is an indication that a greater amount of damage is being done to the biological terrain as a result of the presence of the vaccine contents rather than being an indication that a more enhanced, robust condition of immunological protection is being afforded to an individual.

Immunologists maintain that there are five different kinds of immunoglobulins or antibodies. These are designated as: IgA, IgD, IgG, IgE, and IgM.

The foregoing entities are all correlated with slightly different phenomena that exist at a given time within the biological terrain. However, correlation is not necessarily an indication of causation.

One would have to be able to isolate and purify such molecules. Then, one would have to demonstrate that when they were introduced into certain kinds of conditions within the biological terrain that they consistently had certain clearly demarcated kinds of immunological functions.

The foregoing research has not been successfully done. No one has been able to show that the entities to which the foregoing designations allude are, in fact, actual antibodies that have immunological functions rather than having functions – possibly -- which might only indicate that they have the capacity to communicate certain kinds of information to different parts of the biological terrain in order to help maintain or re-establish a condition of detoxified stability, and all of the foregoing research would need to be done in terms of the stringent requirements surrounding conditions of actual proof rather than through the many degrees of freedom and loopholes that are entailed by language associated with terms such as: "correlated with," "implies," "suggests," or "is consistent with".

One might be willing to concede – and I am not necessarily saying that I do concede -- that both T-cells and B-cells are capable of generating or employing a system of proteins that have some sort of role in helping the body to maintain or re-establish a condition of health. One also might be willing to concede – but not necessarily – that both T-cells and B-cells can only be activated by going through a set of verification procedures which, in some way, ensure that whatever dynamics are set in motion by T-cells and B-cells will not be counterproductive to the health of the body. Nonetheless, none of the foregoing concessions necessarily requires one to adopt an immunological perspective in order to account for such verification behavior.

More specifically, evidence has been presented previously in this book indicating that there is no reliable evidence which is capable of proving that viruses exist. If viruses do not exist, then, there is no need for an elaborate system of antibody production that has been theoretically proposed as a way of explaining how the human body is capable of producing antibodies which have an indefinitely large capacity to generate structural conformations that are capable of uniquely identifying and nullifying a legion of viruses and there alleged multiplicity of variations.

In addition, if, as Béchamp, Enderlein, Rife, and Naessens – as well as many others – have empirically demonstrated (and not just theorized) that the default setting for the biological terrain seems to be one of detoxified stability in which that terrain, together with whatever microorganisms are occupying it, are in symbiotic relationships with one another, then, one might suppose that the tendencies of the biological terrain would be geared toward maintaining such a default position, of health and when necessary – such as instances involving some sort of destabilization event or events which inflame one, or more, aspects of the biological terrain and which, on occasion, induce normally symbiotic microorganisms to transition away from such a status – then under such circumstances, the body might be more likely to engage in activities that are directed toward trying to detoxify and re-stabilize the underlying condition of inflammation that induced microorganisms to transition away from their symbiotic relationships with the terrain than the body would expend considerable resources to go about generating antibodies that are not needed for non-existent viruses, and, in the case of bacteria, have, somehow, resolved the causality issue which has enabled those antibodies to acquire the knowledge that gives expression to how the antigens associated with a given microorganisms are connected to the toxins and poisons which are released by such organisms and which are the actual threat to the body.

If there is a complex system in which B-cells and T-cells are provided with a way to generate an array of morphological characteristics (such as receptor shapes) that give those cells different functional capabilities, and if there is a complex system which requires some sort of verification procedure to ensure that B-cells and T-cells will constructively operate to help return a given biological terrain back to a condition of detoxification, stability, and symbiotic relationships with members of the microbiome that is present in that terrain, then, none of the foregoing considerations need to serve immunological ends. Rather, the communication among, and interaction of, macrophages, neutrophils, dendritic cells, the complement system, the cytokines, T-cells, B-cells, the lymph system, the thymus, the bone marrow, as well as the functions of the liver and kidneys could all be directed toward maintaining and, when necessary, re-establishing a condition of detoxified stability in which symbiotic relationships exist between the biological terrain and the microbiome that exists within that greater ecological context. ... Or is it the other way around?

In short, if one considers the material which has been explored in the present chapter, the notion of an immune system seems rather an arbitrary way of interpreting the available data. On the other hand, what does seem -- at least for me -- to conform with and accurately reflect the available data is a system of dynamics which – either individually, or in combination with, or collectively – is capable, within certain degrees of freedom and constraint ("constraint" refers to modalities of pathology that seem beyond the unaided modalities of the body to resolve acting on its own), to be able to address the conditions of inflammation or destabilization which might have led to the transitioning of some pleiomorphic/pleomorphic microorganisms within the microbiome that exists in the body away from their normal condition of symbiosis with the biological terrain and, as a result, exacerbate the situation by adding to the toxic load that was experienced in the form of the original or initial cause of destabilization and inflammation in the biological terrain.

As was pointed out at the beginning of this chapter, the discussions which followed that opening were never intended to be definitive in character. Instead, the intention was to provide a variety of considerations that might induce a reader to transition away from a perspective that is, to a large extent, purely theoretical (i.e., the notions of an immune system and the correlative notion of immunity) and gravitate more toward a perspective (i.e., similar in scope and orientation to the positions of Béchamp, Enderlein, Rife, and Naessens) that seems to robustly resonate with a great deal of the available data and, in addition, seems far less inclined to build sandcastles in the air in the way that immunology and virology appear inclined to do and, instead, attempts to be devoted --when done properly – to a set of stringent requirements – known as the scientific method – for trying to determine how observation is related to understanding in a concretely demonstrable, or proof-based (and, therefore, not theory-laden) fashion.

Chapter 12: De-stabilizing Vectors of Toxicity

Given that considerable evidence exists (some of which has been presented previously) indicating that viruses do not exist, and given that Béchamp's, Enderlein, Rife, Naessens, and others have put forth evidence indicating that the natural tendency of the human body seems to function in accordance with a set of dynamics that appear to be geared to maintain or re-establish a condition of detoxified stability in which the terrain has a symbiotic relationship with the microbiome that exists within the biological terrain, and given that many microorganisms tend to be pleiomorphic/pleomorphic in character and are only induced to transition away from a relationship of symbiosis with the biological terrain that surrounds it when some other non-microbial cause of inflammation or de-stabilization has taken place, and given that a viable, robust argument can be advanced which indicates that there might not be any immune system in the body (although there are an array of dynamics which are dedicated to detoxifying and stabilizing the body when inflammation of some kind occurs within the biological terrain of an individual), and given that no one has been able to demonstrate that there are proteins which exist which have the sort of morphological and immunological properties that "antibodies" are supposed to have, then there would seem to be no purpose which is served by the administering of vaccines in a great many cases.

For example, measles, mumps, small pox, polio, chicken pox/shingles, RSV (respiratory syncytial virus), viral pneumonia, HPV (human papillomavirus), Hepatitis A, B, and C, Herpes simplex, rabies, influenza, MERS (Middle East Respiratory Syndrome), SARS-CoV-1 and 2, HIV, as well as a number of cancers are believed to be caused by viruses. Yet, if viruses don't exist, then, while one would be willing to acknowledge the existence of pathological conditions that correspond to each of the foregoing designations, nonetheless, any vaccine which is based on the theory that the associated medical conditions underlying the foregoing labels are due to viral infections needs to be able to prove that the viruses which allegedly cause those diseases actually exist, and this has not been done.

Many vaccines contain one or more (usually more) of the following components: Heavy metals such as aluminum or thimerosal (an organomercury compound) and both of which have been proven to have neurodegenerative capabilities (moreover, when these two metals occur together, they have been shown to have synergistic interactions that render them far more toxic than when they used separately); genetically modified organisms (which are synthetic entities that often prove to be disruptive to, or capable of undermining, the dynamics of a person's natural biological terrain precisely because such drugs are synthetic creations that present problems for both anabolic and catabolic aspects of metabolism ... indeed, the adverse side-effects that tend to be associated with different drugs are a direct reflection of the synthetic nature of those drugs since synthetic molecules tend to be incompatible with natural metabolic pathways in a variety of ways, and it is such incompatibility that often underlies the adverse side-effects of a drug); formaldehyde or other kinds of preservatives tend to have toxic properties and also have been shown to have a carcinogenic potential as well (some individuals try to argue that formaldehyde occurs naturally in the body, and, therefore, small amounts of injected formaldehyde are innocuous, but what might be innocuous in one context might be quite problematic in a different biological context ... a molecule can be both beneficial and injurious depending on how it gets into the body and what other components it might cross-react with during such an entry process); stabilizers (such as gelatin to which some people are allergic); surfactants such as polysorbate 80 which often contain contaminants because the actual polysorbate portion of those compounds only constitutes a relatively limited aspect of the overall composition of the compound; PEG or polyethylene glycol (to which many people are allergic); bacteria of one kind or another that are ecological outliers and, as a result, have no established, symbiotic relationship with a person's biological terrain; cells from monkeys, from the brains of mice, or from the kidneys of dogs (all of which often are either in a condition of being, or becoming, cytotoxic -- that is dying and releasing whatever is present in those cells – including an array of foreign proteins that could be toxic to human beings, and, therefore, none of these cells have any business being injected into people); adjuvants such as squalene (which has been shown to have a toxic effect on many people); antibiotics such as streptomycin, gentamicin, and neomycin (each of which might prove problematic for some individuals); potassium chloride which has the capacity to adversely affect the heart and respiratory system (which could be problematic for infants, young children, and anybody with breathing or heart problems); and, peanut oil (which is either capable of adversely affecting people with peanut allergies and their presence in vaccines might be connected to the fact that there has been a veritable explosion of cases involving the emergence of peanut allergies.

People who might be suffering from this or that pathological condition but are not ill because of an entity (i.e., a virus) whose existence cannot be proven, certainly have no need to receive a vaccine that is supposed to protect against a pathogen whose very existence can be credibly challenged, but even more importantly, such people have no need to be injected with ingredients that have considerable potential for introducing toxicity of one kind or another into a person's body. In such cases, all that is being done is that people are being injected with potentially toxic vectors of one kind or another, and none of this is capable of being justified in any viable fashion.

Apparently, there are some people who should know better but who are either ignorant or willfully blind concerning all of the foregoing possibilities but, nonetheless, have bestowed upon themselves the right to poison other individuals and expose the latter individuals to potential toxins. This is done despite the fact that in view of what has been said already – and more will be added to this as we move through the present chapter – viral vaccines are nothing more than de-stabilizing vectors of toxicity which in many, if not most locations within the United States, are being forced – by legal mandates -- to be injected into the bodies of infants, children, and teenagers.

Furthermore, with respect to those vaccines which are not directed toward allegedly countering the presence of some non-viral pathogen (e.g., tetanus, diphtheria, and pertussis), one might want to keep in mind that something called the immune system might not actually exist in the human body and that the dynamics which are present (such as: macrophages, neutrophils, dendritic cells, T-cells, B-Cells, complement system, cytokines) could be operating within the context of a non-immunological oriented system of detoxification and stabilization in which antibodies – which have not been directly observed or proven to exist in human beings but are assumed to exist on the basis of a hermeneutical perspective concerning what some people believe certain surrogate markers tell us – do not have any real-world, non-theoretical immunological role to play, and, therefore, the way in which such non-viral vaccines are made does not accurately reflect what the human body needs.

If antibodies do not exist, and, yet, the alleged presence of antibodies (as determined by questionable surrogate markers) is the index which is used to determine whether, or not, a given vaccine supposedly is working, then vaccines – whether intended to treat viral- or bacterial-based threats – which depend on the idea of such a will-o'-the-wisp are inherently problematic. Moreover, given the rather tenuous, if not non-existent, relationship which immunological theory has with actual reality, then as was true in the case of injections directed toward mythical entities known as "viruses", so too, in the case of vaccines that are used in conjunction with potential bacterial threats, one should reflect on the risk-'reward' trade-off which exists – namely, vaccines based on a theory of immunology which cannot be shown to be true, versus the sorts of potential problems which empirically actually have been shown to be present in those injections in the form of toxins and poisons.

Ironically, the very procedure (a vaccine) which is purported to counter this or that bacterial threat is, in reality, the source of toxins and poisons that are capable of destabilizing the biological terrain and, thereby, inducing pleiomorphic/pleomorphic microorganisms to transition away from their symbiotic relationship with the biological terrain which they inhabit and morph into the very sort of problem against which the original injection supposedly protected an individual. Contagion is not necessarily a function of some external agent infecting a given host, but, instead, might give expression to the extent to which the condition of a given individual's biological terrain is susceptible to the presence of certain kinds of microorganisms which are either endogenous or exogenous in nature.

A healthy biological terrain has the capacity to resist certain kinds of microorganisms transitioning away from a condition of symbiosis. An unhealthy terrain might not be able to resist such transition dynamics and, therefore, might be susceptible to certain kinds of illnesses that might arise through such non-symbiotic transitions, and, as such, the primary causal locus of infectivity might reside with the presence or absence of a condition of susceptibility in a given biological terrain and only secondarily, if at all, be tied to the properties of a given pathogen.

One might want to keep in mind that if a given potential pathogen is pleiomorphic/pleomorphic, not all stages of that entity's life cycle will necessarily release the toxins that constitute the actual threat to, say, a human being. Those toxins might only be released in certain stages of the cycle, but such stages might be induced to become manifest as a result of what is going on in the surrounding biological terrain rather than being a function of something within the microorganism which is taking place in such a microorganism independent of the surrounding terrain.

One also might wonder why the public is being so readily exposed to the potential risks associated with all of the foregoing toxins that have shown to be present in various vaccines directed toward bacterial-related diseases such as tetanus, when this disease is not contagious and is fairly rare. If a person wishes to do the calculus of well-being and try to evaluate actual risk against possible reward and, then, is prepared to expose herself or himself – or children -- to such potentially toxic elements in the hope that some degree of protection against the aforementioned diseases might be afforded, this is one thing, but there is nothing in such a scenario which warrants mandating those kinds of vaccines.

Conducting studies that compare the health of vaccinated children against the health of unvaccinated children are becoming increasingly difficult to do because of the vaccine mandates which are being imposed on parents and children everywhere. One might note in passing that one of the goals of such mandates might be to eliminate the ability to establish any sort of comparison group that could be used to demonstrate the rather stark differences in health that exist between vaccinated and unvaccinated children.

In any event, there are some studies which have been undertaken which provide some rather startling data. Thus, there was a 2017 study which compared non-vaccinated home schooled children with their non-home schooled counterparts and found that: (1) vaccinated children were more than 4 times as likely to experience attention deficit and hyperactivity disorders than were non-vaccinated children; (2) vaccinated children were 22 times more likely to be using an allergy medication of some kind than were unvaccinated children; (3) vaccinated children were 8 times more likely to undergo surgery for purposes of having ear drainage tubes inserted than were unvaccinated children; (4) vaccinated children were more than five times as likely to experience some form of learning disability as were unvaccinated children; (5) vaccinated children were more than 30 times as likely to suffer from the symptoms of hay fever as were unvaccinated children; (6) vaccinated children were more than 4 times as likely to be diagnosed as being on the Autism Spectrum as were unvaccinated children; (7) vaccinated children were nearly 2.5 times more likely to experience chronic disorders of one kind or another than were vaccinated children, and (8) vaccinated children were nearly 6 times as likely to have been diagnosed with a case of pneumonia than were unvaccinated children.

There are other conditions of comparison that could have been added to the foregoing points which tend to indicate that, in general terms, vaccinated children seem to be a lot less healthy than are unvaccinated children. Of course, someone who is a die-hard advocate for vaccines might wish to claim that the foregoing comparisons were not conducted according to relevant conditions of stringency, but such claims need to be backed up by an actual analysis of those studies, and the pro-vaccine crowd tends to distance themselves from anything that has to with comparing the health of vaccinated and unvaccinated children.

Another kind of test that the pro-vaccine crowd consistently avoids has to do with experiments that employ control groups side-by-side with an experimental group that is testing this or that vaccine. The control group should consist of people who have not been injected with whatever vaccine is being tested.

Apparently, pro-vaccine people don't want to run the foregoing sorts of trials because one would be able to determine in a fairly clear manner whether, or not, a given vaccination actually offered greater protection against some disease than is the case in conjunction with people who do not receive such injections. Instead, time and time again they have ignored such experiments and, thereby, missed any number of opportunities to be able to quiet critics of vaccines, hiding behind the excuse that it would be unethical to deny the people in the control group whatever vaccine is being tested, when such an argument has actually placed the cart before the horse because pro vaccine people **have never shown** that being vaccinated constitutes a safer, more effective way, and healthier way to engage life than will be experienced by people who choose not to become injected with such vaccines.

There have been studies other than the one previously cited indicating that unvaccinated children tend to be much healthier than unvaccinated children Every single one of those studies, without exception, came to the same conclusion -- namely, vaccinated children tend to be much less healthy than vaccinated children are, and why should anyone have trouble grasping such claims given the extent of the toxicities that are present in most, if not all, vaccines?

The practices of vaccinology often tend to be firmly embedded and entangled in theories that are more theocratic than scientific. Consequently, those individuals who are inclined to pursue a form of medical evangelism whose adherents believe they have the right to proselytize everybody concerning a system of faith which intent on forcing individuals into submitting to receiving the sacrament of injection along with a surrounding catechism that proclaims, among other things, that vaccines are "safe and effective" when such is not the case, are agenda driven rather than truth oriented.

Consider the following: W.H.O. (World Health Organization), USAID, the World Bank, the Rockefeller Foundation, and the U.N. Population Fund have all supported immunological contraceptive research – that is, research which is focused on finding ways to hijack different capacities of the body that might be engaged in resisting various kinds of disease processes (which tend to be considered to be immunological in character but actually might involve other kinds of dynamics) and leverage those processes (whatever their actual properties might be) in order to serve some kind of a contraception function. Of the three different modalities that might offer venues for inhibiting fertility – namely, anti-egg, anti-sperm, and anti-fetus vaccines – one method that has been pursued revolves about the hormone known as: human chorionic gonadotropin (hCG).

Human chorionic gonadotropin plays an essential role in assisting a fertilized egg or embryo to become implanted. However, hCG has been paired with either a diphtheria or tetanus toxoid and injected into women of child-bearing age in order to prevent pregnancy from moving being able to move forward.

Should the biological terrain become destabilized as a result of the toxins that are introduced into a woman's body via tetanus or diphtheria vaccines that contain hCG, then part of this destabilization process often results in the normal properties of hCG to become compromised and, as a result, the fertilized egg cannot successfully be implanted. Whether, as immunologists might argue, the foregoing sort of destabilization is due to the antibodies which are generated in the wake of the aforementioned injection and are believed to lead to the development of an autoimmune disorder in which those antibodies are inclined to attack hCG as a foreign antigen and, thereby, interfere with the usual manner in which that hormone functions, or whether, hCG becomes dysfunctional in some other non-immunological manner is, for present purposes, irrelevant.

What is important is that components such as hCG can be added to the toxic concoctions that are contained within tetanus and diphtheria vaccines, and, as a result, the activity of hCG appears to become compromised amidst the toxicity that has been introduced into a given woman's biological terrain via those vaccines. Conceivably, hCG might cross react, in various ways, with one, or more, of the toxins that are present in such vaccines and, in the process, undermine the functionality of hCG or, perhaps, the hCG that is paired with a toxoid in the vaccine might engage in some sort of competitive inhibition with whatever normal hCG molecules are induced to come to the location where a fertilized egg exists and is waiting for an opportunity to become implanted – an opportunity that becomes poisoned, blocked, or undermined in one way or another.

For instance, there was a BBC documentary entitled 'The Human Laboratory" which explored a tetanus project that took place in the Philippines. The alleged health campaign was offered only to women of child-bearing age, and instead of receiving only one shot – which, according to immunological theory, should have been sufficient, allegedly, to provide a person with protection against tetanus for a period of ten years, the women who participated in the project were given three shots.

A variety of health care practitioners soon began to observe an increase in miscarriages among the women who were enrolled in the program. When the contents of the vaccine vials being used in the project were analyzed, hCG was detected in approximately 20% of the vials that were examined, and, of course, since the women who were receiving the injections were required to have three jabs rather than just one, the probability that hCG might have been in one, or more, of those injections could have increased with each additional injection.

Not only were there similar problems in other, supposedly, public health initiatives that resonated with the foregoing circumstances and, therefore, also gave tetanus shots only to women of child-bearing age in both Mexico and Nicaragua, but there were also similar issues of concern that arose in other parts of the world. For instance, in 1996, the Catholic Bishops of Kenya requested that the Minister of Health for that country test the tetanus vaccines which were to be administered before the contents of those vials were actually deployed throughout the country.

As was the case in the Philippines, Nicaragua, and Mexico, the Kenya tetanus project was directed toward only women of child-bearing age. Rather than permit the tetanus vials to be tested, the W.H.O. withdrew the vials and suspended the proposed program in public health.

However, nearly twenty years later, W.H.O. returned to Kenya and proposed a new tetanus public health initiative. When someone in Kenya acquired some of the vials that were to be used in the program and had their contents tested, they were shown to contain hCG.

hCG didn't find its way into the tetanus vials that were being used in Mexico, Nicaragua, Kenya, or the Philippines by mistake. The W.H.O., vaccine manufacturers, as well as various organizations that were committed to population control and were providing financial support for such projects were all very likely colluding with one another in order to achieve some of their goals in conjunction with their agenda of population control.

However, the evangelical character of the foregoing program is not just about the issue of population control. Even in the absence of hCG, such vaccination programs are deeply involved in a rather tawdry form of medical evangelicalism which seeks to promulgate doctrines -- despite the absence of anything approaching unimpeachable justification for doing so – that praise vaccines while ignoring their potential for, if not the actuality of their, toxicity and poisoning which are present in the alleged medicinal properties of vaccines that often are promoted through propagandistic strategies of fear-porn in which various kinds of horror stories often are told to parents or are alluded to in order to "persuade" parents to get with the program and vaccinate their children.

To add insult to injury, none of the individuals who were to participate in any of the foregoing programs were being provided with an opportunity to do so with informed consent. Those women had a right to be informed concerning the presence of hCG in the vaccines and to be informed about what its presence might mean with respect to the issue of fertility before they gave – or refused to give – their consent to what was taking place.

Moreover, the women in the different programs that have been mentioned had a right to be informed not only about the potential for toxicity that was present in such vaccines but, as well, they had a right to be informed about the possibility that the theories on which vaccines are based might not be true and that "antibodies" have never actually been shown to exist. All of the foregoing themes are quite independent of, and can be considered apart from, the issue of hCG.

The presence of hCG in vaccines is not an isolated issue of ethical – if not legal – violations concerning the manner in which the vaccine industry conducts itself. The vaccine industry does not consist of just the manufacturers of vaccines, but, it also consists of the universities, journals, research institutions, and government bodies (such as the CDC) that supposedly exercise regulatory control over which vaccines obtain authorization.

On August 27, 2014, Dr. William Thompson, a senior scientist at the CDC made a public confession that he and a number of his colleagues had lied and committed fraud in conjunction with the issue of the nature of the relationship between the MMR vaccine and autism.

The lying and fraud had been going on for approximately ten years and anyone – such as Dr. Andrew Wakefield of England – who might have just suggested or hinted at the possibility of a connection between MMR vaccines and autism often had their lives destroyed in calculated ways by the medical establishment directly or by their surrogates (e.g., people in the media) who have been co-opted by the pharmaceutical and medical industries.

Among the information that had been kept from the public and, in fact, about which the CDC continued to lie for a decade, or so, had to do with an article authored by Thompson and others that had been published in a 2004 issue of the journal *Pediatrics*. The article deliberately omitted data which indicated how African American children who received the MMR injection prior to being 36 months of age were more likely to develop autism.

Interestingly, but quite dishearteningly, the American Academy of Pediatrics whose members make a lot of money through overseeing and administering an extensive vaccine program involving infants and children – and therefore have a deep conflict of interest with respect to anything that they say about vaccines -- decided to double-down on the whole issue. More specifically, despite the existence of evidence to the contrary in cases such as the aforementioned Dr. William Thompson whistleblower affair, the AAP issued a statement in 2015 which asserted that claims linking autism to vaccines were dangerous to the public health and allegedly, all such claims had been demonstrated to be false by different facets of the medical and scientific establishments ... notwithstanding the fact that Dr. William Thompson's testimony directly contradicted what the AAP was saying.

Statistically speaking, one in 10,000 births during the 1970s was associated with an autistic disorder of some kind. Ten years later the incidence of autistic-related disorders had climbed to one in 500 births.

When the 1990s arose, the incidence of autistic-related disorders increased again and was associated with one individual out of every 100 births. Within three years of the turn of the century, autistic-related disorders had become associated with one in 86 births. Finally, in the 2020s, the incidence of autistic-related disorders is, now, calculated to be associated with one in 36 births.

There is only one likely cause for such a rapid increase of autistic-related disorders during the foregoing 50-year timeframe. People are being systematically poisoned by one, or more, environmental toxins, and, perhaps, the form of poisoning that best parallels the increase in the incidence of autistic-related disorders is the precipitous rise in the number of vaccines that children have been required to take during that 50-year period of time.

Despite the fact that viruses cannot be proven to exist, and despite the possibility that there might not even be an immune system, per se, within human beings (although there certainly are an array of capacities within the biological terrain for detoxifying and returning a de-stabilized body to a condition of well-being and symbiotic relationships with the microbiome that occupies many facets of that terrain), and despite the availability of evidence indicating that the notion of an antibody is more theoretical than existential, and despite the many toxicological problems that have been linked to the components that often make up vaccines and whose problematic presence is exhibited in the data that shows the difference in the health and well-being between vaccinated and unvaccinated children, one is supposed to accept the unsupported word of the American Academy of Pediatricians – all of whose members have conflicts of interest concerning the topic of vaccines – that vaccines are safe, effective, and the best chance that infants and children have to not become sick and/or die (fear porn at its best, if not worst).

In 2013 Dr. Suzanne Humphries and Roman Bystrianyk published a book of research – *Dissolving Illusions* -- concerning the forgotten history surrounding the relationship between disease and vaccinations. Much – but not all -- of the data and information that appears in the following 20 pages constitutes a summary and reworded overview of some of their research.

One of the precipitating causes that led to the foregoing book had to do with a graph that Roman Bystrianyk came across while conducting research of his own. The graph indicated that the number of people who died as a result of a diagnosed encounter with measles had declined by 95% prior to the time when a vaccine for measles had come into being.

One ramification of the foregoing graph is that if someone would wish to argue that the reason why people should be vaccinated against measles is because that vaccine was responsible for the decrease in the death rate associated with measles, then such an argument would be based on a false premise. According to the graph to which Roman Bystrianyk is alluding, decrease in the death rate associated with measles apparently had nothing to do with the existence of a vaccine.

Another question that arises in conjunction with the aforementioned graph but which cannot be resolved by means of that graph is whether, or not, similar sorts of things might be said about the relationship between, say, death rates associated with other sorts of diseases. In other words, is it possible that observed decreases in the death rate associated with other kinds of diseases for which vaccinations now exist might have taken place before any sort of vaccine had been developed and/or widely distributed in conjunction with such diseases?

Bystrianyk spent a considerable amount of time in the Yale Medical Library looking through old books, documents, articles and journal articles seeking answers to the foregoing kinds of questions. Eventually, he developed a spread sheet which enabled him to sort and enter data into a variety of categories that presented an array of information concerning disease, vaccinations, mortality rates, and so on that occurred during various time frames.

Not only did he discover that the mortality rate associated with the first disease that he researched -- i.e., measles – actually had declined 98% since 1900 (3% more that the graph mentioned earlier had indicated) and the mortality rate had reached that milestone well before a vaccine for measles had been introduced, he also found out that the mortality rate associated with whooping cough had declined by 90% during roughly that same period of time. This decline also had taken place before the DTP vaccine was introduced.

When he presented the foregoing information to his wife who was a nurse, she resisted what she was being told. In other words, despite not necessarily having any actual evidence with which to refute the information she was receiving from her husband concerning measles and whooping cough, she engaged that information through the frames of reference that had been provided to her by the education and training she had received that not only enabled her to become a nurse but to be able to actively practice what she had learned in different clinical settings.

Studying a variety of references that explored the issue of disease for more than a century – from 1800 to the early 1900s – Bystrianyk began to realize that a great deal of history lived in the shadows. This was especially true with respect to the topic of disease.

Dr. Suzanne Humphries, the other author of *Dissolving Illusions* came to the topic of the lost history surrounding various diseases from a different direction than did Roman Bystrianyk. In many ways, she -- like her co-author's wife -- had been indoctrinated to think in a certain way about what role vaccines supposedly played in the decline of various diseases.

Before she actually engaged in relevant research, Dr. Humphries considered people like Jonas Salk to be a hero for the role they allegedly played in 'defeating' polio. However, in a hospital that sits just a couple of miles away from where I currently live, she underwent a series of encounters that eventually led to her resignation as a nephrologist at the foregoing hospital.

One of the initial set of incidents that induced her to begin to engage in a certain amount of critical thinking concerning the issue of vaccinations had to do with three patients who were in her care. The year was 2009 and there was an on-going push at her hospital to vaccinate patients against the H1N1 strain of influenza.

Dr. Humphries had not prescribed the injections for the foregoing three patients, but they were jabbed anyway and Dr. Humphries was identified on one of the documents in the patient files as being the physician that had authorized the vaccinations. There were a number of problematic, if not unethical, aspects that were present in the foregoing situation, but the issue on which we will focus at the present time is that soon after receiving their respective injections all three patients experienced a complete shutdown of kidney functioning.

All three of the patients had exhibited normal kidney functioning prior to receiving the vaccinations. Following vaccination, all three of her patients were required to undergo dialysis.

Two of the patients eventually recovered. The third individual died a few months later.

Dr. Humphries began to keep track of individuals who were showing up with idiopathic kidney diseases – that is kidney problems which could not be tied to some sort of known causal mechanism. When she came across such individuals, she would ask them about their vaccination history, and, more often than not, she would uncover evidence that such people recently had received some sort of vaccination.

When, during a conversation concerning a variety of issues, she brought up the foregoing cases with the chief of internal medicine and indicated that she believed it was possible that there was a link between vaccinations and different cases of kidney failure, the attitude of the doctor to whom she was talking visibly seemed to change. The doctor asked her why she was blaming the vaccine and, then, put forth a hypothesis that the doctor could not possibly have known whether, or not, what he was saying was true – he suggested that the vaccine simply had not had sufficient time to become actively engaged in protecting the patients against the flu which, obviously, they must have contracted, and, consequently, it was the flu and not the vaccine that should be examined for its possible impact on any subsequent change in the health of those individuals.

At the time of the foregoing conversation, Dr. Humphries might not have been able to prove that vaccines were responsible for the onset of various kinds of kidney failure, but the very notion of "idiopathic" is that the cause of a given condition is not known and, therefore, it would seem that a good doctor would want to explore – as Dr. Humphries was trying to do with the internist -- different possibilities in an attempt to resolve such cases and, thereby, offer her patients a better form of health care. Unfortunately, the doctor with whom she was talking – who also did not know what was transpiring in such cases – merely sought to shut the conversation down while providing vaccines an undeserved presumptive carte blanche get-out-of jail-free-card for whatever happened in connection with those sorts of injections.

Subsequently, Dr. Humphries began to engage in research concerning the issue of safety with respect to vaccines that were given to kidney patients. She was unsettled to discover that there were no safety trials concerning the impact of vaccines on kidney patients because all vaccines were automatically assumed by the medical profession to be safe and effective despite the absence of rigorous studies – such as in cases involving kidney patients – that were capable of proving that such injections actually posed no problems for those patients. The vaccines were being presumed to be safe rather than having been proven to be safe.

As a result of the foregoing kinds of experiences at the hospital where she was working, Dr. Humphries decided to begin to actively investigate and research the relationship between a variety of diseases and vaccines. What she discovered was revelatory.

To begin with, as a nephrologist, Dr. Humphries' job required her to make all manner of judgments about whether, or not, the use of certain drugs could have, or might be having, a deleterious effect upon the kidneys of a patient – irrespective of whether the patient was hers or was in the care of another physician for whom she was serving as a consultant. Her judgments in those cases were always accepted, without question, but, now, when it came to the issue of the possible deleterious impact of vaccines on kidney functioning, her professional judgment was not only resisted but she was criticized for interfering with the hospital's policies concerning vaccines.

Eventually, her research and her clinical experience appeared to point in just one direction. She needed to resign from the hospital where she had been working, and, among other things, continue her research into disease and vaccines, and that is what she did.

The 1800's were tumultuous times. For a variety of reasons, more and more people were leaving rural areas to live in cities, and, as a result, the size of cities began to explode.

Unfortunately, the infrastructure of those cities was not capable of handling those sorts of transitions in population growth. As a result, clean drinking water was hard to come by, and the sewer systems in those overcrowded cities tended to constantly backup into the streets and houses, especially when it rained.

Various kinds of livestock were present in many of the same locations where people lived, and, consequently, a considerable amount of animal waste was being added to human waste in such localities. Neither kind of waste material was being disposed of in a manner that was capable of serving the interests of public health.

In addition, slaughter houses often existed near to tenement dwellings. Among the products of the former factories were all manner of rotting detritus that was left over from the process of slaughtering animals and which, through smell or in other ways, seeped out into the community.

Rats were more than plentiful. They often competed with human beings for available resources involving food and living space and, as well, added to the waste management problem.

Garbage collection programs were often grossly inadequate, for the needs of people. However, vermin of various kinds appeared to thrive in such conditions.

Manufacturing plants also existed in the cities. They were releasing all manner of toxic pollutants and chemicals into the city environment.

Working conditions in those plants tended to be fraught with danger. Moreover, many people worked 12 to 16 hour shifts, and if both parents were working in order to try to make ends meet, children were left to fend for themselves with a minimum amount of supervision which often required older children – who were still children -- to look after their younger siblings.

In addition, as largely semi-automated forms of manufacturing began to increase in prevalence, manufacturers began to hire children to work in their factories to "man" such machines. Child labor was cheaper than adult labor, and there usually were no laws on the books to protect the well-being and health of children from the exploitive practices that were present in any number of industries.

Children as young as three and four – both male and female -- were sometimes employed in those industries. The working hours were long and were frequently carried out in brutal, hazardous conditions (e.g., children were often exposed to chemicals such as lead, mercury, and phosphorous -- all of which have the capacity to debilitate those who handle or breath them in -- that were used during some phase of a manufacturing process).

Good nutritional food often tended to be scarce. Moreover, due to widespread poverty, even when such commodities were available, many people couldn't afford to purchase them.

Furthermore, because of a lack of regulatory laws and/or enforcement, much of the food supply was compromised in one way or another. As a result, people often were forced to eat diseased or rotting food.

Housing was sub-standard. Living conditions tended to be over-crowded and hazardous in a multiplicity of ways as living conditions were frequently over-crowded, cold, damp, improperly heated, and/or poorly ventilated.

In 1750, 85% of the population could be found living outside of cities in most countries. One hundred and thirty years later, only twenty percent of the population lived outside of those same urban areas.

Thus, to give just one example, London, in 1801, had 800,000 people living within its borders. A hundred years later, there were 7 million people living in London.

However, London was not unique. Similar sorts of population growth – and their attendant problems -- were happening both throughout Europe as well as the United States.

The rivers which ran through cities became repositories of all manner of pollutants, manufacturing chemicals, waste materials, and the like. Moreover, individuals that used the water which came from those rivers in order to wash clothes, take baths, obtain drinking water, or have water for cooking, were playing a game of roulette in which they ran the risk of being exposed to all manner of disease-causing pollutants.

All of the foregoing conditions synergistically interacted to create a set of environmental forces that lent support to the emergence of a multiplicity of diseases. However, one should keep in mind that the impact of the foregoing set of interacting conditions on human beings was largely a matter of the extent or manner in which their biological terrains were destabilized. For certain diseases to become manifest, certain microorganism that were present had to be induced to transition out of what, previously, had been a either a symbiotic or non-active relationship with such terrains, and, when this occurred, this led to further complications within bodies that already were experiencing inflammatory conditions as a result of the problematic ecologies or living conditions in which those terrains existed.

As a result, the mortality rate during those times tended to be quite high, and, in different localities, the average length of life for the urban poor was sometimes between 15 and 16 years of age. Moreover, even if one were fortunate enough to dodge the possibility of an untimely, early death, one's life expectancy was frequently not much beyond 30-40 years of age.

Thousands of people died in the 1800s and early 1900s from typhoid fever. It is a disease that is characterized by high fever, abdominal pain, and diarrhea.

Allegedly, the disease is said to be caused by the presence of the Salmonella typhi bacteria. Nonetheless, one might more accurately say that when the biological terrain of an individual is de-stabilized through being exposed to all manner of unsanitary, cold, improperly ventilated, exploitive, impoverished, over-crowded, vermin-invested, hazardous conditions in which proper nutrition, sleep, and clean drinking water were not readily available, then, the aforementioned kind of microorganism could, when the conditions were right, transition into problematic aspects of their pleomorphic/pleomorphic life cycles.

There is considerable evidence indicating that many of us have those same kinds of microorganisms present within our biological terrain, yet they remain inactive within that terrain unless they are induced -- due to the destabilization of that terrain as a result of an encounter with some non-microbial vector – to transition away from such a symbiotic relationship. However, as indicated previously, normally symbiotic or inactive microorganisms sometimes entered into stages of their pleomorphic/pleomorphic life cycle in which toxins might be released by those microorganisms ... toxins which had the capacity to poison a person's biological terrain and lead to illness such as typhoid fever and, perhaps, death.

Such diseases are not autonomous actors. They require the right sort of compromised conditions within the biological terrain of an individual to be present before such microorganisms can be induced to enter certain stages of their pleiomorphic/pleomorphic life cycles that are potentially problematic in one way or another.

Cholera was another form of bacterial-related problem that was running rampant in the severely compromised social living conditions that existed in many parts of the world during the 1800s as well as during the early part of the 1900s. The symptoms associated with the onset of cholera involved debilitating cramps, vomiting, and diarrhea, were quite common, but, in addition, the latter two symptoms tended to lead to a condition of dehydration which brought about a variety of other physiological problems.

There were six cholera epidemics that occurred in different parts of the world between 1816 and 1926. Some 15 million people were believed to have died as a result of cholera outbreaks in India during the period lasting from 1817 to 1860, and thousands of people were said to have died of cholera in Paris, London, Ireland, Egypt, Japan, Spain, Persia, California, and Chicago.

Russia suffered substantial numbers of death on two different occasions. One cholera epidemic resulted in a million deaths, while another, subsequent epidemic cost the lives of a quarter of a million individuals.

Nevertheless, not everyone became sick or died in the multiplicity of locations where cholera surfaced. Whether someone got sick was not necessarily a matter of whether, or not, they had been exposed to the bacteria toxin responsible for the symptoms of cholera.

As with typhoid fever, whether, or not, a person became sick seemed to have something to do with the condition of their biological terrain. Conceivably, in those individuals whose terrains had been compromised due to exposure to other kinds of non-microbial forces which were capable of sufficiently destabilizing the health of that terrain that the bacteria associated with cholera were induced to transition away from an inactive condition or transition away from even some sort of symbiotic relationship with the surrounding terrain, then, perhaps, the pleiomorphic/pleomorphic microorganism associated with cholera might enter a stage in its life cycle that was conducive to the release of the toxins that do the damage which can lead to the devastating symptoms associated with that disease.

One must not only be able to explain why some people become sick. If typhoid fever and cholera are highly contagious – which they are said to be -- then one must be able to explain why other people who live in and around such sick individuals do not necessarily become sick.

Presumably, something more than the presence of the appropriate kind of bacteria is necessary. Contagion is dependent on the condition of the biological terrain that a given bacteria encounters or exists within, and, therefore, infectivity is not necessarily just a function of something that a given bacteria imposes on individuals.

Similar sorts of statements could be made in conjunction with microbial-related diseases such as: Diphtheria, typhus fever (which is not the same thing as typhoid fever), puerperal fever (a post-partum condition affecting mothers), pneumonia, scarlet fever, tuberculosis, and pertussis (or whooping cough). Whether, or not, a given individual becomes ill is a much more complicated affair than merely attributing their pathological condition to the presence of a certain kind of microorganism because one needs to take into consideration not only the state of a person's biological terrain, but, as well, one must factor in the nature of the relationship which exists between that terrain and the microbiome that occupies it and whether, or not, the sort of destabilized conditions exist in that terrain which are likely to induce various bacteria that are present to enter into a stage of their pleiomorphic/pleomorphic life cycle that is capable of releasing the sorts of poisons or toxins that are responsible for the illnesses and deaths that might be associated with the aforementioned diseases.

In all of the foregoing cases, when the environmental conditions that characterized the horrific public health issues that were entailed by compromised conditions of: Sanitation, nutrition, food safety, hazardous and exploitive work environments, sub-standard and over-crowed living conditions, and the inadequate practices for resolving problems surrounding the disposal of garbage and sewage waste that were inherent in the forms of urban living that existed – and proceeded to get worse throughout much of the 1800s and early 1900s – nonetheless, when those living conditions were substantially improved or eliminated altogether, many of the diseases that were prevalent during the 140 years, or so, in which the foregoing sorts of problematic living conditions were at their peak, all dramatically decreased. These decreases were due to improvements in living conditions and had nothing to do with wide-spread vaccination programs that allegedly that were promoted as being safe and effective.

Just to give one example, the Austrian physician, Ignaz Semmelweis, observed that when babies were delivered by physicians, the mothers were three-times more likely to die at the hands of those physicians than were mothers whose babies were delivered by midwives. Dr. Semmelweis also noted that many doctors who tended to mothers about to give birth often went directly from the cadaver dissection labs associated with a medical facility to the expectant mothers without bothering to wash their hands.

He recommended that doctors should employ a solution consisting of chlorinated lyme in order to clean their hands prior to attending to pregnant mothers – either in conjunction with the process of delivery or the process of conducting any sort of internal exam with the pregnant mother. When doctors complied with the directive given by Dr. Semmelweis, the mortality rate went from as much as 32% down to zero.

Dr. Semmelweis was rewarded for the foregoing observations, recommendation, and concern for the health of mothers in a rather ugly manner. Apparently, there were some doctors who, apparently, felt that their reputations had been sullied by the perspective being advanced by Dr. Semmelweis and, as a result manipulated him into going into an insane asylum.

When he tried to escape from the institution, he was badly beaten by a group of guards. The beating, plus the absence of any sort of adequate care, seemed to lead to the death of Dr. Semmelweis several weeks later.

Although different tactics might have been used than were employed in the foregoing Semmelweis affair, similar motivations seemed to prod various scientists and doctors in the 19th and 20th centuries to try to ruin the reputations and lives of people such as Béchamp, Enderlein, Rife, and Naessens, along with the lives of other individuals who either worked with those latter scientists and inventors or who sought to utilize the work of the four aforementioned individuals to improve the lives of clients. Moreover, just as Dr. Semmelweis had demonstrated – on the basis of actual evidence and not on the basis of arguments from authority and unsupported theories – that one could eliminate most, if not all cases, of puerperal fever, if one followed a few simple rules of basic hygiene, so too, scientists and medical doctors such as Béchamp, Enderlein, Rife, and Naessens had demonstrated – on the basis of evidence rather than on the basis of arguments from authority or theories that were nothing more than unproven declarations -- that in contrast to the monomorphic theory of germs which Pasteur had finessed into theoretical existence, the foregoing researchers were able to show that many microorganisms seemed to have a pleiomorphic/pleiomorphic life cycle which tended to be in symbiotic relationships with the surrounding biological terrain unless that terrain were destabilized in such a way that various members of the microbiome were induced to transition away from a condition of symbiosis and, sometimes, enter into stages of their life cycle that might be capable of releasing toxins which poisoned the surrounding terrain and led to one or another kind of disease.

Just as Roman Bystrianyk had come across graphs and documented evidence which he had discovered in old books and journals indicating that the incidence of both measles and whooping cough started to, and, then, continued to, substantially decrease as improvements in infrastructure and public health were made ... improvements that were in place, to varying degrees, long before vaccines for those two diseases came into being, so too were Bystrianyk and Dr. Humphries able to demonstrate that similar decreases in incidence and mortality occurred in conjunction with a variety of other diseases as well – decreases in incidence and death that were independent of vaccines. Smallpox offers an informative case study in this respect.

However, as we run through an overview of their research concerning smallpox, one should keep in mind that unlike some of the other diseases that have been discussed or touched upon during the last seven, or so, pages (e.g., puerperal fever, cholera, and typhoid fever), the medical establishment believes that smallpox is caused by a virus and not a bacterium. Given that a fair amount of information and thought has been presented previously in the present book indicating that viruses might not exist, then, the following discussion will not be about whether, or not, smallpox is caused by a virus, but, rather, the discussion will explore various treatments for smallpox and whether, or not, evidence exists which, on the one hand, suggests that decreases in the incidence of smallpox can be tied to factors other than vaccines, and, on the other hand, that to whatever extent a process of inoculation was available, it was neither safe nor effective.

Smallpox is characterized by very high fevers and skin lesions that leak fluids. If people did not die from their encounter with smallpox, they often had to live with the unsightly scars from the lesions or pox marks that were left in the wake of the disease.

In 1717 Lady Montagu returned from her sojourn into various locations within the Ottoman Empire with knowledge of a practice called variolation which involved taking small scrapings from the active lesions of individuals who were ill with the disease and transferring that material to human beings who were not, yet, ill. The theory underlying the practice (which carried an uncertain empirical pedigree) was that by following the foregoing protocol, one could induce a mild case of smallpox in healthy people and save them from the more severe ravages of that disease in the future.

There were two caveats concerning the practice. The people to whom such scrapings were transferred didn't necessarily have only mild cases of smallpox and, they sometimes, died (2-3 people per hundred people inoculated), and, moreover, the practice of variolation tended to spread the disease rather than contain it.

Consequently, approximately 11 years after being introduced into Europe, the foregoing practice was discontinued for a time. Fast-forward another 10-15 years, and it resurfaced as a popular treatment for those who had the money to pay for it.

There was evidence, based on events in Boston, which seemed to demonstrate that those who underwent variolation were less likely to die than people who became ill with smallpox in the "normal way" – whatever the latter term might mean given that no one really understood what caused the disease. Nonetheless, whether, or not, the process of variolation was successful often depended on a variety of factors – such as the skill of the individual who performed the procedure and/or the ingredients that were used in the produces – both of which were, for a variety of reasons, difficult to assess.

The Boston "evidence" notwithstanding, there also was a growing parallel body of evidence indicating that irrespective of whatever protection such a practice might provide, variolation was responsible for the spread of the disease into areas where, previously, it had not been present. Furthermore, there was also evidence to indicate that when one compared the rates of death -- as measured against either births or burials in a given area -- prior to the introduction of the technique with the rates of death – as, once again, measured against either births or burials in a given area – then, following the introduction of the practice, there was a substantial increase in death rates of between 27 and 41 percent, depending on which of the foregoing measures one used as a baseline.

A form of treatment for smallpox that began to be pursued in the last quarter of the 18th century involved a sort of variation on the process of variolation. Instead of taking scrapings from the active lesions of a person ill with smallpox, an alternative way of proceeding involved something that many milkmaids of the time claimed offered some degree of protection against smallpox, and, as a result, Benjamin Jesty, a farmer, decided to try to protect his wife and children from the ravages of smallpox, by taking scrapings from the lesions in cows that were suffering from cowpox. Apparently, or so the story goes, when his two sons were placed in the vicinity of some people with smallpox, the two boys did not come down with the disease.

In 1796, Edward Jenner also had heard about how, apparently, milkmaids were able to avoid smallpox by using scrapings from cowpox and decided to put the underlying theory to a further test when he induced an 8-year old boy to undergo the same sort of procedure that Benjamin Jesty applied to his wife and two sons, and, as a result, took scrapings from what he believed were cowpox lesions on the back of the hand of a milkmaid he employed and, then, transferred them to the boy. Like Jesty, Jenner deliberately exposed the subject of his experiment to an individual who was believed to have smallpox, and, once again, as also appeared to be the case with the sons of Jesty when they were exposed to someone with smallpox, the 8-year old did not contract smallpox.

Initially, the foregoing treatment was believed to confer a lifetime of protection. However, soon differences of opinion arose as to how long a person who had received such cowpox scrapings might be protected against smallpox, and the period of alleged immunity ran anywhere between one and ten years.

Jenner's experiment involved just one individual. Moreover, there was no control "group" to determine whether another individual who had not been treated with cowpox would, or would not, develop smallpox if exposed to someone who was ill with smallpox.

In 1799, a year after Jenner published an article which claimed, among other things, that his method of inoculation would protect people against smallpox for life, a surgeon from Stroud, England, by the name of Drake sought to replicate Jenner' original experiment. Consequently, he used inoculation materials that were obtained directly from Jenner and proceeded to inoculate three children who were 15 months old, four years old, and 17 years old in accordance with the protocol that had been established by Jenner.

All three of the children went on to develop high fevers as well as other symptoms associated with smallpox. Like many, if not most, manufacturers of vaccines today, Jenner ignored experimental results which ran counter to his claims.

There was an additional question that might be asked. How could one be certain that if someone were treated with the scrapings from either cowpox or smallpox that it was the scrapings that had been incorporated into a person's body which was the reason why such a person did not, subsequently, become ill?

Although many people who were exposed to individuals who might have been ill with smallpox did also become ill, nonetheless, there were many others who had not been inoculated but had been exposed, in one way or another, to people with smallpox and, yet, did not get sick at all, or who did get sick but survived, or who only had mild cases of the disease. What was the reason, or what were the reasons, for such differences in disease dynamics?

Moreover, if viruses don't actually exist, then, what actually is going on when a person exhibits symptoms of smallpox? Variolation – that is, the process of using scrapings from humans, cows, and so on --

seemed – possibly -- to be doing something in some cases, but no one knew exactly what the nature of that 'something' might be or exactly what induced the body to respond with the symptoms that it did when the smallpox disease seemed to be actively present in some manner.

In 1810, a publication known as the *Medical Observer* released information indicating that among a group of 535 individuals who had received an inoculation against smallpox, there had been 97 people who had died from smallpox. There also were another 150 people in that same group who had experienced injuries of one kind or another that could be related to their inoculation process (and there were a variety of illnesses which showed up in some individuals shortly after undergoing the Jenner protocol).

Thus, nearly half of the individuals in the inoculated group being described either died or suffered an inoculated-related injury. There also were many other medical articles which indicated that claims causally linking cowpox exposure to a lifetime of protection were not, yet, proven.

In 1817, an article appeared in the *London Medical Repository Monthly Journal and Review* which stipulated that many people who had undergone the Jenner procedure had not been protected against the on-set of smallpox. The following year, Thomas Brown, a surgeon from Scotland, reported that of the 1,200, or so, individuals which he had inoculated using the Jenner method, many of them still became sick with smallpox, and a not insignificant number of those inoculated individuals died.

During a smallpox outbreak that occurred between 1820 and 1822, many people who had been inoculated, became severely ill. Moreover, there were large numbers of people who had smallpox earlier in their lives and, yet, became sick once again.

In 1822, the British government provided Jenner with a grant of some 20,000 pounds for purposes of furthering his research and work involving smallpox. Seven years later in 1829, William Cobbett, a full-time farmer and part-time journalist, indicated that many of the individuals whom Jenner, himself, had inoculated later became ill with smallpox, and quite a few of those individuals died.

In addition, some thirty years after Jenner performed his experiment, there was an article which appeared in the *Lancet*, a medical journal, which claimed that before he died, Jenner had confessed that the lymph materials he used in his experiment were from a horse, not a cow. Apparently, Jenner claimed that the material taken from a horse was pretty much the same as what was taken from a cow.

Subsequently, there was an aura of mystery which surrounded the process of inoculation. One could not be sure where the materials came from that were used in the inoculation procedure.

Some of the materials might have come from cows or horses. However, apparently, some of those materials were, on occasion, drawn from other animal sources as well.

There was a further consideration related to the foregoing mystery that no one seemed to be pursuing. More specifically, did the people who died after having been inoculated die from smallpox or did they die from some other sort of disease process that might have been connected to the mystery substances that were being used in the inoculation process, and, as a result, while they might have **died with** smallpox, they didn't necessarily **die from** smallpox.

For example, there is a bacterial-based disease known as erysipelas which, sometimes, seemed to be connected to different animal scrapings that might be used during the inoculation protocol. Some medical doctors believe that the aforementioned disease arises when a given bacterium (namely, Streptococcus pyogenes) is induced to release a toxin as a result of the impact which a certain kind of phage or bacterial virus has on such a bacterium (similar sorts of events have been documented in conjunction with both diphtheria and tetanus), but the phenomenon of toxin release can also be engaged through a pleiomorphic/pleomorphic perspective in which toxic substances are released during a stage of the bacterium's life cycle which tends to take place when the surrounding biological terrain has been destabilized sufficiently (due to, say, malnutrition, unclean drinking water, environmental pollutants, stress from overcrowded living conditions and exploitive labor practices) to induce such a bacterium to transition away from either an inactive or symbiotic relationship with the terrain in which it resides and assume a non-symbiotic dynamic in which toxins are released into the biological terrain and a disease process ensues.

In addition to erysipelas, there are several other diseases which also might arise in conjunction with the smallpox inoculation process. For example, both syphilis and tuberculosis have emerged following smallpox inoculations.

Any number of other kinds of maladies might have been introduced into the people being inoculated because the preparation process which collected the animal scrapings that were to be used in the inoculation process often included an array of microorganisms which were not in symbiotic relationship with the biological terrain into which they were being introduced. Furthermore, there was no means to keep the scrapings from undergoing cytotoxic events and, (due to the absence of refrigeration) therefore, begin to rot prior to being transferred to an individual, and, in addition, the same needles tended to used in person after person without any interim attempt to sterilize the instruments which were being used to transfer scrapings and create small wounds in the skin of the individuals and into which such scrapings were being pushed.

Notwithstanding such considerations and unable to hide from the considerable evidence indicating that inoculated individuals still got sick and died, a number of medical doctors who were earning a pretty good income stream from allegedly inoculating well-to-do people against smallpox asserted that while the inoculation procedure might not prevent people from becoming sick with smallpox, nevertheless, what the inoculations could do is reduce the severity of the disease should one become ill with it. During the 1844 outbreak of smallpox, 8 percent of those who had received the Jenner procedure died, and a further two-thirds of people who had undergone the procedure experienced severe forms of the disease.

No matter what unsubstantiated claims were made on behalf of the Jenner inoculation process, the actual experiences of many people who had been inoculated tended to contradict those claims. For example, following the 1844 smallpox outbreak in England someone remarked that there had been more admissions to hospitals for treatment of smallpox than there had been during the 1781 smallpox outbreak which had occurred prior to the introduction of the Jenner method.

A hundred years after Jenner introduced his smallpox protocol, more evidence came forth indicating still other kinds of problems that were associated with the inoculation protocol. For instance, during the serious outbreak of smallpox that took place between 1871 and 1872, a Dr. Wilder observed that people who had received the Jenner protocol seemed to be more susceptible to, or more vulnerable to, the disease because those who were inoculated often experienced severe forms of the disease long before the unvaccinated did.

Apparently ignoring the considerable amount of evidence which had been accumulating for a number of decades that the Jenner protocol for smallpox was neither necessarily safe nor effective, a number of governments began to mandate the protocol. For example, England introduced its first mandate of this kind in 1853 and, then, doubled-down and put in place an even more draconian form of mandate some 14 years later in 1867, while Massachusetts passed a set of laws in 1855 which compelled parents to have their children inoculated prior to their second birthday and, as well, stipulated that any child who had not been inoculated would not be permitted to enter the public school system.

Despite such mandates, empirical data was beginning to surface during the smallpox outbreaks which took place in: 1859-1860, 1864-1865, 1867, and 1872-1873 (the worst of the aforementioned series of smallpox outbreaks) that the foregoing kinds of laws did not improve the situation. People – including children – who had undergone inoculation got severely sick nonetheless, and many of them also died, and, therefore, one can't help but wonder what the rationale might be for enforcing such mandates when empirical data showed that they served no purpose other than tyranny, oppression, and a complete lack of understanding concerning the many unknowns that surrounded the phenomenon of smallpox.

Only one-third of the individuals who had received the Jenner inoculation seemed to come away completely unscathed. However, there is no way to determine whether the reason for their good fortune was due to the inoculation they received or it was because they didn't have any sort of close contact with people who were ill or whether, possibly, people still might have been able to escape becoming ill with smallpox if they had not been inoculated.

In Boston, there were far more individuals who died from smallpox during a twenty year period following the aforementioned inoculation mandate of 1855 than had died in the twenty year period prior to such mandates. The period prior to the institution of such mandates was not free from outbreaks of smallpox, and, in fact, one might wish to argue that it was because such pre-mandate smallpox outbreaks had taken place that mandates came into being, but, the reality was that mandates seemed to exacerbate the problems involving smallpox rather than resolve them.

More than 95% of the inhabitants of Chicago were inoculated against smallpox by the beginning of 1869. Furthermore, following the Great Chicago Fire of 1871 (initiated, some said, when Mrs. O'Leary's cow kicked over a lantern), people were only able to receive relief supplies if they underwent inoculation.

Nonetheless, a year later, in 1872 when Chicago was hit by a severe outbreak of smallpox, nearly two thousand of the inoculated individuals became ill with smallpox, and approximately 500 of those individuals died.

The situation in many other parts of the world was similar, if not worse, than what took place in Boston and Chicago. For example, according to an entry in the *Encyclopedia Britannica* written by Dr. Charles Creighton, 60,000 people died during the 1870-1873 outbreak of smallpox despite stringent laws in Prussia governing smallpox inoculations. Moreover, despite the existence of such laws, approximately one million people inoculated individuals died from smallpox between 1870 and 1885.

High rates of smallpox inoculation had taken place in Italy, yet, nearly 20,000 people died during the 1899 smallpox outbreak in that country. In England, the *Lancet* reported in July of 1871 that among the 9.392 smallpox patients who were occupying beds in London hospitals, 6,854 of those people had undergone the inoculation procedure for smallpox, and roughly 17% of the inoculated group died.

The French enforced a strict policy prior to, as well as during, the Franco-Prussian war -- which lasted from July of 1870 to May of 1871

– that required everyone who became a member of the military to undergo the smallpox inoculation procedure. During the aforementioned war, there were 23,469 cases of smallpox within the military.

Japan implemented compulsory smallpox inoculation laws beginning in 1872, and, then instituted even more stringent inoculation laws in 1885 which required, among other things, that every child must be inoculated against smallpox. Records indicate that 25 million Japanese people were either inoculated for the first time or re-inoculated over a seven year period running from 1885 to 1892, and, yet, during that seven year period, nearly 40,000 people died from among the 156, 175 people who became ill with smallpox, and, in addition, during a five year period between 1892 and 1897, another 40,000 people died from among the 142,032 cases of smallpox that were recorded.

Could one argue that the millions of people who were inoculated with the smallpox procedure were saved because of the inoculation process? Yes, one could, but, perhaps, one could more easily argue that clear evidence existed which showed that not only were such inoculations neither safe nor effective for hundreds of thousands of people (i.e., the people who had been inoculated but still got sick, as well as the people who had been inoculated but died), but, as well, one really had no idea why people who were inoculated didn't get sick.

Would such people have remained illness free even if they had not been inoculated? Since there was no control group to explore such a possibility, a person would merely be assuming – i.e., one had no way of proving what was transpiring -- that inoculations worked for some people but not others.

Moreover, if viruses do not exist, then, what is the nature of the disease process to which smallpox gave expression? Why do some people become ill while others do not?

Compulsory inoculation laws were being instituted. However, the people who were doing this not only had absolutely no idea why they were doing what they were doing, but there was an accumulating body of evidence from around the world that inoculations were neither necessarily safe nor effective.

As late as 1948, one encountered instances when, in a given area, only one person might have died from smallpox who had not been inoculated. Yet, hundreds of people in that same area died who had been inoculated.

The only data surrounding and permeating the issue of smallpox inoculation which cannot be refuted is that thousands of people who did get inoculated, nonetheless, still got sick and, sometimes, died. Concluding that people who did not get sick were protected by the inoculations they received is pure speculation because correlation (i.e., the fact that x-number of people who were inoculated did not become sick with smallpox) does not necessarily mean causation (i.e., there is evidence which can demonstrate that the cause of smallpox is 'y" and, as well, there is evidence which demonstrates that the process of inoculation is capable of nullifying such a causal dynamic by way of the following set of concrete, biological dynamics).

The mortality rate associated with smallpox began to go down after 1872. In some places –- for example, England – smallpox seemed to disappear, for the most part, in the first few years of the 20th century.

As the mortality rates began to decrease after 1872, the rates of inoculation also began to wane. Yet, despite a sharp drop in inoculation rates, the incidence of smallpox did not rise, and, in fact, the evidence seemed to indicate that cases of smallpox tended to rise in lockstep with the extent to which people received inoculations.

An historic manifestation of the foregoing realities took place in Leicester, England in the late 1800s. The saga begins with the fact that England implemented a series of laws in 1840, 1853, and 1867 concerning the issue of smallpox inoculation that, among other things, required all children to be inoculated by their third month of existence.

Refusal of parents to abide by the foregoing sorts of laws could result in imprisonment and/or fines. If those fines couldn't be paid, government officials came into the homes of the offenders and sold whatever furniture might be present that could cover the costs of those fines.

Notwithstanding the high rates of inoculation which were engendered by the foregoing laws, Leicester, among other places in England, was beset by a massive outbreak of smallpox in 1871 and 1872. Some 3,000 cases of smallpox occurred in Leicester, and over 350 of those individuals died during the outbreak.

The government doubled-down on the enforcement of the inoculation laws following the foregoing outbreak of smallpox. Over a twelve-year period, more than 6,000 people were caught up in the legal net which had been cast to punish those who were non-compliant with the inoculation mandates, and, as a result, more than 60 people were imprisoned, while nearly another 200 individuals were hit with fines that they could not pay, and, as a result, government compliance officers entered their homes and sold off all, or some of, the furnishings of the people who could not afford to pay the indicated fines.

The foregoing practices -- together with concrete evidence that compulsory laws of inoculation had not prevented people in Leicester from becoming ill with smallpox or from dying – led to the fermenting of a great deal of anger and resentment concerning the government's ineffective and punitive mandates. Consequently, in 1885 a massive protest (which has been estimated to involve anywhere from 20,000 to 100,000 people) took place in Leicester which denounced government policies concerning smallpox, and there were representatives from more than 60 English towns that were present on the speaker's dais.

Following the foregoing protest, there was a concerted movement that ensued over the next 60 years which ran in opposition to the inoculation laws governing smallpox. This movement was assisted by the election of a new set of officials who, unlike the previous members of local government, were in agreement with the principles of non-compliance, and within two years of the aforementioned protest demonstration, the rate of inoculation had declined by 90 percent.

Instead of inoculating people, the people of Leicester established a different set of protocols for engaging smallpox. More specifically, when smallpox occurred, the patients were quarantined immediately in a hospital while the homes of such individuals underwent a thorough process of disinfection,

The foregoing set of procedures came to be known as the "Leicester Method." When it was followed, cases of smallpox soon disappeared.

The vested interests of medicine which were pro-inoculation despite all the evidence that existed indicating how the process was neither a safe nor effective way of dealing with smallpox were very vocal in their prognostications about what was transpiring in Leicester. They boasted that the people of that city were going to rue the day when they stopped requiring people to be inoculated.

In 1893 there was an outbreak of smallpox in a number of communities in England. Mold is a city that is about 128 miles distant from Leicester and which, for the previous 18 years, had been requiring all infants to be inoculated with the smallpox protocol, whereas in Leicester, virtually all children under ten years of age had not been inoculated.

The city of Mold experienced a mortality rate that was 32 times higher than that of Leicester during the 1893 smallpox outbreak. The high rate of inoculation seemed to work against the people of Mold, whereas the low rate of inoculation appeared to benefit the people of Leicester, and, in fact, the morality rate in Leicester that was associated with the outbreaks of smallpox between 1892 and 1894 was considerably less that a number of other cities in England – such as: Middlesbrough, Birmingham and Warrington – all of whom had populations that were highly inoculated.

Compulsory inoculation in conjunction with smallpox came to an end in England by 1948. At that point, Leicester had been observing a policy of non-compliance with the inoculation laws for nearly 60 years, and, yet, despite a substantial decrease in the process of inoculation, among the residents of that city, there had been only two deaths that might be linked to smallpox over the previous four decades.

Generally speaking, many other localities in which the rate of smallpox inoculation sharply plummeted also experienced similar results. In other words, when the rate of mortalities which occurred in childhood decreased one could also see that rates of smallpox inoculations decreased simultaneously.

Mortality rates were not dropping because of a high inoculation rate. Rather, death rates were dropping at the same time as inoculations were also substantially in decline.

High inoculation rates were not correlated with falling rates of mortality. Higher mortality rates associated with smallpox tended to be correlated with higher rates of smallpox inoculations, and, therefore, the myth that smallpox was eradicated through programs of inoculation just doesn't stand up to the evidence of history.

Supposedly – at least according to the theory-laden hindsight of some virologists -- smallpox was, and is, due to the presence of a virus. However, if, as substantial evidence indicates (some of which has been presented in the present book), that viruses do not exist, then, the issue of herd immunity becomes a rather awkward topic for conversation in conjunction with smallpox because no one has actually been able to isolate and purify the alleged smallpox virus and, as well, proceeded to demonstrate that such a virus not only causes the smallpox illness but can be lethal, as well demonstrate why some people who have not been inoculated, never become ill with the disease.

Furthermore, given that proteins have never actually been discovered that not only can be shown to have the shape and structure accorded to them by the theory of antibodies, but, as well, such proteins have never been proven to have a clearly delineated immunological function, and given that the alleged presence of such antibodies is considered by many medical doctors and vaccine manufacturers to be the sine qua non of whether a given vaccine has "taken" and, therefore, is able, allegedly, to offer protection against a given disease, then, one has difficulty understanding how one can talk about herd immunity in such a context of claims that lack empirical credibility when it comes to the issue of causality.

In addition, if the existential status of an immune system can be subjected to a range of questions that do not seem to have been adequately addressed because most, if not all, of the components (e. g., macrophages, neutrophils, dendritic cells, lymph system, complement system, cytokine molecules, T-cells, and B-cells,) associated with such a theoretical system can be understood as serving other kinds of ameliorative, but not necessarily immunological, functions, then, one can't really claim that vaccines boost an immune system which might not exist -- especially given that one of the most fundamental points of contact that vaccines allegedly have with the biological terrain has to do with the alleged stimulation of antibody production, and, as indicated previously, the latter entities have not been shown, in any independent and direct manner, to actually exist apart from the surrogate markers that are used to claim – based on assumptions that cannot be vindicated precisely because the existence of antibodies remains questionable -- that antibodies of a certain titer are present in a given sample.

If antibodies in the foregoing sense do not exist, then, the Rube Goldberg mechanism known as a vaccine (whose primary claim to efficacy has to do with increases in the levels of certain molecules said to be antibodies) serves no constructive purpose. Or, stated in another way, given that antibodies and an immune system in any traditional sense have a questionable existential status, then, one has difficulty understanding how vaccines have any function other than to introduce a litany of poisons into a person's biological terrain which either individually, or in concert with one another, have the capacity not to protect a person but to undermine the well-being, or detoxified stability, of that person's biological terrain.

If the nature of the biological terrain is geared not toward the sort of immunological functioning that involves an array of automatic dynamics (involving the alleged adaptive learning capacity of antibodies which might not exist and which, supposedly, protect an individual against all future encounters with certain kinds of pathogens – such as, possibly, viruses that might not exist), but, instead, one were to argue that the biological terrain is geared toward maintaining, or struggling to re-establish, a detoxified form of stability in which the biological terrain remains in symbiotic relationship with the microbiome that occupies such terrain (something that only can be accomplished on a case by case basis in conjunction with events -- such as environmental poisoning or internal, biological dysfunctions of some kind-- that destabilize the biological terrain), and that members of the microbiome which occupy a person's terrain can only assume a problematic status if they are induced to transition to a non-symbiotic stage of their pleiomorphic/pleomorphic life cycle as a result of prior events that have destabilized an individual's biological terrain and, thereby, rendered the terrain vulnerable to various kinds of disease processes, then, the notion of herd immunity seems to have no meaningful place in the latter way of engaging human illnesses.

Although individuals might not be susceptible to viral diseases that do not seem to exist, human beings can be susceptible to the disease process that are being attributed to the presence of a virus but actually appear to be due to some other set of idiopathic or unknown pathological factors.

However, if the foregoing claims are true, then, attempting to proactively protect people by injecting them with materials that cannot possibly protect against a non-existent virus would seem to be a rather dubious enterprise. Presumably, it makes no sense to use anti-viral injections or medications to treat conditions that are not caused by viruses, and, therefore, one must set about trying to discover what the actual cause of the diseases are that are said, without real proof, to be viral in nature, and until one establishes actual causality, talk of herd immunity begins at no beginning and works toward no reliable end.

Moreover, while one can be susceptible to the toxins that are released by bacteria in diseases such as diphtheria and tetanus, these diseases (despite all the fear porn) are so rare, that they might be better handled when people actually have the disease or when the conditions through which one might have been exposed to the requisite bacteria (such as having a puncture wound where animals have been evacuating their bowels) suggest that receipt of an anti-toxin might be -- but, then again, might not be – prudent – depending on what the actual nature of the risk versus reward calculus might be in any given situation. Notwithstanding the foregoing sorts of considerations, one might contemplate the possibility that processes (i.e., vaccines) which pump all manner of toxicity into a person's body would seem to accomplish little more than to be contributing to the body's existing toxicity load – a load which, given the right conditions, might have the capacity to destabilize the biological terrain and lead to other kinds of disease processes as normally symbiotic microorganisms are, sometimes, induced to transition into non-symbiotic stages – and, therefore, potentially, more problematic expressions -- of their pleiomorphic/pleomorphic life cycles.

In addition, until one knows why some people become ill when exposed to certain kinds of bacteria while others do not become ill, then one has no baseline against which to measure what is needed to identify some sort of rigorous and verifiable notion of herd immunity. Indeed, to talk about the notion of herd immunity would appear to become meaningless with respect to illnesses such as tetanus which do not seem to be contagious. If contagion of some kind does not enter into the equation (and what the process of contagion might involve will be discussed in a later chapter), then, whether, or not, other people might be protected, in some way, against tetanus will have absolutely no bearing on whether another person who is not protected will ever encounter, let alone, succumb to the toxins that might, or might not, be released by such a pathogen under the right set of circumstances.

A hundred years ago, in 1923, a group of researchers from the University of Manchester began to explore the notion of herd immunity while studying issues of immunology in conjunction with mice. Based on certain epidemiological ideas which had been advanced through the Rockefeller Institute in America, the foregoing University of Manchester researchers were inclined to believe that scientists could study a process of immunity which might exist in a group or herd of animals independently of the notion of immunity in any given individual.

Epidemiology – which formed the creative spark for the ensuring perspective of the researchers at the University of Manchester, cannot tell a person what causes a disease. All that such a methodology can do is try to identify where a given phenomenon might have begun, or how quickly or slowly the phenomenon seems to have or be spreading, or how long it lasts or might last, or when it might reach its zenith, as well as when and where it might go into or have gone into decline.

Different diseases often give expression to characteristic epidemiological profiles. For instance, diseases that are due to some kind of environmental toxicity often exhibit certain kinds of clustering patterns that can demarcate the area of toxicity, whereas, so-called contagious diseases tend, supposedly, to give expression to different kinds of dynamic patterns, but while the manner in which a given disease spreads might indicate that some sort of process of contagion (via direct contact, air-borne transmission, bodily fluids such as blood, or some other modality) is present, the precise venue of such contagion cannot always be determined ... although some possibilities for transmission might be eliminated.

If a disease such as smallpox spreads, one could have a theory that the vector for the spread of the disease at issue might involve a virus of some kind. Nonetheless, if one cannot prove the existence of such a virus, then, what is actually generating the spread of the disease is idiopathic in nature or unknown, and, conceivably, some form of environmental poisoning could be taking place. If the foregoing possibility turns out to be true, then what one might have believed to be a matter of contagion could actually have been due to the properties of some unknown form of poisoning to which various people appear to be vulnerable while other individuals do not necessarily seem to be susceptible. As such, the poison seems to spread like a contagious diseases does, but, in reality, what one is observing is a clustering phenomenon and not a contagion phenomenon.

While the researchers at the University of Manchester believed that it is possible to separate and study issues of alleged immunity in a group or herd independently of alleged immunity phenomena in individual human beings, nevertheless, until one actually understands the nature of a given disease process which one is studying, then, one has no idea if one is dealing with a problem of environmental toxicity or a problem of contagion of some kind. More specifically, given that smallpox, herpes simplex, mumps, measles, chicken pox/shingles, polio, influenza, SARS, MERS, and a host of other diseases are considered to be caused by the presence of certain kinds of viruses, and given that the existence of such viruses have not, yet, been proven to exist, then one has no basis for saying that such diseases have something to do with immunological dynamics rather than environmental poisoning of some kind, and, therefore, it is presumptuous to talk about issues of either group immunity or individual immunity.

Surviving some sort of environmental toxicity – say, a gas leak -- on one occasion provides no immunity against having to deal anew with similar gas leaks in the future. Similarly, there is no guarantee that if it turns out that so-called viral diseases are not actually viral diseases because viruses don't exist, then, surviving one of the aforementioned idiopathic non-viral diseases on one occasion does not necessarily mean that one will be required to deal with the problems associated with surviving such a disease all over again should such a disease process manifest itself in the future.

Even if one should never experience such a disease process again after having it once, this does not necessarily demonstrate that one is demonstrating some form of natural immunity concerning such a disease process. Instead, the foregoing situation could merely indicate that the circumstances which led to the de-stabilization of one's biological terrain previously (and induced certain kinds of symptoms associated with a given disease to be expressed) never re-occurred, or if those circumstances did re-occur, the condition of one's biological terrain might have been sufficiently different to not render one susceptible to whatever caused such symptoms to occur originally – and such 'sufficient differences' might have nothing to do with the alleged dynamics of immunity.

Could there be cognitive and/or non-viral physical forces at play in diseases like chicken pox, mumps, and measles? For instance, if one were to have a gathering of young people with the intend of inducing them to become ill with a given disease in the hope that that such an illness will never manifest itself again in the lives of those who become ill with the indicated disease process (and such gatherings were often held), can one be sure that the children who became ill contracted a contagious virus of some kind? Is it possible that the children who attended the party had been exposed to a certain set of cognitive and physical frequencies (communicated in some way by both parents as well as the other children at the party) that helped de-stabilize their respective biological terrains in a manner which rendered them susceptible to the emergence of certain kinds of symptoms and an accompanying disease process (This possibility will be explored in a little more depth in a later chapter involving the issue of resonance)?

An article appeared in a 2011 edition of a journal entitled *Clinical and Infectious Diseases* in which three scientists from the London School of Hygiene and Tropical Diseases claimed that although the notion of herd immunity has been in existence for quite some time, nonetheless, the issue of herd immunity didn't really start to become well-established until various pharmaceutical companies, immunologists, and medical doctors began to try to tie decreases in the incidence of certain allegedly contagious diseases to the increased use of vaccines while implementing different vaccine campaigns which were supposed to bring about the complete eradication of this or that pathogen-caused disease. However, if, for instance, the diseases that are attributed to viruses are not caused by viruses – since they have not, yet, been proven to exist – and, therefore, we don't actually know what is causing those diseases, then, such pharmaceutical companies, immunologists, and medical doctors would appear to be pushing a false, if not delusional, narrative which holds that vaccines based on viral theories will be capable of eradicating those sorts of diseases.

If viruses do not exist, then, there can be no herd immunity in relation to such non-existent entities. Moreover, with respect to the conditions to which illnesses such as tetanus, cholera, botulism, and so on, give expression, there also can be no such thing as herd immunity because those illnesses are a function of the presence of toxins that are released by different kinds of bacteria in conjunction with circumstances that are have to do with the nature of the relationship between an individual and the bacteria that has the capacity to release those sorts of toxic molecules.

Herd immunity cannot be established with a nail that is present in environmental conditions that are conducive to the emergence of tetanus. Everyone who steps on that nail runs the risk of being poisoned, and what other people have done to protect themselves has absolutely no bearing on what will happen to any individual who steps on the same nail.

Similarly, herd immunity cannot be established in relation to an improperly canned food within which botulism toxins have arisen. Everyone who eats the food from the problematic can will run the risk of being poisoned irrespective of what other people do to protect themselves, and, thus, the only form of protection is to not eat the contents of such a can.

Herd immunity cannot be established with a polluted water source that gives rise to conditions that are conducive to the onset of cholera. The best protection is not to drink the contaminated water, and even if other people have been given some sort of treatment to counter the effects of such contaminated water, anyone who drinks such water runs the risk of becoming ill.

As is the case with all toxin-laden and poison-laden dynamics, safety depends on being able to avoid the circumstances that are likely to give rise to such circumstances of toxicity or poisoning. Providing materials that are capable of countering a given toxin or poison does nothing to generate herd immunity against the source of those poisons and toxins, and as long as the source of such poisoning and toxicity remains active, people will continue to be vulnerable to the pathologies that might arise via those source vectors irrespective of what the majority of people might do to protect themselves.

There are other kinds of bacterial illnesses – such as pneumonia or meningitis – that might be a function of the condition of someone's biological terrain. In other words, individuals with destabilized terrains might become vulnerable to certain kinds of bacteria that are transitioning away from an inactive or symbiotic stage of their pleiomorphic/pleomorphic life cycle and, in the process of doing so, give rise to some sort of illness, but there can be no sort of herd immunity protection for individuals whose biological terrains have become compromised and, as a result, becomes ill in one way or another.

Measles, mumps, and a variety of other diseases have all been shown to have gone into decline prior to the time when vaccines came into existence. In addition, smallpox seemed to begin to go into decline following periods in which smallpox inoculations also began to go into decline.

While the use of vaccines might be correlated with further declines in the incidence of the foregoing diseases in a manner that is somewhat – but often only marginally so -- above and beyond the declines in incidence and mortality with respect to certain diseases that occurred independently of the presence of vaccines, how does one know that the sort of further declines which are being alluded to were due to the use of vaccines rather than due to any number of other public health factors (such as: More ready access to nutritious foods, cleaner drinking water, better sewage systems, improved systems of garbage collection and disposal, more stringent laws concerning the dumping of toxic wastes into the environment, more effective means of reducing different kinds of environmental pollutants, enhanced standards in personal hygiene, expanded forms of suburban living as opposed to urban living that distanced one from manufacturing processes, decreased use -- at least for a time -- of toxic vaccines and pharmaceuticals). How does one prove that whatever statistical correlations might exist between certain kinds of decline in the incidence of certain diseases and the use of vaccines reflects the causal impact of the latter practices upon the incidence of certain diseases rather than reflects the causal character – taken individually or considered collectively – of the many other environmental factors that also can be correlated with such declines? To identify vaccines as the cause of such declines seems entirely arbitrary.

\

Chapter 13: Epigenetics, An Adaptive Learning System

In 1974, the Sloan-Kettering Institute, as well as the medical/scientific world, was rocked by a major scandal that took place within that organization. Some people might say that the scandal was precipitated by the unethical activities – masquerading as science – of a person by the name of William Summerlin who not only had been appointed to oversee a clinical department at the hospital (Memorial) which is associated with the Institute, but as well, had been made a full member of the Sloan-Kettering Institute.

Full membership at the Institute was, and is, something that is difficult to achieve and usually involves a long period of apprenticeship of sorts before it can be realized. However, Summerlin seemed to be something of a 35-year old wunderkind and, somehow, had acquired his lofty status fairly quickly.

Earlier, an indication was given that some people might wish to claim that Summerlin was solely responsible for the scandal that occurred in 1974, but this is only true to a certain extent. The reason for putting forth such a qualifier is that what Summerlin did was done while being supervised – allegedly -- by a senior member of Sloan-Kettering, namely, Dr. Robert Good who had been brought in the year before from the University of Minnesota to serve as head of the Sloan-Kettering Institute.

Summerlin had been able to ascend through the ranks of the Institute as a result of various innovations that he had introduced to the methodology of tissue culturing. His work had potentially fundamental implications for the entire field of transplantation which involved taking some biological component (tissues, organs, etc.) from one person and transferring that component to another person without the latter individual rejecting what was being transferred.

The standard way of describing the foregoing process is that Summerlin seemed to have discovered a way to assist a transplant recipient to avoid the so-called immune response in which the body of the person who is receiving, say, new skin tissue from another human being tends to treat the new tissue as non-self and, therefore, would initiate processes that were intended to reject that tissue as foreign or other. On the other hand, one also could understand such a rejection phenomenon as being part of a detoxification process that was not necessarily immunological in character but, instead, might give expression to the manner in which the body of a transplant recipient was attempting to re-establish some sort of detoxified stability amidst the set of biological traumatic events entailed by the foregoing sorts of procedures that had de-stabilized the biological terrain of the recipient. As a result, various symbiotic relationships which the individual's biological terrain had with different facets of the microbiome occupying that terrain have been altered or destabilized, in one way or another, and, in the process, various elements of the person's microbiome have been induced to enter into stages of their pleiomorphic/pleomorphic life cycle that are no longer symbiotic with the surrounding biological terrain and which, as a result, are capable of leading to a multiplicity of inflammation processes that need to be resolved.

The foregoing dynamics of inflammation are not necessarily signs of an immune response of rejection between self and non-self. Rather, perhaps, the network of inflammation processers that are occurring in connection with a given instance of transplantation constitute signs that different parts of a person's microbiome have become non-symbiotic as a result of being induced to transition out of a normal state of symbiosis with the surrounding biological terrain and, consequently, different non-symbiotic stages of the pleiomorphic/pleiomorphic life cycle of such endogenous microorganisms have begun to create detoxification issues that an individual's body might not be able to properly address on its own or might not be able to resolve even with clinical intervention of some kind.

Summerlin had begun his research on tissue culturing techniques in 1970 while at Stanford when he was a teaching fellow. He claimed to have developed a special solution of some sort which -- following the immersion of the tissue that is to be transplanted within Summerlin's allegedly innovative medium for a period of between 4 and 6 weeks – supposedly would enable tissue taken from one body to be transplanted to another without any rejection phenomenon ensuing.

He used mice to demonstrate the alleged effectiveness of his culturing technique. More specifically, he took mice that were genetically unrelated to one another and obtained skin tissue from black mice and transplanted that tissue to white mice which would, continue to be white with the exception of the black skin tissue that had been transferred from the black mice to the white mice, and all of this would occur without any rejection phenomenon arising.

If the alleged principles inherent in Summerlin's tissue culturing technique could be applied to organ transplants, then, among other things, doctors would be able to avoid giving all of the anti-rejection drugs that tend to be administered to transplant recipients. Such drugs have a potential, all on their own, for generating medical problems in the transplant recipients (such as an increased likelihood of cancer as well as leaving the biological terrains of the recipients vulnerable to other kinds of destabilizing pathologies).

Dr. Good, the new head of Sloan-Kettering, took on the responsibility of supervising and supporting Summerlin's research. They wrote papers together on the topic of the tissue culturing technique which supposedly had been developed by Summerlin. However, beginning in 1973, Good was receiving communications from researchers outside the Institute who indicated that they were having difficulty replicating the results which had been published by Summerlin and Good.

Summerlin was asked by Dr. Good to reproduce the aforementioned results by means of another demonstration involving white and black mice. Subsequently, Summerlin brought forth the requested donor and recipient research subjects (i.e., black and white mice) to confirm what he, supposedly, had demonstrated previously.

He showed the foregoing results to Dr. Good. Unfortunately, Dr. Good failed to exercise any sort of due diligence with respect to what he was being shown.

Shortly thereafter, when a technician who handles the experimental animals was in the process of returning the mice to their cages, he noticed something peculiar concerning the white mouse. In order to more closely examine the anomaly he was sensing, the technician took a cotton ball which had been dipped in alcohol and proceeded to wipe the black area of the transplant recipient with the cotton swab, and, lo and behold, the black area began to disappear because it had been created with ink rather than with skin tissue that had been miraculously transformed by means of Summerlin's special medium.

As many institutions are inclined to do, when word of the foregoing scientific fraud was revealed to the people in charge of the Sloan-Kettering Institute (including Dr. Good), the latter individuals did not immediately denounce the research as fraudulent, unethical, and unacceptable, but, instead, they sought to cover it up. The fraud was only made known to the public when approximately three weeks later, Barbara *Yuncker*, a reporter for the *New York Post*, received a tip from a whistleblower that such an incident had taken place at the Institute.

Once the fraud became public knowledge, Dr. Good assembled a committee of five individuals who had been working at Sloan-Kettering for quite some time and tasked them with writing a report on Summerlin's research. When that report finally was issued, Summerlin was identified as being solely responsible for the fraud, and although Dr. Good was chastised for his hasty promotion of Summerlin, Dr. Good was cleared of any wrong doing in the actual fraud.

While, technically, it might have been true that Dr. Good did not actively and knowingly participate in such a fraud, that sort of scientific fraud was only able to be perpetrated because Dr. Good had failed to exercise any kind of rigorous oversight with respect to Summerlin's "research." When Dr. Good began to receive communiqués from other researchers that they could not replicate Summerlin's results, he did not exercise due diligence and conduct his own investigation of the matter, and, moreover, even when shown the living participants (i.e., the mice) that were being used to serve as confirmation that the original experiments were capable of being replicated, Dr. Good failed to detect what a technician, using only observation and some alcohol, was able to uncover.

Summerlin's time at Sloan-Kettering was terminated, but he received a severance package that amounted to one year's salary. He was described as being mentally unbalanced by members of the Institute, and, yet, he was able to practice as a dermatologist for 35 years without any apparent signs manifesting themselves in relation to the mentally unstable behavior with which he had been labeled by various individuals at the Sloan-Kettering Institute.

The foregoing saga has been narrated for a variety of reasons. One of those reasons has to do with research that was discussed somewhat during chapter five of the present book when the work of Gaston Naessens was being explored.

More specifically, Naessens, apparently, had been able to actually accomplish what Summerlin only fraudulently had led other people to believe had been accomplished. However, Naessens worked with rabbits rather mice.

Like Summerlin, Naessens was interested in whether one could conduct a skin graft without encountering the phenomenon of rejection. In contrast with Summerlin's research, Naessens wanted to see if he could induce a patch of fur and skin from a white-furred rabbit to take root, so to speak, in a genetically unrelated black-furred rabbit.

Naessens was not just engaging in the foregoing research arbitrarily. There was a certain theoretical understanding which led to his experiments.

As outlined in chapter five of the present book, Naessens believed that somatids, not cells, were the basic units of life and that, in fact, he was of the opinion that while life was not possible without the presence of somatids, nonetheless, those entities, like Béchamp's microzymas and Enderlein's endobionts, had the capacity to exist independently of living organisms. Naessens stipulated that somatids were viral-like in size and, therefore, were measured in nanometers that were toward the lower end of the scale.

Naessens also was of the opinion that somatids were pleiomorphic/pleomorphic in character, and, therefore, under the appropriate circumstances, he claimed that they could transmogrify functionally as well as structurally and also indicated that his claims in this respect could be verified if one were to examine somatids with his Somatoscope which was capable of capturing the nano-dynamics of those entities. In addition, while acknowledging that further research was needed, he maintained that the species of somatids varied with the nature of the tissues and organs one might be examining and, consequently, that not only did different kinds or species of somatids uniquely regulate what was transpiring in given organs or tissues, those different species of somatids could be found throughout the extensive networks entailed by the circulatory systems of both blood lymph.

Finally, he felt that genetic activity of some kind went on within the different species of somatids. However, because somatids seem to be virtually indestructible (e.g., they have been exposed to acids, 50,000 rems of nuclear radiation, temperatures as high as 200 degrees Centigrade, and diamond-tipped drills without any of this seeming to affect, or be able to penetrate, their physical structure), discovering what, precisely is taking place within somatids tends to be shrouded in mystery.

Nonetheless, on the basis of his experiments with rabbits, he believed that somatids were capable of some sort of genomic activity. In other words, when Naessens isolated and purified the somatids which were present in the skin tissue out of which fur grew, and, then, he transferred those somatids (at the rate of one cubic centimeter per day for two successive weeks into the bloodstream of the transplant recipient), he found that when skin from a white-furred rabbit subsequently was transplanted to the area of a black-furred rabbit from which black fur had been removed and to which the appropriate sort of skin somatids had been transferred earlier, then a white patch of fur grew in the area from which black-fur had been removed and did so without any kind of rejection phenomenon taking place.

Apparently, the transplanted skin from the white-furred donor rabbit was able to survive without rejection because of the presence of the somatids from the skin of the white-furred donor rabbits that previously had been transferred to the black-furred rabbit. Thus, on the basis of the results of the foregoing experiments, Naessens was led to entertain the possibility that somatids seemed to have a genetic role to play which involved some kind of capacity to organize what transpired in the skin of the transplant recipient.

Previously, I have put forth some considerations indicating that there is no immune system, per se, but, instead, the body has an array of different ways through which it defends itself against various kinds of destabilizations of the biological terrain and the latter's normally symbiotic relationship with the microbiome that occupies that terrain through a network of various kinds of cells (e.g., macrophages, neutrophils, dendritic cells, T-cells and B-cells), and molecules (e.g., cytokines, 30-plus members of the complement system) that do not have immunological functions so much as they have detoxification functions. The foregoing perspective was buttressed by an overview concerning the notion of antibodies and some relevant evidence indicating that antibodies might not actually exist, or if they do exist, they do not necessarily have immunological functions.

The theory of antibodies is what, supposedly, provides the body with a system of adaptive learning which allows the biological terrain to match up an indefinite number of possible antigen receptor shapes with the structural properties of this or that antibody. Aside from raising questions in passing -- such as what is the precise nature of the dynamics that enable a particular antibody structure to be identified from among an indefinitely large number of such antibodies so that an appropriate match can be made with a given antigen structure (and how long would this take?) -- one might wish to argue that while there is an adaptive learning system within the biological terrain that enables that terrain to improve -- within certain limits -- the speed and efficiency through which detoxification takes place as well as to find ways to deal with an environment that is often changing, nonetheless, the nature of this adaptive learning system is not immunological in character but is epigenetic in character.

Furthermore, one might advance a hypothesis at this point which suggests that what organizes and regulates the aforementioned epigenetic set of dynamics resides in the different species of somatids which reside in various kinds of tissues and organs and that are constantly circulating throughout the blood and lymph systems. While I don't intend to prove such a hypothesis during the course of the present chapter, I do wish to put forth a variety of considerations that might help to place such a hypothesis in a context that could lend credence to it.

Although Susumu Ohno popularized the notion of "junk DNA" in 1972, the term actually had been kicking around since, at least, the 1960s. However, the phrase did not actually come into wide-spread use until the Human Genome Project indicated that only a relatively small portion of the DNA (2%) that was present in the genome seemed to code for identifiable proteins and, at the time, no one seemed to understand why the other 98% of the DNA was present.

I first came into contact with the idea of "junk DNA" during the 1980's when I was involved in exploring a variety of sciences that might have some sort of applicability to my dissertation topic. Moreover, without trying to claim, at the time, that I had any understanding of what junk DNA actually entailed, I intuitively felt that it had some sort of organizational role to play in various organisms, and, therefore, was not really junk or non-functional in nature.

Unfortunately, all too many individuals were using that term because they were projecting their ignorance on to something that as far as they could see (which turned out not to be very far) didn't appear to serve any known function. Furthermore, in the process of using that sort of ignorance to frame part of their existential world, and rather than actually scientifically studying the phenomenon, many of those "scientists" just proceeded to prematurely generate a number of theories (usually of an evolutionary nature) about why junk DNA might be present in the genome.

Inexplicably, there were life forms (e.g., worms) that were much simpler than human beings which actually had roughly the same number of coding genes as humans did. In addition, there was even a considerable overlap in the kinds of genes that showed up in the two species that were quite similar to one another despite the considerable morphological and functional differences that differentiated or separated those two life forms.

If two such different species had roughly the same number of genes and seemed to hold many genes in common, then, how could one explain the obvious structural and functional differences between them? An early clue that might help scientists address the foregoing question actually had to do with the so-called "junk DNA."

More specifically, researchers discovered that the complexity of an organism often ran in parallel with the amount of non-coding or junk DNA which was present. In other words, organisms that were categorized as being more complex, in some sense, tended to have a greater amount of junk DNA than organisms that were considered to be less complex in some sense.

Over a period of time, there were a number of different functions which were discovered that appeared to be regulated by so-called junk DNA. For example some of that DNA seemed to have what might be termed a structural support role which helped DNA to not unravel, while other sections of the mysterious DNA appeared to help to structurally anchor chromosomes during the process of cell division.

Notwithstanding the foregoing sorts of structural roles, researchers also began to discover that a considerable amount of the DNA that had been written off as not having any function actually coded for RNA, and such RNA turned out to give expression to an array of different functions, including the transporting of materials that are needed to be able to generate proteins (transfer-RNA) as well as part of the dynamic platforms (ribosomes) where amino acids are strung together to make proteins.

More recently, scientists have found that so-called non-functional DNA – i.e., junk DNA – also can serve different kinds of regulatory functions. In other words, this sort of DNA has the capacity to, among other things, turn genes on and off, and, in fact, various kinds of diseases tend to arise when regulatory responsibilities are rendered dysfunctional through the occurrence of one or another kind of mutation such that genes are turned on or off in problematic ways.

For example, there is genetic disorder known as myotonic dystrophy which entails a form of atrophying or wasting away that takes place across three generations within a family. Usually, a grandparent might have cataracts, and one, or more, of the children of that grandparent might experience regular bouts of muscle stiffness as well as cardiac problems, while one, or more, of the grandchildren that are affected by the disorder tend to exhibit various kinds of learning disabilities and muscle floppiness.

Both males and females run a risk of incurring such a genetic disorder from an affected parent. Although only one of the two copies of the relevant gene that is passed on might be problematic, nonetheless, the disorder is said to be dominant because the gene that is associated with the mutation is able to nullify or prevent the normal gene from being expressed.

Usually speaking, dominant disorders tend to be fairly stable with respect to whatever dysfunctional property is being passed on to a child. Thus, if the affected parent has problem 'x,' then the affected child will have the same problem 'x.'

This is not the case in myotonic dystrophy. As one goes from grandparent to child to grandchild, the disease becomes progressively worse and is manifested earlier in each generation -- from cataracts, to muscle stiffness and cardiac problems, to learning disabilities and floppy muscles. However, the severest form of the disorder that occurs in affected grandchildren tends to be passed on by the mother of those children.

Affected individuals are found to have multiple copies of a sequence of three DNA molecules – namely, cytosine, thymine, and guanine. Multiple copies (ranging from 5 to 30) of this sequence are also found in individuals without the disorder, but the number of copies of the foregoing DNA sequence occur more than 35 times in affected individuals, and under certain circumstances when the sequence repeats 50 times or more, then a parent – who normally passes on the same number of sequence repeats to a child as the parent has – might pass on a set of sequences which are greater than the number of such sequences that are present in the parent.

What is anomalous about myotonic dystrophy is that the gene which is involved in the disorder has not mutated. What has mutated is the number of the DNA sequences (C, G, and T) of "junk DNA" which are associated with that gene.

Myotonic dystrophy is not the only kind of genetic disorder in which a given gene associated with the disorder is left intact (i.e., is passed on without any mutation). Instead, what changes in these different kinds of genetic disorder (e.g., Fragile X syndrome, which gives expression to learning disabilities) are the character of the sequences of so-called junk DNA that are associated with the non-mutated gene (cytosine, cytosine, and guanine in the case of Fragile X syndrome) and/or the number of multiple copies of that seemingly superfluous DNA that are associated with the gene that has not undergone any sort of change in the sequence of amino acids that give expression to the protein for which the latter gene codes.

Another genetic disorder – known as FSHD ("facioscapulohumeral muscular dystrophy" if you wish to either punish yourself or impress/annoy people on the subway) -- entails a wasting away of muscles that help operate one's upper body and face. However, what differentiates this particular disorder from the two previous maladies which were touched upon earlier is that while people who do not have this disorder exhibit multiple sequences (between 11 and 100) of a block of DNA which consists of more than 3,000 letters (A, C, T, G), those who suffer from the disorder tend to have ten or fewer blocks of the foregoing set of 3,000 genetic letters.

More than ten years of research were required to put the foregoing information together. One of the primary reasons why such a lengthy period of research was needed to accomplish that task is because the blocks or sets of repeats of the 3,000 DNA sequence do not occur anywhere near the gene that it affects.

Somewhere around 40% of the human genome consists of what are known as "interspersed repetitive elements.' There are believed to be four primary classes of those sorts of repetitive elements – namely, (1) LINEs (long interspersed elements); (2) DNA transposons; (3) SINEs (short interspersed elements; and (4) LTRs (elements with long terminal repeats0.

Some individuals have advanced various kinds of evolutionary hypothesis to account for why they believe the foregoing classes of repeating sequences exist. However, what the actual function, if any, of the aforementioned classes of repeating sequences might be seems to remain something of a mystery.

Furthermore, not all repeating sequences necessarily involve large sets of genetic letters like the foregoing genetic disorder known as FSHD. There are many repetitive sequences which consist of only a couple of genetic letters that tend to be quite characteristic of a given individual's genetic material, and, therefore, vary from person to person in ways that enable one to differentiate whether such a pattern of sequences comes from one person rather than another.

The foregoing property functions like a genetic fingerprint. That property can be used to establish paternity, rule out someone as having committed certain crimes, or help facilitate various kinds of research projects which are seeking to understand how different parts of the genome might operate.

Enough has been said over the last several pages to begin to ask some questions. For instance, one might ask about how the foregoing sorts of short sequences come to be so uniquely tied to individuals.

Alternatively, in the case of FSHD, someone might be interested in discovering why most people who possess anywhere between 11 and 100 blocks of a set of 3,000 letters do not seem to have any dysfunctional features associated with such an arrangement, whereas individuals who have ten or fewer of those blocks incur a disease? After all, other than the number one, what is the difference between having 11 such blocks versus having 10 such blocks?

One might also be interested in learning how the foregoing sorts of lengthy blocks -- which appear to be quite distant from the gene they influence -- communicate with, or alter the functioning of, their target genes? Are there any functional differences in allegedly "normal people who possess, say, 11 or 15 of the aforementioned set of 3,000 genetic letters, and those individuals who have 90 or 95 of those sets, and, in addition, what determines how many of those sets of 3,000 letters will be produced?

Given that most mutations consist of just a single letter difference in the DNA code, what sort of change is necessary to prevent a human being from developing eleven or more blocks of the 3,000 genetic letters? What determines how many of those blocks are produced, and what, exactly, are those sets of 3,000 letters communicating?

Similar sorts of questions could be raised in conjunction with the repeat of certain sequences of "junk" genetic material in relation to myotonic dystrophy (5 to 30 copies in "normal" human beings versus 35 or more such repeated sequences in genetically affected individuals). Why does the genetic disorder seem to become worse as it goes from grandparent to grandchild, and why do different systems appear to be affected as the disease progresses in severity across generations? What is the difference between someone with 30-34 copies of the repeated sequence and someone with 35, or more, such copies? What is the nature of the mutation which leads to such differences in functionality? When the norm is for parents to pass on to their children the same set of repeated sequences as they themselves have, why does this change in the more severe cases, and why are such departures from the "norm" usually passed on only by the mother?

All of the foregoing sorts of questions could be summarized by asking just one question. What is the source (sources) that regulates or (regulate) the foregoing events?

This is a question that will continue to be asked throughout the following discussion. Something appears to have regulatory oversight concerning so-called "junk DNA" which is not only independent of the 20,000, or so genes that normally are thought of as constituting the genome of a human being, but, in addition, that sort of regulatory functionality seems to be directing "junk" genetic material to regulate – at least to a degree -- what does or does not transpire in relation to the 20,000 genes that were uncovered during the Human Genome Project.

One could, of course, argue that the 98% of the genetic material that is found in human beings and which does not code for the 20,000, or so, genes that comprise the basic human genome is somehow self-regulating and, therefore, there is no need to posit the existence of some sort of regulatory system that oversees what is transpiring in the allegedly "junk" sector of genetic material. However, there seems to be quite a lot of evidence (some of which will be covered in the present as well as subsequent chapters of the present book) to suggest that the 98% portion of genetic material that, previously, was considered to be non-functional -- and, therefore, something of a genetic junk yard – actually might be receiving its marching orders (concerning when, for example, to turn certain genes on or off) from something other than the aforementioned 98% of genetic material ... such as Naessens somatids, or Enderlein's endobionts, or Béchamp's microzymas.

Initially, the DNA which exists in the nucleus of a eukaryotic cell is transcribed via a process that translates DNA into a form of RNA known as mRNA. The latter leaves the nucleus and makes the journey to ribosomes where the genetic message inherent in mRNA gets converted, with the help of tRNA -- or transfer RNA -- into amino acids at ribosome factories in the cytoplasm.

The genome of a human being consists of two sets of 3 billion base pairs. A base pair consists of either cytosine connected to guanine (both of which constitute nucleic acids), or thymine connected to adenine (both of which are nucleic acids).

One of the foregoing sets of 3 billion base pairs is from the mother, while another set is from the father. If one were to straighten out either set of the foregoing string of base pairs as well as take into consideration that any given base pair is separated from the base pairs on either side by a distance of 25 centimeters, then, the length of each set of base pairs would extend to more than 46 million miles.

The nucleus is the largest organelle in a cell. It takes up about 10% of a cell's volume and has a diameter of about 6 microns or micrometers. Yet, it contains 2 times 46 million miles worth of information.

While the size of any given instance of mRNA varies with the nature of the message that has been transcribed, nonetheless, such molecules are relatively miniscule compared to the aforementioned sets of 3 billion base pairs. When reflecting on the foregoing information, I've often wondered what induces mRNA to leave, rather than stay, in the nucleus.

Moreover, one wonders how the mRNA "knows" where to go. The size of the nucleus is much larger than any of the messenger molecules (which run about 50 nanometers but become somewhat larger when certain modifications are made), and the size of the cytoplasm into which mRNA molecules venture is larger still since the cytoplasm contains 90% of the cell's overall volume, and, consequently, finding ribosomes – which vary in size, depending on the organism, but generally run between 20 and 30 nanometers – is, seemingly, not necessarily all that easy.

Given the foregoing considerations, one can't help but ask how a given instance of mRNA "finds" its way to a given ribosome. Moreover, one – at least this is true for the one represented by me -- has a hard time believing that all of the foregoing dynamics is just a matter of a random series of events involving processes of trial and error that, somehow – eventually – gives expression to an organism that can quickly adjust to both changing environmental conditions as well as the variable biological needs that those sorts of changing conditions engender.

Perhaps, there is some sort of guidance system which regulates what mRNA molecules do and how they get to where they need to go in order to be able to deliver their message. The basic genome of 20,000 genes codes only for proteins, and those genes are turned on and off by different facets of the remaining 98% of the genetic material (previously known as junk DNA) that constitutes the full genome, and the activity of that 98% of the genome seems to be induced into action by something other than itself. Just as the basic genome of 20,000 proteins doesn't turn itself on and off, so too, the remaining 98% of the genetic material doesn't necessarily activate itself but might be activated by something other the remaining 98% of the genetic material.

There also seems to be various evidential indications which allude to the possibility of some sort of independent system of regulation that might be related to the foregoing processes of activation. This involves the capacity of mRNA, with the help of tRNA and ribosomes, to generate sequential strings of some 20 amino acids whose molecular structures are nothing like the molecular structures of DNA, RNA, mRNA, or tRNA, and, thus, this sort of disconnect raises the question of how did a genetic coding system arise which enables nucleic acids, of one kind or another, to generate totally dissimilar amino acids.

How did certain kinds of nucleic acids come to mean or stand for various amino acids? How did different sequences of three nucleic acids come to mean one amino acid rather than another? How did some sequences, rather than others, come to serve as start and stop signals?

Genetic dynamics seem to give expression to a language-like process in which certain combinations and sequences of letters give expression to words known as amino acids, which, in turn, can be arranged in ways that constitute different kinds of functionalities like nouns, verbs, prepositions, adverbs, and so on that when organized in the right sequences give expression to sentences that constitute complete thoughts in the form of metabolic processes of one kind or another. What are the woof and warp or syntax and semantics of such a language-like system, and does it suggest the existence of some sort of regulatory system that is responsible for keeping the biological terrain in a condition of detoxified stability with the microbiome that occupies that terrain?

One can introduce further complicating factors into the foregoing scenario by noting that genes rarely, if ever, come in a form in which they contain nothing but the sequences that will code for various proteins. Sprinkled throughout a gene are bits and pieces of genetic material that don't seem to have anything to do with the final protein that is to be put together via ribosomal, mRNA, and tRNA activity.

Such interstitial genetic entities are known as introns. Those introns are removed so that nothing but the genetic sequences that are needed to code for a given protein will be taken out of the nucleus via mRNA.

Again, one would like to know what it is that performs this sort of editing process. What determines whether certain sequences are essential or are unessential components for any given mRNA message, and are there functional reasons why such introns exist at all?

Again, such questions seem to raise the possibility that there is some regulatory system that might not be under the operational control of either the basic genome of 20,000 genes in human being (and this also would seem to be true in other organisms as well) or under the operational control of the other 98% of the genetic material as well. If this is the case, then, such questions would seem to allude to the existence of some sort of regulatory operating system that is present which might be responsible for making those kinds of determinations and, thereby, be responsible for overseeing various kinds of regulatory dynamics.

Of course, being able to ask such questions or, as a result of trying to resolve those mysteries, proceeding to posit the foregoing sort of regulatory system which is not a function of either the basic genome of (in humans) of 20,000 genes or the 98% of the extra genetic material that seems to be present, does not really prove anything. However, rather than trying to prove something, all I am trying to do is induce readers to begin to critically reflect on such possibilities.

In one sense, introns do seem to have a functional significance, at least in a negative manner. The repeated sequences of genetic letters which are associated with genetic disorders such as myotonic dystrophy and Fragile X syndrome are to be found among the interstitial sequences within a gene that are known as introns.

For example, in Fragile X syndrome there are a series of repeats (consisting of the nucleic letters CCG) that occur before the initial coding area that constitutes what will be the first of a series of amino acids that will make up a fully functional protein. So-called "normal" people will have anywhere between 15 and 65 copies of the foregoing three-letter sequence, whereas the gene of the individual who has the Fragile X defect will have anywhere from 200 to several thousand repeating sequences.

What sort of mutation might cause such sequences to go from between 15 and 65 repetitions up to between two hundred and several thousand repeats of that three letter sequence? What, if anything, is keeping track of how many of the repeated sequences are present, and what terminates the set of repeats at one number – say 200 – rather than some other number such as one or two thousand?

When the number of repeated sequences becomes very large, production of mRNA is discontinued. What determines what constitutes a sufficiently large number of repeated sequences to discontinue production of mRNA and what is responsible for the shut down directive?

If repeated sequences of the three-letter nucleic sequence that are sufficiently large are problematic, what function, if any, is served by the presence of between 15 and 65 repeated sequences, and why are the "normal" set of repetitions so variable, and in any given "normal" individual what is responsible for determining what the number of repeated sequences will be? One has difficulty reconciling the idea that while 200 to several thousand repeated sequences means trouble, nonetheless, the presence of 15 to 65 repeated sequences has no "meaning" and simply needs to be excised from the gene that is coding for a particular protein.

Researchers have discovered that the "normal" range of repeated sequences (15 to 65) apparently has remained fairly stable for a considerable period of so-called evolutionary time. This suggests to those who are inclined toward evolution, that such a set of sequences must have some kind of function – and, therefore, is not just nonsense genetic material -- but what the nature of the function of such a range of repeated sequences might be in so-called normal individuals is not entirely clear.

One might note in passing that the way in which some evolutionists travel about in their conceptual domain resonates with a travel technique that is, sometimes, used in a Muppets movie. Given that such movies tend to be about an hour and a half long, should the need arise in such movies to make a lengthy journey that normally would take a great deal of time, then, a "travel by map" device is introduced in which one can traverse great distances between different cities on Earth by simply drawing a line between one's starting point and the desired end point of the trip, and, without having traversed actual distances, one arrives at one's destination.

Many evolutionists do something which is very similar. One might call their technique "travel by conjecture" during which a person is able to arrive at the desired conceptual destination without having to actually slog through any intervening empirical miles at all.

In any event, the fact that the aforementioned set of "normal," repeated sequences has remained quite stable across thousands of years, does not necessarily demonstrate that such stability has evolutionary significance. What is important is that the range of repeated sequences which is considered normal has remained stable and this remains so irrespective of whether, or not, researchers can identify which set of forces (evolutionary or something else) is served by such a conserved condition.

The conservation of such regions of interstitial genetic materials does seem to indicate that normal regions of repeated sequences do have some role in shaping or modulating the manner in which mRNA is used. If so, this would suggest, in, yet, another way, that there might be some sort of regulatory dynamics taking place that is not necessarily a function of either the basic genome of 20,000 proteins or the more extended genome which involves the remaining 98% of genetic material.

More specifically, the function of the gene with which Fragile X syndrome is associated not only serves as a sort of shuttle system for an array of RNA molecules that enables the latter molecules to be delivered to various locations within the biological terrain, but, as well, the gene which is associated with the Fragile X syndrome also plays a role in shaping how the RNA molecules that are being transported will be involved in the process of protein construction. So, if, as result of the presence of a sufficiently large number of repeats of the CCG base sequence, mRNA production is discontinued, and, therefore, the gene does not become properly functional, then a series of important biological tools will not be built.

Neurons appear to become impaired as a result of the absence of the protein that is coded by the foregoing gene. The specific nature of how the neurons are adversely affected by the absence of the protein at issue is not, yet, known, but the bottom line is that the learning capacity of a person with such a disorder becomes dysfunctional in various ways, and, therefore, one of the differences between a properly functioning system of neurons and a dysfunctional system of neurons has to do with whether the "junk" regions that are present as introns within the DNA sequence that constitutes the gene associated with Fragile X syndrome are, or are not, normal in character with respect to the number of repeats that are contained in such introns.

If one compares certain genes -- in, say, a worm -- that are fairly similar to genes in human beings and which serve similar functions, the genes in the simpler organism tend to be fairly straightforward sequences of DNA that can be transcribed into mRNA which, in turn, will be translated into a string of amino acids when processed by a ribosome that result in a specific protein. However, comparable genes in human beings tend to be much longer than their counterparts in simpler species, and the factor of length is a function of the introns that are present in human genes but which are not present in the simpler organisms.

This feature of greater length that is tied to the presence of introns actually entails the possibility of arranging genetic information in a multiplicity of ways that are capable of leading to the production of proteins that are other than what a given gene normally codes for if all – or most -- of the introns were removed or edited out. Although the set of 20,000, or so, genes which constitute the basic complement of genes with which all human beings start their lives – notwithstanding, of course, certain variations in the character of those genes as one goes from one person to the next – some of the introns that are contained within any given gene actually provide those genes – which usually code for specific proteins – with the degrees of freedom that allow the genetic material in a given gene to be edited and assembled in any number of ways, depending on what introns are retained and what introns are removed.

Some researchers have indicated that 60% of the fixed genes in the human genome have the capacity to generate multiple kinds of proteins depending on how they are edited. This means that 12,000 standard, fixed genes in the basic genome (60% of 20,000 genes) have the capacity for giving rise to a multiplicity of genes other than what such genes normally would code for if all, or most, of the introns in such a gene were edited out.

While the 98% of the genetic material that previously had been thought to be non-functional in character (i.e., junk) might be responsible for the **mechanics** of gene editing that takes place as the DNA sequences for one kind of protein, rather than another, are selected from the genetic material in a gene (consisting of both introns and the sequences that entail the coding for the protein that normally is associated with a given gene -- say, the same protein that serves a similar function in simpler organisms), one cannot argue that the regulatory directives that determine which kind of protein will be assembled in conjunction with a given gene is necessarily a function of the editing process per se, as much as it might be a function of an independent system of operational regulatory activity that is calling for one kind of protein rather than another to be generated in response to changing environmental conditions to which a given biological terrain must respond.

The human genome in any given cell (consisting of both the sequences for the 20,000, or so, genes that make up the basic genetic package of the genome as well as the remaining genetic material that makes up 98% of the overall total of the genome) is not necessarily aware of what is transpiring in either the surrounding biological terrain considered as a whole or aware of how that terrain is being affected by changing conditions within the environment in which such a biological terrain resides. On the other hand, presumably, there might well be some sort of capacity for awareness which is present in a given organism or biological terrain that is engaging, as well as being engaged by, the surrounding environment ... a complex, dialectical dynamic which generates the need for different kinds of directives or communications to be sent to various cells that induce the latter to start producing or stop producing various kinds of proteins, or to start (or stop) assembling one kind of protein rather than another modality of protein (depending on how the introns in a given gene are edited or parsed).

In the human genome, there are almost 1,300 gene families that exist in the human genome which are comparable to gene families that exist across most branches of biological life. However, in vertebrates, there are about 100 gene families that are engaged in an array of intricate sorts of dynamics that have responsibility for, among other things, helping to maintain a condition of detoxified stability in the biological terrains of such vertebrates.

To be sure, having a system of operational oversight concerning the aforementioned 1,500 gene families (which are largely held in common by most species of life) would be important in order that dynamics governing those biological systems would start and stop the production of the proteins associated with the foregoing sorts of gene families in ways that are conducive to the continued well-being of different kinds of biological terrain. Nonetheless, there are other gene families that would seem to need to be even more responsive to what is transpiring throughout the biological terrain of a given species of vertebrate and its interaction with the surrounding ecological environment and, as a result, such a need might suggest the possibility of the existence or presence of some sort of sophisticated system of operational oversight.

This is because this smaller set of 100 gene families involves complex operations of detoxification and stabilization that are crucial for, among other things, helping to maintain or, when necessary, attempt to re-establish a condition of detoxified stability in the biological terrain that gives expression to a given kind of organisms. This sort of operational control would be able to regulate, among other things, the relationship between the biological terrain and the microbiome that inhabits that terrain remain in a state of symbiosis and try to prevent that relationship to become destabilized to the point where different microorganisms within the microbiome are induced   to   enter   into   non-symbiotic   stages   of   their pleiomorphic/pleomorphic life cycles which have the capacity to further destabilize the biological terrain and, in the process, give rise to different kinds of diseases depending on the nature of the destabilization that takes place and depending on what sorts of transitions are induced to take place in different segments of the microbiome which constitute a retreat from symbiotic behavior in conjunction with the surrounding biological terrain.

Among the sorts of functions to which the foregoing set of 100 gene families might give expression might involve many of the processes that were explored in a previous chapter of the present book which sought to argue that an immune system, per se, does not exist in human beings. More specifically, biological dynamics involving such components as: Macrophages, neutrophils, dendritic cells, T-cells, B-cells, the complement system, cytokines, and the lymph system might all be connected with the aforementioned set of 100 gene families which are capable – when properly regulated – of helping to contribute to the detoxified stability of a given biological terrain or organism.

With each passing year, more and more of the 98% of the genome which previously had been considered to be non-functional, and, therefore, junk, is being shown to have the capacity to influence the manner in which the basic complement of 20,000 genes in the human genome can be expressed. Nonetheless, what seems to be missing from the developing biological portrait that is being drawn is the presence of some sort of oversight capacity which communicates with that 98% of the genome concerning how the 2% of the genome that constitutes the basic set of 20,000 proteins will be turned on, off, and parsed, or edited, and my candidate for this command and control center resides within the somatids of Naessens, or the endobionts of Enderlein, or the frequencies with which Rife dealt, or the microzyma of Béchamp.

In essence, what is being referred to in the foregoing paragraph has to do with the epigenetic dynamics that occur in a given biological terrain. Such dynamics constitute a system of adaptive learning which is set in motion when the human genome (consisting of both the 98% and the 2% of genetic material) is directed to stop, start, or be edited by some sort of operational control center that is capable of interacting with the entire biological terrain as well as the surrounding environmental ecology with the speed, efficiency, and finesse that is necessary to maintain or -- when necessary -- help a given biological terrain to re-establish a condition of detoxified stability that preserves the symbiotic relationships that exist between such a biological terrain and the microbiome that occupies it.

Epigenetics entails the biological dynamics that are needed to help a system to maintain or recover, if necessary, a condition of stability without altering the nature of the genetic material that makes up the genome. Epigenetics is about processes that control and affect how genetic information is used in conjunction with changing circumstances both within a given biological terrain as well changes in the surrounding environment that pose both opportunities for, and challenges to, the capacity of an organism to be able to maintain, or recover, stability or well-being.

Epigenetics entails various degrees of freedom as well as degrees of constraint concerning the capacity of a biological system to engage in different forms of adaptive learning that are geared toward helping a given biological terrain to be able to deal with changing conditions. However, the system of adaptive learning that is being expressed here is different from the system of adaptive learning that is proposed by those who believe in the existence of antibodies and an immune system.

All of the components (e.g., macrophages, neutrophils, dendritic cells, complement system, cytokines, and so on) which are being mentioned by immunologists and those who are influenced by those individuals do not necessarily serve any sort of immunological function (and evidence for this was presented in earlier chapters) that provides continuous or semi-continuous forms of automatic protection that is mediated, to a large extent, by the presence of antibodies. Instead, the focus of the epigenetic adaptive learning system being proposed here has entirely to do with the dynamics of detoxification and stabilization which need to be performed, in whole or in part, on each occasion that a given biological terrain is destabilized in some fashion and, as such, there is no sort of on-going immunological memory associated with the kind of epigenetic dynamics that are being suggested in the present chapter.

The sort of epigenetic adaptive learning system which is presently being proposed concerns creative uses of existing genetic tools to counter any given set of changing conditions that destabilizes or threatens to destabilize the well-being of an organism. Well-being is a condition of detoxified stability which preserves the set of symbiotic relationships that exist between a given biological terrain and the microbiome which occupies that terrain.

The foregoing sense of adaptive learning is not rooted in a monomorphic theory that entails relatively fixed and static forms of antibody-mediated responses to hostile pathogens (e.g., various kinds of microorganisms including viruses) that are "remembered" (in some collective sense) by a set of antibodies. Instead, the aforementioned epigenetic adaptive learning system is rooted in a pleiomorphic/pleomorphic understanding concerning the capacity of microorganisms to change their morphological and functional capabilities in response to an ever-changing set of environmental conditions that impinge on the capacity of a given biological terrain or organism to be able to respond to such changes in unique ways while seeking to maintain – or recover – a condition of detoxified stability through which well-being is established.

There is a set of genes known as the HOX group which plays an array of crucial roles during the process of development. That group of genes needs to be turned on and off in a particular order of expression if development is to unfold in a fully functional matter.

The margin of error for the successful, sequential expression of the HOX genes is pretty-much zero. Consequently, one might expect that the epigenetic system of adaptive learning that is being suggested here would be fairly silent when it comes to potentially creative ways to parse the genes that make up the HOX group of genes, but, at the same time, something is turning the genes in that group on and off in a very precise sequence, and, therefore, one might propose that the same system that is responsible for the epigenetic regulation of the sort of gene parsing that offers creative ways for handling certain existential challenges also has the capacity to oversee forms of gene expression that are governed by few, if any, degrees of freedom while simultaneously being restrained through various dynamics of necessary constraint.

Both kinds of epigenetic adaptive learning (relatively free and relatively constrained) serve the overarching process of maintaining, or recovering, the sort of condition of detoxified stability which gives expression to well-being. In other words, both of the foregoing kinds of epigenetic dynamics that are being suggested here would seem to allude to, or give expression to, the existence of a system of command and control that oversees what transpires within a given biological terrain or organism.

Such a system of epigenetic command and control seems to operate in accordance with an endogenous gyroscope-like dynamic that "knows" what constitutes a condition of detoxified stability and continuously measures and balances what is transpiring within the given biological terrain that it oversees against an internal dynamic or model of well-being and makes adaptive adjustments according to what is needed to maintain a condition of well-being or detoxified stability or what is needed in order to try to recover a condition of well-being that might have become destabilized in some fashion. I believe that such an epigenetic system of oversight and adaptive learning is contained within the somatids of Naessens, or the endobionts of Enderlein, or the frequencies of Rife, or the microzymas of Béchamp, and, as well be delineated in later chapters, I believe that somatids or endobionts or microzymas constitute transducers which have the capacity to convert one kind of energy (a field energy of some kind) into another kind of energy (the capacity to operationally direct what transpires in a given biological terrain or organism).

There are a number of components which are involved in the process of editing genes to generate various kinds of proteins other than the one which normally would be produced if the introns present in such a gene were removed. There also are a number of components involved in the starting and stopping of any given version of a given gene that is to be expressed.

For example, whether, or not, a given gene can be turned on depends on a sequence of so-called "junk DNA" that is known as a "**promoter**". The promoter sequence needs to be located prior to the first string of DNA that, together with many subsequent strings of DNA, will collectively constitute the genetic message that is present in such a gene and which will be converted into mRNA

If the promoter sequence is absent, then, the gene cannot be turned on. Moreover, if that promoter sequence were to somehow become reversed, then even though it might occupy a space at the beginning of the gene sequences that are to be transcribed into a mRNA molecule, nonetheless, the gene could not be turned on.

There are, however, other kinds of components that need to be active in addition to the foregoing sequence of promoter "junk" DNA if a given gene is to be expressed. For instance, there are a number of proteins known as "**transcription factors**" which need to be present in order that a certain kind of enzyme which is crucial to the process of generating an mRNA copy of a given gene can be bound to, or bound by, the aforementioned transcription factors.

Furthermore, promoter sequences can be influenced by various kinds of molecules that have modulating properties. These properties often determine whether a given gene will be expressed or suppressed and will determine the extent to which a given gene will be expressed or suppressed.

The molecules that can have a profound effect upon whether, or not, a given gene is expressed can be quite small. For instance, methyl groups – which consist of just one carbon atom and three hydrogen atoms – are at the center of a range of modulating forces that operate in conjunction with many genes.

More specifically, when a methyl group is juxtaposed next to a cytosine base and the foregoing two molecules are followed by a guanine base, then such a sequence is able to serve as a locus of modification when enzymes of one kind or another are added to the complex. What makes such an arrangement especially interesting is that the process of adding of a methyl group (known as methylation) does not appear to be a function of either DNA or RNA activity, and, yet, methylation can have a considerable impact on what happens genetically.

For example, identical twins each have precisely the same set of genes. Nonetheless, over time, and, sometimes even beginning when the twins are in the womb, subtle differences might begin to emerge that are a function of processes like methylation that will alter the way in which certain genes function. For whatever reason, some of the genes that are found in each and every cell of the bodies of the twins begin to be used in slightly different ways, and methyl groups are one of the non-DNA and non-RNA molecules which are involved in the mediation of those sorts of differences.

Whereas methyl groups tend to be involved in shutting off or dampening down the expression of a gene, there are other molecules that have the capacity to help certain genes to be turned back on or which can help to dial up the extent to which, given various circumstances, those genes can be expressed. Histones – which are proteins, and there are many kinds of histones – are often involved in the foregoing sorts of genetic transactions, and given that there are more than 60 kinds of chemical groups that can be brought into modulate histones via one, or another, of the amino acid components that make up a histone, there are a huge number of combinations which are possible when one, or more, of the foregoing sorts of chemical groups interact with different kinds of histones and, when acting in concert with one another, can affect the expression of genes.

Among other things, histone protein molecules can not only determine the extent to which a gene might be expressed, but some of those proteins can determine the state of readiness with which a given gene might be processed in the future. As a result, the presence of histone proteins can help enhance the efficiency and speed with which a given gene operates under different circumstances.

A wrinkle, or two, of complexity can be introduced into the foregoing scenario by keeping in mind that certain histones can do more than just dial up the extent to which a given gene is expressed or, alternatively, prepare a given gene to be ready to be expressed given the right sort of circumstances. Some histones interact with certain kinds of enzymes (known as "**major repressors**") that, in turn, interact with long segments of so-called "junk" or non-coding segments of RNA (non-coding in the sense of not being a part of the genetic material that codes for the standard set of fixed proteins which, in humans, consist of some 20,000 genes).

The foregoing kind of interaction will result in suppressing certain modalities of gene expression. There are many degrees of freedom which exist with respect to how histones, major repressors and the aforementioned long segments of non-coding RNA can interact and affect which genes are expressed and how they are expressed.

Finally, promoters are not necessarily assigned to a specific gene. They tend to be involved in turning on whichever gene happens to be sufficiently close and only if, relative to the gene being turned on, such promoter sequences have the right sequential relationship in conjunction with that gene (in other words, a gene might be sufficiently close to a given promoter sequence to be a candidate for being turned on, but if the promoter sequence has a reverse sequence orientation relative to that gene, then the gene will not be turned on).

So, in order for a gene to not only be turned on but in order for a needed gene to be turned on at a given time, a number of conditions have to be satisfied. Thus, a promoter gene with the appropriate sequential orientation must be found at the beginning of the gene that needs to be transcribed according to the needs of the biological terrain that exist at that time, and, in addition, the right sort of transcription factors must arrive ahead of, in order to be able to be ready to bind, the enzyme that is to generate a given sequence of mRNA, and, finally, the appropriate sorts of methylation, histone proteins, major repressors, and long segments of non-coding must be present to ensure that the gene is either not expressed in a certain way or that it is expressed in one way or another.

Different kinds of promoter sequences require certain kinds of transcription factors. Usually speaking, different cell types will tend to express the sorts of transcription factors that are needed by a given promoter sequence which operates within such a cell type.

To further complicate matters, there is another set of allegedly junk DNA sequences that are known as "**enhancers**". Enhancers tend to be several hundred base pairs long, but they are highly variable in the nature of their sequences.

Unlike promoters, they do not have to possess any particular sequential orientation relative to a given gene in order to be operational. However, there are forms of enhancers which are referred to as "**latent enhancers**" which are variable in whether, or not, they are active at any given time. Such latent enhancers have to be activated in order to begin to influence or modulate what is transpiring within any given gene.

Enhancers, themselves, seem to be functionally dependent on the presence of another kind of so-called junk DNA. As previously indicated, there is a class of sequences involving "junk RNA" that is known as "long non-coding RNA."

Sequences of long non-coding RNA interact with a group of proteins that interact with one another and, collectively, are referred to as a "**Mediator**." This dynamic between the Mediator and the long non-coding RNA sequence has the capacity to modulate what happens in a given proximate gene that codes for a particular protein.

The aforementioned Mediator complex of proteins also plays a role in the nature of the activity that takes place in conjunction with a collection of enhancers that are known as "**super-enhancers**" which can be as many as times the size of regular enhancers that usually consist of a few hundred sequences of "junk" DNA.

The Mediator and super-enhancer dynamic appears to play a key role in the manner in which embryonic stem cells manifest themselves. In other words, whether a given kind of embryonic cell stays embryonic, and, therefore, pluripotent (i.e., has the capacity to become any kind of cell), or become specialized (and, therefore, moves away from pluripotency) can be affected by how the Mediator protein complex and super-enhancer region of so-called junk DNA interact with one another.

In connection with the foregoing considerations, there also are a group of proteins known as "**master regulators**." This concerns four proteins that when they are highly expressed, the pluripotency of embryonic cells seems to be retained but when the foregoing proteins are not highly expressed, specialized cells of one kind or another come into being, and which outcome will occur in any given instance will depend on the activity of the super-enhancers that are present.

Promoters, transcription factors, enhancers, latent enhancers, super enhancers, the Mediator complex, and the master regulators are all involved in a dance of exquisite timing, precision and varying degrees of freedom. In addition, components such as methyl groups, histones, various kinds of enzymes, and long segments of non-coding RNA also are present which expand the complexity of how all of the foregoing components will interact with one another.

Moreover, to add to the cauldron of complexity that presently is being stirred, there are certain genes that operate with anywhere up to 20 separate so-called "junk DNA/RNA" regions. In addition, there are certain regions of such "junk DNA/RNA which are able to engage anywhere from one to ten different genes.

While the term "epigenetics" is often restricted to the way in which, say, histone molecules and methyl groups turn different genes on and off or modulate the way in which they are expressed, a case might be made for considerably expanding the notion of what constitutes epigenetic activity. More specifically, epigenetics seems to involve processes of adaptive learning that are a function of a great many modalities of biological activity which determine how, when and where different genes are expressed in various cells of the body.

As such, epigenetics should not be limited to just the non-DNA and non-RNA molecules (such as methyl groups or histones which are modified in different ways) that are involved in affecting the way in which the genome is expressed. Epigenetics seems to encompass all of the forms of adaptive learning that take place during the process of gene expression or suppression.

Consequently, the notion of epigenetics, when considered in an expanded sense of the term, seems to point in the direction of some kind of over-arching system of control that is independent of both the 2% of the genome that generates a set of fixed proteins, as well as the 98% of the genome which involves the activity of an array of DNA and RNA sequences that constitute the surface of the dynamics which are being regulated by some sort of underlying or overarching system of operational control concerning what takes place in the biological terrain under different circumstances of contingency. As such, the operational system that regulates how, and when, and where the 98% and the 2% of the genome interact with one another would seem to reside in something beyond those two segments of the genome, and, as stated previously, my candidate for the location of such a operational control system is in the guise of the somatids, endobionts, or microzyma that seem to be essential to life and, yet, as Béchamp, Enderlein, Rife, and Naessens all maintained, are, simultaneously, independent of those same life-forms.

The nature of the epigenetic control that somatids, endobionts, or microzymas have with respect to the way in which the 98% of the genome interacts with the 2% of the genome is not captured by the specific dynamics that are entailed by, among other components: Promoters, transcription factors, enhancers, latent enhancers, super enhancers, the Mediator complex, the master regulators, methyl groups, histone proteins, long sequences of non-coding RNA, and so on. These components are the workers that serve as the means through which certain kinds of biological tasks are carried out, but the heart or essence of epigenetics resides in the operational control center that instructs those, and other, molecular workers how, when, and where to perform their functions.

As such, the scope of epigenetics goes beyond whatever sorts of nuances are introduced to modulate the dynamics that are being carried out by the aforementioned components. Epigenetics really refers to the processes of operational control that govern when things are to be done, or in what order they are to be done, or in what combinations they are to be done, or where they are to be done, or how such processes are to be modified so that the biological terrain can effectively respond in a timely and appropriately adaptive manner to the changing conditions of life.

Epigenetics doesn't change the nature of the tools which are to be used to carry out various functions. Epigenetics changes how those tools will be used in response to changing conditions, and such operational capabilities appear to go to the very heart of what constitutes adaptive learning.

Moreover, the foregoing sort of adaptive learning would seem to be present in the Naessens transplant experiment which was discussed toward the beginning of the present chapter. In those transplant experiments, rabbit-skin from a white-furred rabbit was observed to give rise to a certain amount of white fur in a black-furred counterpart without encountering any sort of rejection phenomenon -- provided that somatids from the white-furred donor were first transferred to the black-furred recipient prior to the process of transplantation. The donor somatids seem to have responsibility for the kinds of adaptive learning that had to occur in the recipient rabbit in order for the subsequent transplantation to be able to occur without initiating a rejection phenomenon.

If the foregoing is true, then, the issue of rejection is not a self versus non-self issue. The rejection occurs if the recipient organism is not provided with the sorts of epigenetic operational controls that are present in the donor organism, and, as such, rejection is really a matter of the epigenetic process breaking down due to the absence, for whatever reason, of the right kinds of operational control capabilities, and, as a result, the necessary sorts of adaptive learning cannot take place which normally enable the biological terrain to detoxify the poisons or toxins that give expression to the sorts of strong allergic reactions that emerge when transplantation takes place without the appropriate capacity for adaptive learning being present.

Earlier, mention was made about how histones can affect the manner in which genes are expressed, including the sorts of modifications to genes that enhances or enables the readiness of those genes to be expressed under certain kinds of circumstances. Given that histones seem to be involved in many kinds of allergic responses, it is not that much of a reach to suppose that something has gone wrong with those aspects of epigenetic control which are responsible for certain kinds of histone dynamics, including a readiness to respond (problematically) to the presence of certain kinds of molecules (poisons or toxins) to which the individual has become sensitized as a result of a breakdown in epigenetic functioning.

Conceivably, many of the diseases that are considered to be autoimmune in character are, instead, what results when the operational control capacity of the system of epigenetics is poisoned in some fashion. As a result, various aspects of metabolism (whether anabolic or catabolic) become dysfunctional.

One might even say that all of the foregoing sorts of dysfunctional dynamics are variations on one theme – allergic reactions of one kind or another. More specifically, the body develops allergies – which are processes of inflammation or destabilization – in response to the presence of poisoned or dysfunctional chemical pathways that are occurring in different parts of the body.

As indicated earlier, allergies are a form of inflammation within some aspect of the biological terrain. Such inflammation has the capacity to induce various aspects of the microbiome to transition away from symbiotic relationships with the terrain.

Consequently, allergies, of whatever kind, give expression to a breakdown in the dynamics of epigenetics in which poisoned or dysfunctional processes of one kind or another cannot be properly detoxified. As a result, the biological terrain cannot be returned to a condition of detoxified stability in which that terrain continues to have an on-going symbiotic relationship with the pleiomorphic/pleiomorphic microbiome that occupies the terrain.

Unless the underling process of epigenetic poisoning or dysfunction can be detoxified, then, allergies tend to become chronic in nature. This is the case irrespective of whether such maladies occur in the guise of normal allergies, or they occur in the guise of more complex forms of dysfunction such as so-called autoimmune diseases.

Therefore, the condition of being chronic is a symptom of the way in which the epigenetic system of operational control continues to be poisoned or rendered dysfunctional. Just as the adaptive learning that occurs in conjunction with epigenetic processes had become stagnant or static or fixed in a constructive fashion when, for instance methylation takes place in relation to the suppression of certain genes, to too, there is a negative counterpart to the foregoing in which the adaptive learning process becomes stagnant or static in a problematic way, and, this results in the emergence of one, or another, kind of pathology.

Consequently, so-called autoimmune diseases might not necessarily have anything to do with issues of immunity in which parts of the self supposedly attack other parts of the self because the latter components are, somehow, perceived to be operating in ways that are not consistent with what is considered to be the self's way of conducting genetic business. Instead, autoimmune diseases might be just another set of symptoms that arise when the epigenetic system is poisoned in one fashion or another, and, as a result, some portion of operational control is lost or becomes dysfunctional because what is normally a process of adaptive learning is being prevented (through absence or dysfunction) from properly governing the manner in which the 98% of the genome which encompasses a high degree of non-coding DNA and RNA modulating capacity will interact with the other 2% of the genome that codes for fixed proteins.

Chapter 14: Resonance and Frequency Following Behavior

The dynamics of protein receptors has dominated a great deal of medical and biological research over the last five, or so, decades. The dominant role which the theory of protein receptors has come to occupy during that period of time might not be warranted.

In 1994 Harold Hillman wrote an article entitled "New Considerations About the Structure of the Membrane of the Living Animal Cell." Within the Abstract which precedes the paper's main body of text, Dr. Hillman puts forth the proposal that cell membranes are unlikely to be populated with an array of receptors and channels, and he proceeds to indicate that the biochemical and physiological properties which tend to be attributed to such channels and receptors take place independently of whatever structural, anatomical, or morphological properties that might be present.

While he also points out in the Abstract of his article that researchers have been cognizant of the fact that small ions are able to cross cell membranes since at least the 1940s, nonetheless, generally speaking, physiologists appear to believe that channels in membranes only become open within nerve and muscle cells which have become excited in some fashion, and, otherwise, when channels exist in other kinds of non-excitable cellular membranes, the status of those channels seems to be one of always being closed.

During the main body of the foregoing paper, Hillman indicates that the trilaminar (three-layered) character that is often assigned to the structural character of any given membrane is likely to be an artifact. An artifact refers to changes that are induced in a tissue structure – such as a membrane -- that are the result of the process of generating a micrograph of some kind and which cannot be reconciled with what can be observed with other kinds of microscopy that are capable of showing properties of living organisms rather than the lifeless samples that are viewed, say, via electron microscopes.

For instance, in actual living organisms, there tends to be a certain amount of water which is present in the membranes. That water disappears as a result of dehydration during the process of producing an electron micrograph, and as a result various kinds of properties (e.g., shape and thickness) of a cell membrane might be distorted.

In addition, the heavy metals that are used to stain the object being "photographed" via an electron microscope are likely to distort the appearance of such membranes, and, in the process, will affect the measured thickness of any given sample. For instance, the thickness of membranes is usually considered to be somewhere between 7 and 10 nanometers, but this measurement cannot necessarily be considered to be reliable because heavy metal salts are deposited on both sides of the membrane that is being measured and, therefore, constitute an obstacle to being able to accurately measure the membrane which is between such heavy metal deposits.

Furthermore, the angle at which an electron microscope engages an object that is to be captured in the form of an electron micrograph is very limited. As a result, one's impression of the object tends to be driven by the foregoing angle of engagement which prevents one from seeing other facets of the object at the same time and, thereby, provide a person with variable sight lines that could alter the way one perceives what is being depicted.

In addition, there are many alleged macromolecular transmembrane proteins (molecules that supposedly span the thickness of a membrane) which have been identified following isolation and sequencing. The width of these macromolecules tend to be two or three times the thickness of any given membrane, and, yet, according to Hillman, although the thickness of a membrane is within the capacity of an electron microscope to resolve, nonetheless, the foregoing sorts of macromolecules tend to be rarely seen when transmission microscopy is being used.

Notwithstanding the foregoing considerations, a potentially relevant observation has been made in conjunction with a scanning microscope (but not an electron transmission microscope) that has encouraged some researchers to claim to have seen the receptor for the acetylcholine molecule. However, whether such a receptor was actually seen or whether what had been observed was a function of artifact generation during the process of fixing a given sample seems to remain an open question.

Furthermore, while many explanations (rationalizations?) have been given by various researchers for why there has not been more evidence uncovered that reveals the existence of transmembrane proteins, one should keep in mind that what constitutes much of the available evidence concerning transmembrane molecule tends to be a function of why there might an absence of evidence in support of their existence rather than being a function of the presence of evidence in support of their existence. Until evidence is forthcoming that positively demonstrates the existence of those kinds of macromolecules is readily available, the existential status of such molecules remains theoretical rather than having been confirmed as being real.

Later, during the course of the 1994 article currently being discussed, Hillman puts forth a hypothesis which he believes might account for why there are many experiments that have been performed which demonstrate how various kinds of drugs, amino acids, and other kinds of molecules are able to rapidly affect what transpires within a cell, and that such a dynamic can be considered quite independently of theories which propose that mediator for such effects must be via some sort of transmembrane protein. More specifically, Hillman claims that all living organisms are inherently inclined to be able to interact with a wide variety of hormones, chemical molecules, drugs, proteins, and toxins that might be in close proximity to a given cell membrane.

However, the foregoing proposal comes at the end of his article. As a result, he doesn't elucidate the nature of the foregoing, endogenous feature that supposedly characterizes all living organisms and which would enable molecules that are proximate to, but external to, the membrane of a cell to be able to interact with molecules in the interior of the cell that is enclosed by what Hillman believes is a relatively sold membrane, devoid (with previously noted exceptions) of open, active channels and transmembrane protein molecules.

One candidate that bubbles to the surface at this point and is consonant with Hillman's foregoing suggestion has to do with research that Royal Rife pursued and concerning which an overview was given in Chapter 5 of the present book. The Universal microscope that Rife invented in the 1920s and subsequently improved upon over the next 10-15 years, had the capacity to observe living (not dead) microorganisms in resolutions that extended down to the sub-micron level of size (1/30th of a micron).

The method Rife used for staining specimens was via a process of resonance. By fine-tuning the frequency to which the microscope was attuned at any given time, Rife discovered that he was able to detect the presence of entities that resonated with the frequency which his microscope was using to search for entities and objects that radiated with frequencies that were resonant with his probe.

Consequently, there is a sense in which Rife's research resonates with Hillman's aforementioned proposal. In other words, the endogenous property of all living organisms to which Hillman alluded might have something to do with the way in which different components of any given cell have frequencies associated with them, and, therefore, when drugs, proteins, hormones, toxins, or other molecules are near to the perimeter of a cell membrane, one might suppose that various kinds of resonance phenomena could take place between the different kinds of frequencies that are given off by components of a given cell as they interact with various kinds of frequencies that are given off by molecular components outside of, but proximate to, such a cell.

Although Carolyn McMakin didn't invent Frequency Specific Microcurrent (FSM) therapy, she did develop this form of therapy in extraordinary ways. As the foregoing therapy name indicates, the focal center around which FSM gravitates involves finding the right frequencies that are able to help detoxify and stabilize a given biological terrain which has become dysfunctional in some way.

Early in her 2017 book: *The Resonance Effect: How Frequency Specific Microcurrent is Changing Medicine*, Carolyn McMakin informs readers of her book that just as an electronic fob (a short-range radio transmitter which sends out a specific frequency) is used to unlock or lock a particular device (such as a car) but is not keyed for any other kind of electronic device, so too, the same principle can be used to help treat various kinds of diseases. In a sense, FSM treatments seem to be directed toward elements that interfere with one, or more components, in specific tissues or cells and prevent those tissues or cells from being able to operate at their proper modes of resonance or frequency.

Just as microorganisms that normally are in a symbiotic relationship with the biological terrain within which they reside can be induced to transition away from such stages of their pleiomorphic/pleomorphic life cycles, so too, different processes within the body can be induced (due to the emergence of various forms of interference) to transition away from, or be blocked from, operating at frequencies that are necessary for the well-being of the body. FSM therapy is about finding modes of resonance that assist an individual to be able to return to the sorts of operating frequencies that are consonant with a state of health.

Like Rife, Carolyn McMakin was able to discover forms of treatment that were able to remove elements which were interfering with proper resonance functioning within human beings. She also discovered treatment techniques which could help reset the resonance properties of dysfunctional tissues or cells and return them to functional forms of resonance as well.

However, whereas Rife developed his own system for identifying functional and dysfunctional resonances on the basis of his work with his Universal microscope, Carolyn McMakin appeared to enter into the realm of frequency treatments through a different route. Although she had earned a degree in psychology, for the next 16 years she worked as a sales representative for a pharmaceutical company before deciding to change career directions in 1986 and began to take courses that eventually would lead to studying for a degree in chiropractic medicine when she was 42 years old and, along with her husband, raising two young children.

As life is wont to do, some existential contingencies came into her life which required her to interrupt her chiropractic education for a time. Eventually, she returned to school, but due to an array of stresses and the toll which those stresses took on her marriage, she and her husband divorced in 1992.

At a certain point after returning to school, she taught a course at the chiropractic college, and during this period of time she was receiving treatment, from time to time, for a skiing injury to her shoulder that had occurred several years earlier. As a result of her skiing accident, her shoulder was unable to move through a full range of motion.

The supervisor who was overseeing – but, initially, was not directly involved in -- her treatment was a guy by the name of George Douglas. He was a doctor of chiropractic medicine.

After watching someone else treat her shoulder for a month but not have much success, Douglas asked Carolyn McMakin to come to his office. When she arrived, he took out an old single-channel Microcurrent machine.

Next, he consulted an acupuncture chart and proceeded to attach one of the two probes emanating from the aforementioned microcurrent machine to her hand and, then, attached the other probe to a certain place on her face, before turning on the current for a short time. When she was asked to move her shoulder, the shoulder did not exhibit any increase in its range of motion.

Douglas repositioned the two probes. One was placed at a point that was on the inside of her wrist, while the other probe was positioned near her armpit but still on her chest.

The machine was turned on for six seconds, and, then, turned off. Again, she was asked to try to move her shoulder. Surprisingly, she was able to move her shoulder a full 90 degrees and do so without the sort of pain that had been plaguing her for two years.

Dr. Douglas continued on and tried a number of other placements of the probes before turning the microcurrent machine on again for just a short time. On each of these subsequent occasions, the shoulder was not able to rotate to a position of 90 degrees, and the pain returned.

At that point, he positioned the probes at the two points which, previously, had met with success. He turned the machine on and off several times for 6 second bursts each time.

Following the foregoing treatment, her shoulder could rotate to 90 degrees. Once again, she could do without any pain.

Once the treatment session ended, she began to get some of the back story pertaining to how Dr. Douglas had come to practice such energy work. He had learned about the treatment process from an osteopath by the name of Harry Van Gelder who originally came from Australia but had migrated to the United States in 1946 by way of England.

Once Van Gelder arrived in America he bought an osteopathic practice that came with, among things, a microcurrent machine that had been made in 1922 as well as a chart of frequencies that could be used in conjunction with the aforementioned machine in order to try to resolve issues of dysfunction that were identified as being tied to specific frequencies that appeared on the chart.

Through a process of trial and error, Royal Rife also had developed a chart of frequencies that could be used to resolve various kinds of maladies. Frequencies refer to the number of pulses per second (often measured in units of Hertz) that occur in a given waveform referred to as a current, and current refers to the flow of electrons past a given point in space that takes place within a given time frame (often measured in units of amperes).

When Rife identified the frequency at which a microorganism operated when it had been induced by conditions in the biological terrain to transition away from a symbiotic relationship with that terrain, he would employ an electronic device he had invented which could be set to a frequency that would eliminate such rogue microorganisms. By operating in the foregoing manner, the procedure helped to bring a person back to health, and, in fact, this was the treatment technique that he used when he helped to cure people of advanced cancers in the clinical trials that had been run at the University of Southern California in 1934 that was being supervised and overseen by a number of prominent medical doctors and microbiologists.

What is intriguing about the list of frequencies which Van Gelder inherited when he bought the practice of a retiring osteopath is that it didn't seem to have any discernible connection to the research which Royal Rife had been conducting during the late 1920s. The origins of the list of frequencies that Van Gelder and taught to Dr. Douglas and the story of how someone, prior to Van Gelder, had come to know that certain frequencies worked for specific maladies appears to be a complete mystery.

In part, perhaps, one can blame the foregoing mystery on the Flexner Report which had been released in 1910, because once that report was issued, a great many non-allopathic approaches to medicine began to be extinguished. Furthermore, due to the self-serving actions of non-doctor "doctors" like Morris Fishbein who was the head of the American Medical Association for several decades, many people – such as Royal Rife – were hounded into obscurity, and, as a result, there were many discoveries – such as the Universal Microscope and, apparently, the aforementioned mysterious list of frequencies -- that became buried beneath the multiple layers of ignorance, greed, and desire for control that "guided" people like Morris Fishbein who was able to remove the medical licenses of anyone who did not bow down to the allopathic system of medicine ... a practice that continue to the present day.

Eventually George Douglas and Carolyn McMakin married. She completed her requirements for a chiropractic degree in 1993, and the following year she was able to buy a small practice.

To help launch his wife's new practice, George purchased a microcurrent device which had been invented by Glenn Smith in 1992 that like the old microcurrent device had two channels. George wondered if the new instrument would be able to make use of the frequency chart that he had been using with the older microcurrent machine.

He soon had an opportunity to resolve his curiosity. His wife was treating a client to help rid the latter individual's calf muscles of some knots that had been formed, but instead of relieving the pain associated with those knots, her treatment led to a significant increase in the pain felt by the client.

She phoned her husband at his place of work, explained the situation, and, then, asked for his advice. Because he had been exploring the capabilities of the new machine which he had purchased for his wife, he counseled her to use the new machine that had been set up in one of the rooms in her office complex and also informed her about what frequency settings to use and where to place the electrical probes on her client's body.

She followed his instructions, and 15 minutes later, her client was free of pain. Later, he explained to his wife that the initial form of treatment employed by his wife might have broken a small blood vessel and that the bleeding which resulted from that injury is what might have increased the pain felt by the client.

One of the settings which appeared on the old frequency chart addressed the issue of bleeding. The other setting was directed toward healing the arterial tissue that was connected to that bleeding.

The specific cause of the inflammatory pain which was caused by bleeding had been resolved through the use of one frequency. The specific facet of the biological terrain that was injured during the earlier treatment was resolved through the use of another specific frequency.

Although the specific frequencies that are used vary from condition to condition, the general structure of the microcurrent treatments seem to remain the same across all treatments involving FSM therapy. More specifically, one channel of the microcurrent machine is set to a frequency that is directed toward a specific kind of inflammation, while the other channel seems to be set to a frequency that focuses on a more fundamental level of tissue dynamics or functioning in the biological terrain.

The foregoing descriptive summary seems to resonate with Dr. McMakin perspective when she indicates in her book, *The Resonance Effect*, that one of the channels for the microcurrent machine was dedicated toward inflammations generated by such conditions as toxicity, scarring, concussion, and various microorganisms. She also indicates in her book that the second channel of the microcurrent machine was reserved for issues that addressed problems concerning what caused the underlying dysfunction that led to whatever sort of inflammation that was being addressed by the first channel of the microcurrent machine.

She approached the more fundamental issue by trying to identify what prevents a given kind of tissue from operating in a normal or healthy fashion, and, as a result, inflammation of one kind or another takes place. Like Rife, she came to believe that if one removes the source of interference in the more fundamental tissue dynamics -- that is, if one were to engage the source for a given kind of frequency interference which is undermining proper functioning with an appropriate counter frequency -- then, that tissue would be able to return to a condition of well-being.

Given Gaston Naessens previously discussed transplant experiments (Chapter 5) and the importance which the transfer of specialized skin somatids had for the rabbit that was receiving a transplant if one were to avoid a rejection phenomenon, and given Naessens contention that every kind of tissue has its own species of somatids operating within that kind of tissue which helps regulates that specialized tissue, and given the notion of epigenetics that was introduced in the last chapter which hypothesized that the task of epigenetics is to maintain, or to help re-establish, detoxified stability within a given biological terrain so that the microbiome residing in that terrain is in a symbiotic relationship with the surrounding biological terrain, then, an appropriate course of inquiry might be to seek answers involving the following issue: Is it possible that the second microcurrent channel setting that directs specific frequencies toward resolving problems with aspects of tissue functioning that appear to involve more fundamental dynamics than some presenting symptom of inflammation (which is what the first channel of the microcurrent machine is directed toward)? In other words is it possible that the second frequency setting of the microcurrent machine which is directed toward deeper problems of tissue functioning beyond inflammation might be helping to either re-establish or reset the frequency with which somatids should operate within a given tissue, or could the channel that is directed toward resolving deeper problems of tissue functioning be removing various forms of interference which are preventing those tissues in the cell from being able to clearly receive what is being communicated to them by the specialized somatids that populate that tissue?

Of course, there could be a third possibility which amounts to a variation on the foregoing scenario. More specifically, the counter frequencies that are being generated by Dr. McMakin's microcurrent machine might not be resetting the tissue somatids directly but, instead, those counter frequencies might be resetting the pleiomorphic/pleomorphic life cycle of a given microorganism and, thereby, helping to return such an organism to a condition that was, once again, in a symbiotic relationship with the surrounding biological terrain.

Whatever role, if any, which the foregoing considerations play in the processes of pathology and health, Carolyn McMakin was very clear that figuring out what might be causing certain kinds of inflammation as well as what might be causing the deeper, underlying conditions out of which certain kinds of inflammation arose is not always straightforward or easy to determine. There are organs and metabolic pathways in the body which can affect relatively distant, and, seemingly, unconnected events within the biological terrain.

For instance, the portion of the brain stem that is known as the medulla connects up with one end of the vagus nerve which can involve: Emotional states; various components that are connected to different aspects of the body's network of detoxifying and stabilizing processes; as well as, digestion. Consequently, when a person suffers a concussion that traumatizes, among other things, the medulla, then, the fallout from such an event can trigger downstream problems – such as dysfunctional emotional states -- that one might not immediately be able to identify as having something to do with damage to the medulla or the vagus nerve that connects with the medulla.

Another example which illustrates some of the complexity of the body involves what are known as trigger points. These are regions of sensitivity within a given muscle knot that are capable of triggering pain in other parts of the body.

Without an understanding of how trigger points in one part of the body are connected with the generation of pain in other parts of the body (and there is a document known as *The Trigger Point Manual* which maps out such relationships), then treatment can be ineffective. Dr. McMakin actually discovered a way to engage such issues by intuiting a form of practical innovation in the use of the microcurrent machine.

In her book, *The Resonance Effect,* she describes a client who had been in an auto accident several years before that she had been treating for more than a month with traditional forms of thumb massage applied several times a week. At a certain point during the treatment process, there were some trigger points that had emerged in his sternocleidomastoid which made him dizzy when he moved his head and neck in certain ways.

The aforementioned traditional chiropractic treatment was not resolving the problem. In fact, the dizziness was becoming worse when he merely turned his head.

While she was reflecting on the problem, her eye was caught by a pair of graphite current-conducting gloves that were resting on top of the microcurrent machine which was situated in a room across from her. Normally speaking, cosmetologists used the gloves in order to try to reduce or remove wrinkles and other age-related lines from the faces of clients.

She knew, on the basis of various animal studies, that microcurrents in and of themselves increased energy generation within cells by as much as 500%. She wondered what might happen if she were to send specific frequencies through those current-carrying graphite gloves in order to direct or focus such energy.

The foregoing image seemed to resonate with her. She brought her client into the room that was located across from her, attached the gloves to the microcurrent machine, adjusted the frequencies on the machine to the settings recommended by the manufacturer of the gloves, put the gloves on, turned the machine on, and, then, placed her gloved hands on the neck of her client.

As her gloved hands became, first, warm, and, then, hot, she could feel the trigger points in her client's sternocleidomastoid disappear. Within ten minutes, the hardness in the muscles had dissolved, and as this occurred, the pain and dizziness that had been endured by her client for such a long period began to dissolve as well.

The trigger points in her client's sternocleidomastoid were connected to the client's experience of dizziness. The use of frequencies had dispelled the presence of trigger points, and this in turn had led to the disappearance of the client's experience of dizziness ... a sense of dizziness which, on the surface, might not seem to have anything to do with knots in the sternocleidomastoid.

Consequently, using the microcurrent machine is not just a matter of applying sets of frequencies. First, one has to understand how the different facets of the human body connect with one another, and, then, one must try to work out what the actual nature of a given instance of inflammation is as well as how that inflammation could be rooted in underlying issues of function and dysfunction.

One might agree with a contention which Dr. McMakin makes in her book that, for the most part, allopathic medications tend to only reduce, eliminate, or mask different kinds of symptoms rather than offer a cure for the underlying problem out of which such symptoms have arisen. However, there seems to be a dimension of her work involving resonance in which although cures do take place and although specific resonances are used to bring about those cures, nevertheless, exactly what the foregoing frequencies are actually engaging, or impinging upon, is not actually clear.

Knowing how to counter inflammation without adversely affecting the biological terrain with so-called "side-effects" (which often are mislabeled as 'side-effects' but, in reality, are among the direct effects of those drugs) is an important accomplishment for Frequency Specific Microcurrent therapy and this is something that many allopathic medicines cannot do. In addition, knowing how different parts of the body are connected to other parts of the body so that one is in a position to grasp what underlying tissues or organs need to be targeted with certain frequencies in order to be able to effect a cure and not -- as much of allopathic medicine does – just engage in endless rounds of managed care that never results in an actual cure is also an important accomplishment.

Notwithstanding the foregoing considerations, one still would like to be able to know the precise nature of the dynamics which are taking place so that one could understand exactly how the frequencies that are being used interact with the biological terrain. One would like to know: What is being countered by such microcurrent frequencies, and/or what is being cancelled through the use of those frequencies and/or what is being changed through the use of such frequencies, and/or what is being reset when those frequencies are applied?

For instance, Royal Rife maintained that a microorganism which he referred to as "BX" was the cause of carcinoma forms of cancer, whereas "BY" was the name given to the microorganism that caused sarcoma forms of cancer. When he used different frequencies to destroy the presence of those microorganisms – as he did in the 1934 clinical trials held in conjunction with the University of Southern California -- cancer disappeared in most, but not all, cases.

Rife maintained that certain other diseases also could be traced to the presence of certain kinds of microorganisms that had been induced to transition away from a symbiotic relationship with the surrounding terrain as a result of some sort of toxicity or poisoning or trauma incurred by the body. When he zapped those microorganisms with the appropriate frequency, those sorts of pathologies also appeared to be cured, and this also was the experience of a number of doctors who used the technology which he had invented to cure their clients of a variety of disorders before those medical practitioners were eventually shut down by Morris Fishbein and the AMA.

The term "destructive interference" is a phrase that Dr. McMakin uses as a way of trying to account for what is transpiring during the microcurrent treatments. That term might be, to varying degrees, an accurate description of what is taking place when certain frequencies are applied to a given person's body, but the term also lacks a certain amount of specificity because it still doesn't provide one with a clear account of the dynamics that are involved in that kind of process since one doesn't know just what it is that is being interfered with or how that process of interference works.

When Dr. McMakin conducts her microcurrent therapy, she can generate genuine cures. However, as noted previously, one is not really sure what has transpired to make such a cure possible, and, in this respect she is somewhat like medical clinicians who have discovered uses for off-label drugs in the treatment of certain medical problem without necessarily understanding how those drugs – which were not manufactured to resolve such off-label uses -- achieve what they do.

None of the foregoing comments should be construed as a criticism of Dr. McMakin's approach to medicine. She has been able to successfully treat all manner of pathologies – including many kinds of maladies (such as asthma, fibromyalgia, complex regional pain syndrome, Crohn's disease, and Post traumatic Stress Disorder) that allopathic medicine tends to either ignore or with respect to which it has had a long history of failure (and a constant record of failure is often why they end up ignoring those sorts of medical issues).

Be that as it may, I am fairly certain that Dr. McMakin would be among the first individuals who would welcome the efforts of anyone who might be able to work out what, exactly, the frequencies from her microcurrent devices were affecting, or changing, or resetting, or eliminating within the biological terrain. Are those frequencies operating on various microorganisms – as Rife believed -- that might have transitioned away from a symbiotic relationship with the biological terrain and, in the process, are creating forces of interference with the ability of somatids to be able to epigenetically organize the activities of the full genome? Or, is it possible that the frequencies emanating from the microcurrent devices are somehow impacting somatids, or endobionts, or microzymas more directly in some way? Or, could it be some combination of the foregoing set of possibilities?

What is the nature of the interference which specific frequencies of microcurrents are acting upon? What are the underlying dynamics of that interference?

Although Dr. McMakin had the frequency chart used by Van Gelder that specified what frequencies to use with respect to surface conditions such as bleeding, bruising, inflammation, and scarring, there were many underlying conditions that were not addressed by the Van Gelder chart. Through a process of trial and error she had to discover how dysfunction in a given tissue would lead to various kinds of symptoms, and through a similar process of trial and error she had to figure out not only what frequencies needed to be used in conjunction with those symptoms in order to be able to treat the underlying condition, but she also had to determine the order in which various frequencies should be delivered.

A certain amount of time was spent varying treatment conditions during the aforementioned trial and error process in order to be able to rule out the possibility that whatever might be taking place was not a matter of the placebo effect. She wanted to be certain that is was the resonance established between the microcurrent therapy and a given medical issue that was responsible for resolving a problem as opposed to some sort of placebo phenomenon.

There was one form of feedback that helped guide her journey of trial and error and, among other things, helped her to differentiate between, on the one hand, the possibility of a placebo effect being responsible for treatment success and, on the other hand, the presence of a form of resonance being responsible for such successes that had nothing to do with the former phenomenon. More specifically, she learned that if the frequencies she selected to treat a given medical issue were correct, those frequencies would lead to changes in the pertinent tissue within seconds, but if the frequencies selected were incorrect, the problem remained as it had been prior to a given treatment during the trial and error process.

Microcurrent therapy was all about the match between the frequencies applied and the frequencies that were needed by a given kind of tissue needed in order for it to begin to healing. When resonance was established, physical problems got resolved, and when resonance was not present, those problems tended to persist.

Thus, if the nature of a given medical problem had to do with an injured or inflamed nerve, and the frequency appropriate to such a condition was applied, then, the pain and inflammation disappeared. On the other hand, if the foregoing problem was due to some sort of injury or inflammation involving a joint, or muscle, or bursa (a small sac of fluid that helps to reduce friction as well as cushion the interfacing of soft tissue and a bone), then, applying a frequency that was appropriate for, or capable of resonating with, a certain nerve would not resolve the problem.

Dr. McMakin also indicates in her aforementioned book that the process of trial and error she pursued was not only helped by the immediate feedback she got from whether, or not, an appropriate form of resonance had been established between therapy and the medical problem being addressed, there was something else involved as well. More specifically, she maintained that she had to learn how to be quiet or still within herself so that she could listen to what her intuition or the other person's body, or the universe, or God was communicating to her concerning the nature of the medical issue which was to be treated.

One is entitled to question just what was happening when various ideas, images and the like arose within her concerning how to proceed with a given form of treatment, but she could observe and keep track of those instances when there was a definite link between her trying to remove whatever factors (e.g., ego, beliefs, etc.) might be interfering with her ability to grasp what was taking place in another person's body and being able to find successful forms of treatment or therapy. The foregoing phenomenon was especially valuable when she began to treat much more complicated medical issues.

In order to try to find ways of removing aspects of her being that might be interfering with discovering the right kind of resonance treatment to apply to a given physical problem, she joined a Theosophical–based meditation group in 1991 that had been started by Harry Van Gelder in the late 1950s. The group met every Friday night, and she participated in those meetings for about eight years.

At a certain point during those meetings, she underwent a transcendent sort of experience of Oneness in which not only did she experience everything as being connected, but, as well, there was an internal stillness at the heart of that experience. Subsequently, whenever she made breakthroughs concerning how to treat a given condition which had been resistant to whatever therapeutic measures might have been taken previously, the foregoing sort of stillness often was at the heart of those kinds of epiphanies.

Over time, she developed a set of protocols for treating different conditions. Moreover, she found that individuals suffering from the same kind of malady could be treated with the same set of frequencies.

As word of mouth began to spread concerning the many successes that were occurring in conjunction with treating various kinds of pain and injuries at her clinic with FSM therapy, she was contacted in early 1999 by a medical doctor who wanted to establish a pain management facility in Northwest Portland. The doctor wanted his group to be able to offer an array of treatments (including the use of medications and injections) and, consequently, felt that the resonance/energy therapy in which Dr. McMakin was engaged should be added to the mix.

For quite some time, she had hoped that the very opportunity which was being offered to her might come along, and, therefore, she agreed to participate in the program. As a result, she worked at the Northwest Portland facility for several days a week, and, then, worked with other clients for three days a week in her own clinic.

After a period of time, she shared some of her successes with other members of that pain clinic during one of the weekly sessions that were held by the medical professionals who were participating in the program. Although the doctor who initially had recruited her was quite happy with the success which her Frequency Specific Microcurrent therapy was chalking up, one of the other "professionals" at the table was unhappy with what he was hearing.

When his opportunity to speak arrived, he stated that he was concerned about what sort of reputation their clinic would have in the medical community if that clinic became known as a pain facility that actually resulted in people's health becoming better. Four of the other "professionals" who attended the meeting shook their heads in approval in relation to what that "doctor" was saying.

Apparently, if one actually cured problems or substantially improved the quality of life of someone without having to entangle that person in an endless series of treatments and potential side-effects, then, the rest of the medical community might take a dim view of what their clinic was achieving. After all, the gold standard of allopathic medicine seems to be one of continuous managed care rather than actual resolution of the medical issues that are present in a given individual, and, here was Dr. McMakin treating people in a way that threatened the aforementioned gold standard of on-going, never-ending, side-effect-prone managed care. As a result, she resigned from the group.

At some point following her resignation from the Northwest Portland Pain Clinic, Dr. McMakin became interested in whether, or not, three might be ways to measure changes in pain levels that occurred in clients following certain kinds of resonance treatments. This would add a quantitative dimension to her clinical treatments.

Following one of her public workshops that were held to demonstrate to a wider audience various facets of her Frequency Specific Microcurrent therapy, she was approached by a member of the National Institute of Health. His name was Terry Phillips, and he was a specialist in what is referred to as "micro-immuno-chemistry" which enabled him to detect the presence of even very small amounts of molecules that were present in the bloodstream.

Furthermore, if we leave aside the issue of whether anything that was present in the bloodstream actually has something to do with some sort of immune function rather than, possibly, being components of processes involving detoxification and seeking to restore destabilized regions of the biological terrain to healthy working order, then, one might say that Terry Phillips, the NIH researcher, specialized in micro-chemistry of the bloodstream. In either event, he indicated that he would be willing to try to see if he could identify anything in the bloodstream of Dr. McMakin's clients that might be used as a measure which could serve to help quantify the issue of pain.

One should note that the individual from the NIH specializes in micro-chemistry. However, as Béchamp elucidated in his last written work – *Blood and Its Third Element* – there was an element in the blood (as well as in other organs, tissues, and cells of the body) that Béchamp considered to be the most fundamental unit of life and which he referred to as microzymas.

According to Béchamp, one could not reduce microzymas to some underlying set of chemical reactions. Instead, those entities were involved in the generating and shaping of many chemical reactions that took place in the body.

Like Naessens, Béchamp maintained that there were different kinds of microzymas operating in different organs and species of organisms. When conditions in the biological terrain were destabilized in some manner, microzymas were induced to undergo pleiomorphic/pleomorphic changes.

Consequently, whatever the nature of the techniques might have been that were being employed by Terry Phillips to aide his analysis of blood and, thereby, enable him to detect the smallest of chemical molecules that might be present in the blood, apparently, those techniques did not allow him to identify the presence of microzymas in that fluid. As a result, on the basis of his techniques in micro-chemistry, he would have been able to gain only a limited insight into the fundamental dynamics of the blood which, according to Béchamp, Naessens, and others, were largely shaped and regulated by the potentials associated with microzymas (Béchamp), somatids (Naessens), and endobionts (Enderlein).

Notwithstanding the foregoing considerations, Phillips sent special blotter paper to Dr. McMakin with instructions about how to use that paper. As a result, everybody who came to her clinic was asked to donate a few drops of blood to help further the study.

When the analysis of the blood samples came back from Terry Phillips, the data seemed to highlight the presence of cytokines. These small molecules were encountered previously in an earlier chapter of the present book during the exploration of various issues involving immunology and, in the process, arguments were put forth indicating why someone – for example, me -- might claim that human beings do not necessarily possess an immune system even though we do possess a biological defense system of sorts that does not operate in accordance with immunological principles as generally understood.

Since Dr. McMakin didn't know much about cytokines, she asked a friend of hers who she might contact to find out more about those molecules. Her friend suggested that she contact a guy by the name of Michael Ruff who, with Candace Pert, had written the book *Molecules of Emotion* because, apparently, he was one of the leading experts in the United States concerning the topic of cytokines.

Before moving on Michael Ruff's contributions to Dr. McMakin's resonance therapy, several points seem worth mentioning. First, one of the functions of cytokines seems to involve serving as messengers of one kind or another. Conceivably, pain causes such messengers to be sent out, or, alternatively, cytokines constitute a surrogate marker that is capable of detecting the presence of pain, but in neither of these cases, can one necessarily suppose that the cytokines are what constitutes pain. Secondly, and following from previously comments concerning what the techniques of micro-chemistry blood analysis are capable of identifying and what such techniques of analysis might be missing (i.e., the issue of microzymas, endobionts, or somatids), whatever Michael Ruff has to say about the nature of the relationship between cytokines and pain, like Terry Phillips, he might not have the full picture of what is transpiring in conjunction with the phenomenon of pain.

Given the presence of cytokines in the blood, one does not necessarily understand – based on their mere presence -- what causes their levels to go up or down. For instance, is it possible that when the levels of certain kinds of cytokines change that this has something to do with the way in which the underlying epigenetic system of adaptive learning for the body is seeking to regulate various aspects of the biological terrain or, alternatively, could the changing levels in certain kinds of cytokines be a function of the activity of microzymas, somatids, or endobionts? Or, perhaps, epigenetic activity gives expression to the manner in which such entities regulate the dynamics of the biological terrain.

In the book: *Cancer and the New Biology of Water*, Dr. Thomas Cowan indicates that whatever cancer is, it seems to be a metabolic disorder of some kind rather than a condition which gives expression to a genetic form of pathology. To lend credence to the foregoing perspective, he refers to research conducted across a number of years which continuously demonstrated that when the nuclei of cancer cells are transferred into healthy cytoplasm, then the daughter cells that arose from those cells were free of any sign of cancer-related issues, but when the nuclei of healthy cells are transferred to cancerous cytoplasm, the daughter cells that arise from the latter arrangement are cancerous.

Béchamp, Enderlein, Naessens and others all indicated that different kinds of microzymas, endobionts, or somatids were present in the organs, tissues, and cells that make up the body, and, as well, those entities flowed throughout the body via the bloodstream. Consequently, just as the foregoing experiments involving the transfer of healthy and cancerous nuclei into, respectively, cancerous and healthy cytoplasm might allude to the possibility that whatever metabolic problems which underlie the condition of cancer could be a function of destabilizing changes in the biological terrain that are inducing microzymas, somatids, or endobionts within the cytoplasm of some of the foregoing cells to pass on certain kinds of dysfunction in metabolism to daughter cells, so too, one might entertain the possibility that changes in levels of cytokines have been set in motion by the underlying activities of microzymas, endobionts, or somatids that are present in the bloodstream.

Dr. McMakin reports that when she modulated her ESM form of therapy by adding the aforementioned graphite current-carrying gloves and, then, subsequently sent to Terry Phillips -- the micro-chemistry expert working at the NIH -- blood samples from clients who had been treated by means of the foregoing protocol to Terry Phillips, she received back reports that, among other things, the level of endorphins went up as the level of cytokines went down which occurred in conjunction with reports from clients of experiencing significantly diminished pain or no pain at all.

Many of her clients experienced a sort of dreamy, drugged-like state during treatment which often led to them dozing off when pain from their condition began to subside. However, just as cytokines levels might serve as surrogate markers for the rise and fall of pain rather than constituting the pain itself, so too the presence of endorphins in the blood or their increase following FSM therapy does not necessarily mean that endorphins are the cause of the dreamy, drugged-like state which was experienced by many of her clients during certain protocols of therapy treatment.

One of the problems surrounding the issue of endorphins is the same as the questions that arise in conjunction with cytokines. More specifically, how do the activities of those molecules generate – if they do – the phenomenology of, respectively, pain relief and pain, in relation to various kinds of inflammation?

As previously noted, Michael Ruff was one America's foremost experts on cytokines. During a phone conversation between Dr. McMakin and Michael Ruff, she was asked by the latter individual to state what the cytokine readings had been for a certain patient, she indicated that the levels of interleukin-1 cytokines (which are associated with, but do not necessarily cause, conditions of inflammation) had gone done from a high of 392.8 down to 21.4. When Michael Ruff asked, and was told, that this downward transition had taken place within a period of 90 minutes, he was inclined to disbelieve what he was being told and responded by claiming that the levels for a given cytokine – such as interleukin-1 – were quite difficult to change, and if those levels changed at all, they tended to do so slowly.

Michael Ruff was further nonplused when he was informed by Dr. McMakin that it was not just the levels of interleukin-1 which had changed during the course of FSM treatment, but the levels of other cytokine (all of which tend to be associated with various forms of inflammation) had gone down precipitously as well. Interleukin-6 dropped to 15.6 from 204.3, while Interleukin-8 went from 59.9 to 4.8, TNF-alpha dropped from 299.1 to 20.6, and interferon gamma descended to 11.4 from 97.2.

There were other molecules, as well, that are related to issues of pain and inflammation that were present in the blood of the client being treated by Dr. McMakin. For example, substance P which is associated with increased levels of pain and arises in the spinal cord, as well as calcitonin gene-related peptide, or CGRP -- which seems to have some role in conjunction with the experience of pain -- both went down in response to FSM therapy.

The foregoing cytokine levels, along with the levels of other molecules that were detected in the blood of a client undergoing FSM treatments all served as objective measures for the presence or absence of pain being experienced by a given individual. However, were the Frequency Specific Microcurrents acting directly on the aforementioned molecules, or were those molecules merely the metabolites that precipitated from some other kind of dynamic taking place in the biological terrain. Were those objective measurements surrogate markers or were they the cause of pain?

As indicated previously, the measured cytokines that dropped in levels over the course of a 90 minute treatment were all associated with inflammation in some way. What is the nature of the message that is being sent by those cytokines?

Are they signaling for substance P and CGRP to go up when the former molecules increase in level, as well as signaling that levels of substance P and CGRP should drop when the levels of such cytokines drop? Or, do increases in P and CGRP induce the levels of certain cytokines to go up, while decreases in the two former molecules lead to a decrease in the presence of cytokines, along with an increase in endorphins, that are, in different ways, associated with the dynamics of inflammation?

Alternatively, perhaps the activity of some third element – say the activity of microzymas, somatids, or endobionts – cause levels of cytokines, together with levels of substance P and CGRP, to go up and down as a function of the activity of the entities being alluded to above. Conceivably, the various kinds of cytokines, as well as substance P and CGRP, all constitute information that is generated by, and used by, microzymas, endobionts, or somatids to induce the epigenetics of the biological terrain to move in one direction rather than another.

What is cause and what is effect is not always easy to parse out in any given context of biological functioning. Similarly, trying to determine exactly what FSM therapy is cancelling, changing, resetting, or the like with respect to the dynamics and metabolic pathways of specific cytokines and related molecules is not necessarily a straightforward matter.

Michael Ruff indicated during the aforementioned phone conversation that levels of cytokines are difficult to change, and if those levels changed at all, the tendency of those sorts of changes – prior to the presence of FSM therapy – was to take place slowly. What makes it so difficult for the levels of cytokines to change or why is it that when they do change, the transition, at least independently of FSM therapy, the levels of those molecules appear to occur slowly?

Perhaps whatever is holding cytokines in place under normal circumstances or whatever is resisting a change in the levels of those cytokines is what is being engaged by FSM therapy. When that form of dysfunctional interference is treated, then, cytokine levels drop because whatever messenger role they might be serving in the larger epigenetic dynamic is no longer relevant.

The fact that FSM therapy worked is not in question. What is still in question is how it accomplished what it accomplished, and the notion of destructive interference that is used by Dr. McMakin really doesn't explain what is actually taking place.

In passing, she does note during *The Resonance Effect* that we should all remember that on a quantum level we are probably more spatial than we are material, but, nonetheless, the material is held together by a network of electrochemical bonds that resonate at specific frequencies. Like the electronic fobs that are used to open and close various kinds of devices, the frequencies used in FSM therapy have the capacity to affect what is transpiring in conjunction with the foregoing electrochemical bonds.

She contends that frequencies are better able to change cell membrane receptors than are medications, and this is the model that she uses in conjunction with her FSM therapy. However, if Hillman's research – along with the research of others -- concerning the nature of the cell membrane is correct, then, conceivably, there might not be any receptors on, or in, most – perhaps all -- membranes and, as well, there might not be any active channel ways (except in certain kinds of excitable cells) present in most cells.

If various aspects of the considerable research put forth by individuals like Harold Hillman concerning, among other things, membrane dynamics – and some of his work has been introduced during the present chapter, -- or Gilbert Ling prove to be correct (e.g., among other things Ling re-imagined the nature of the sodium-potassium pump which operates within the body and also indicated that the water in our cells is unlike the water with which we are generally familiar and the former is crucial to the proper functioning of a cell ... this fourth phase of water will be explored in a subsequent chapter), then quite a few of the theories involving modern cell biology might prove to be problematic if not false, and, if this is the case, there could be quite a few issues in biology that remain something of a mystery. Among these remaining mysteries would be the research of Dr. McMakin because while she has put forth a extensive body of evidence to demonstrate that Frequency Specific Microcurrents do effect cures in relation to many different kinds of maladies – some of which defy the capacity of allopathic medicine to deal with successfully – nevertheless, irrespective of whether resonance operates through cell receptor membranes or through some other kind of undiscovered form of resonance dynamic, we still don't know precisely on what it is that the frequencies of FSM therapy – specific though they might be – are actually cancelling, changing, resetting, and so on.

We know that specific frequencies or resonances work. We just don't know what it is that they are working on.

In 2006, Nick Begich wrote a book entitled: *Controlling the Human Mind: The Technologies of Political Control or Tools for Peak Performance*. As the title indicates, Dr. Begich was concerned about both the constructive as well as destructive sides of a certain kind of technology, and since the technologies in which he was interested had to do with issues of frequency and resonance, it might prove to be an instructive follow-up to the work of Dr. Makin.

Dr. Begich began his public service by going to work for the school district that regulated educational issues in the city of Anchorage, Alaska. Some ten years later, he continued to work within the same school district, but he began to complement the day job with intensive research into various aspects of science and technology.

One of the first topics that he began to investigate was HAARP, the High-Frequency Active Auroral Research Project located in Alaska that was experimenting with what might happen if one probed the ionosphere with high-frequency wave forms. In 1994, he co-authored a book with Jeane Manning titled: *Angels Don't Play This HAARP: Advances in Tesla Technology*. The documents, articles, and other research materials that were critically reviewed in order to prepare for the writing of the foregoing book have served as the foundation of many of the other research projects in which he has been involved following the publication of the foregoing book.

The purpose of his books was to help educate the public. Moreover, the nature of the foregoing initial research project was to alert people to both the destructive, as well as, constructive potentials inherent in the manipulation of frequencies and the generating of resonance phenomena.

If all of life entails biological dynamics that give expression to, are shaped by, and, in one way or another, are governed by frequencies, and resonance then, the ideas, thoughts, feelings, emotions, desires, understandings, perceptions, interpretations, dreams, sense of identity, motivations, attitudes, interests, choices, behaviors, and languages which characterize human life also give expression to, and, to varying degrees, are functions of, frequencies and have a potential for involving resonance phenomena. Frequencies are not only involved in modulating what transpires internally within us as we experience the phenomenology of life but, as well, frequencies, when integrated into various kinds of technology, have the potential to manipulate all of the foregoing, internally generated features of the human psyche.

Every kind of naturally occurring frequency within the human body – or, indeed, within any form of life – can be interfered with or destabilized. As has been indicated on many occasions during the foregoing pages of the present book, different forms of destabilization or inflammation (including electromagnetic forms of interference) can, in turn, induce pleiomorphic/pleomorphic microorganisms to transition away from their normally symbiotic – or, at the very least, their inactive – relationships with the biological terrain of an organism.

Dr. Begich uses a traditional sort of biological vocabulary in order to illustrate the omnipresence of frequencies. In other words, he talks about: Cells, metabolic processes, genetic codes, proteins, receptors, cell membranes, organic chemistry, and so on in order to indicate how frequencies are present in governing day-to-day life within any given biological terrain (human or otherwise), and he points out that just as there is a genetic code, there is also a frequency code that is operative with living organisms.

While introducing various terms that are to be used to provide his research with a context that is intended to facilitate the understanding of anyone how might read his book, Dr. Begich does refer to the notion of liquid crystals which are forms of organized energy that are characterized by properties that combine qualities of both liquids as well as solid matter. Although he doesn't mention the idea of the fourth state of water when referring to the idea of liquid crystals, nonetheless, that notion resonates with some of the characteristic of structured water that will be explored in the next chapter of the present book.

Biological dynamics takes place through the phenomenon of resonance. Resonance is the way in which, or through which, different components of the biological terrain interact with and affect one another.

Consequently, frequencies are one of the common currencies that are exchanged in any given biological or ecological economy. In addition, as noted previously, frequencies also have the capacity to either help stabilize or destabilize those types of economies and, in the latter case, frequencies help set in motion conditions involving the life cycles of pleiomorphic/pleomorphic microorganisms that have the capacity to be pathological in nature.

However, there is a potential mystery which lies at the heart of all of the foregoing sorts of frequency transactions. This has to do with the unknown dynamics that take place within, and through, the basic units of life – whether referred to as microzymas, endobionts, somatids, or by some other term (e.g., the bions of Wilhelm Reich notion of biogenesis).

According to Béchamp, Enderlein, Rife, Naessens, and others, the events that occur within any given biological terrain are governed by the dynamics of different species of microzymas, endobionts, somatids, and the like. This means that the spectrum of frequencies which are present in any biological terrain are modulated, regulated, shaped, and give expression to the dynamics inherent in the aforementioned, basic non-cellular unit of life.

However, whether, or not, the dynamics of those basic units of life are a function of the sorts of frequency phenomena with which we are familiar, or whether the microzymas, endobionts, or somatids serve as transducers which transform one kind of energy into another form of energy is not, at the present time, at all clear. Consequently, conceivably, the frequencies that populate any given species of life could be regulated by something that can give rise to those frequencies but do so by transducing another kind of energy or information to generate the frequencies with which we are familiar that occur in the cells, molecules, and metabolic pathways of biological life forms.

Leaving aside, for the moment, the foregoing sorts of considerations concerning the basic unit of life, one should mention that Dr. Begich indicates how the electromagnetic spectrum consists of an array of frequencies ranging from those that are ultra low, but which also proceed on up through much higher frequencies that involve frequencies that give expression to more familiar forms of electromagnetic energy involving visible light, microwaves, radio waves, X-rays, and so on. He goes on to stipulate that while most of the natural frequencies that reach us tend to be scattered rather than coherent in form, there are pulsed forms of coherent energy that can be used to impact the resonant frequency of any particular object or process.

The technology associated with the structuring of energy is referred to as a process of 'electronic coupling' in which a pulsed, coherent form of energy can be tuned to vibrate at any particular frequency one might wish and, then, that wave form can be directed toward this or that aspect of biological functioning. Such processes of electronic coupling can alter the behavior of whatever process or object that is operating at a frequency which is resonant with the directed form of coherent energy and results in what is known as "frequency following behavior" – that is, the behavior of the targeted entity will begin, in different ways, to follow, comply with, or reflect, the frequencies that are being directed toward it.

Bioelectrical and biomagnetic fields are continuously being propagated through the human body. The presence of biomagnetic fields were not detected in the human body until 1963 when researchers discovered that the magnetic field of the heart operates at a level that is one-millionth the strength of the Earth's magnetic field. Eight years later, biomagnetic fields were detected in the brain, and these were several orders of magnitude weaker than the biomagnetic strength of the heart and 100 million times weaker than the strength of the magnetic field of the Earth.

Although the strength of the foregoing biomagnetic currents which take place in the heart and brain are very weak, nonetheless, they still can be affected by certain kinds of directed forms of energy. For instance, transformers can be used to transfer energy from one point to another by means of a process of magnetic induction which does not alter the frequency of that which is receiving such energy, and, therefore, once resonance is established, many kinds of inductive forms of energy manipulation are possible.

Electromagnetic fields consisting of high-end forms of energy that are directed toward living organisms tend to have the capacity to ionize the biological processes that go on within the organism or organisms toward which such energy might be directed. When this occurs, high-end forms of energy have the ability to damage tissue by creating biological havoc through the destructive ions that are generated by means of that kind of radiation (and, thus, is known as ionizing radiation).

However, there are forms of electromagnetic fields which are non-ionizing in character. These wave forms also are capable of establishing resonance relationships with different facets of biological functioning and, thereby, effect changes in that functioning by means of various bioelectric and biomagnetic phenomena.

Many Western standards of safety concerning the potentially debilitating and harmful effects which pulsed forms of electromagnetic energy can have on organisms, including human beings, tend to be focused on the capacity of those fields to generate thermal and ionizing effects that can inflict tissue damage and disrupting cellular dynamics. Such safety standards rarely, if ever, involve the many harmful effects (emotional, psychological, cognitive, cellular, metabolic, and genetic) that can be caused by non-ionizing forms of radiation.

When electromagnetic waves of a certain frequency are transmitted to a television, those waves have the capacity to carry information involving images and sound. As a result, such waves are known as carrier waves.

Carrier waves can be used to deliver all manner of signal waves. They can carry electromagnetic codes involving whatever information or effects someone might wish to communicate in such a context – including information that is capable of affecting biological phenomena.

When signal waves are mixed with carrier waves, this has the potential to give expression to the phenomenon of modulation. Modulation involves processes that affect either the height (amplitude) of a waveform or the frequency of those waveforms, and, therefore, alters the nature of the information which is being transmitted through carrier and signal waveforms.

Receivers – whether in the form of electronic devices or in the form of the human body – translate the information that is present in the signal wave, while energy can be transmitted to a given receiver by way of the carrier wave. Although Dr. Begich describes the frequency modulation dynamics that might occur in connection with living organisms (which serve as antennae) as processes that involve protein receptors which, supposedly, are present on, or in, cell membranes, nonetheless, as noted previously, Herbert Hillman and others have raised questions about whether proteins receptors are actually present on, or in, cell membranes.

Therefore, even though the research of Dr. McMakin -- which was explored somewhat toward the beginning of the present chapter -- indicate there can be no doubt that frequencies are capable of penetrating to the inner workings of organs, tissues, and cells, nevertheless, how those frequencies are able to engage different facets of a human being's biological dynamics is not necessarily known. The forgoing sort of caveat, however, should not be construed to be an attempt to deny that processes of frequency modulation can be used to transfer information and energy to the organs, tissues, and cells of human beings, as well as affect biological processes in other organisms.

During his discussion involving issues of frequency and resonance, Dr. Begich introduces the term "nanotronic nutrient effects." This phrase refers to those dynamics which are engaged in the transmission or delivery of either some form of dietary nutrient or some kind of device which is intended to have a frequency modulated impact on a biological system.

Exchanges of energy (involving carrier and signal components) constitute a fundamental part of biological dynamics. Nanotronic nutrient effects refer to forms of delivery or transmission that have the capacity to shape, modulate, facilitate, undermine, as well as interfere with the aforementioned sorts of exchanges.

One of the cautionary statements which Dr. Begich makes with respect to the whole issue of nanotronic nutrient effects is to raise concerns about the possible extent of the adverse impact on human beings and other life forms which: (a) Tens of thousands of chemical compounds that have not been properly tested (either individually or in congress with one another), along with (b) the ever-growing smog of electronic frequencies (which increase every time someone sends up another satellite to beam signals back to Earth) in which we all are immersed are having. Harmful nanotronic nutrient effects can be transmitted via both malevolent intent and willful neglect.

Dr. Begich quotes from a document entitled: "New World Vistas: Air and Space Power for the 21st Century – Ancillary Volume" which was published in 1996 by the United States Air Force Advisory Board. The foregoing document advocated for the development of technologies involving frequency modulations of signal and carrier waves that would have the capacity to: Disrupt existing memories of human beings, as well as undermine the ability to form new memories; impede movement; plant ideas or suggestions in the minds of human beings; and generate hallucinatory states which were considered by those experiencing those states to be reliable experiences that took place in the so-called "real" world.

The Air Force, together with: Other branches of the military, the CIA, DARPA (Defense Advanced Research Projects Agency), as well as any number of intelligence agencies have had nearly three decades of access to billions of dollars in black-bag budgets to be able to bring the foregoing ideas to fruition. Anyone who supposes that if and when the foregoing sorts of ambitions are realized that they will be applied only to people who live elsewhere has not been paying attention to what has been transpiring in America for quite some time.

For instance, if were to leave out critically reflecting on the assassinations of John Kennedy, Martin Luther King, Robert Kennedy, along with the events surrounding 9/11, together with the wars in Vietnam, Iraq (I and II), and Afghanistan – not to mention the invasions of Grenada and Panama – all of which government officials lied about and tried to hide the truth concerning those events, one might consider an article written in a September 29, 1994 edition of *The Washington Times* in which the authoress, Karen MacPherson, recounted how the United States government abused and terrorized at least 500,000 Americans and deliberately exposed various segments of that set of a half million citizens (many of whom were poor, homeless, institutionalized, physically or mentally challenged in some way, or were members of minority groups) to all manner of chemical, radiological, psychological, biological, and eugenics-oriented experiments. Alternatively, one might also recall that such stalwarts of democracy and the "rule of law" as Madeline Albright and Bill Richardson publically stated that while the decision might have been difficult, nonetheless, killing 500,000 children during the Iraq war was a worthwhile thing to do.

MKULTRA is not a conspiracy theory. It constitutes an American government operation (involving hundreds of different research projects) that helped to undermine, damage, and, then, set loose, on the American public, people such as Theodore Kaczynski (the so-called Unabomber).

'The Senate Select Committee to Study Governmental Operations With Respect to Intelligence Agencies' that was convened in 1975 and chaired by Frank Church, revealed that for more than 25 years, the CIA, along with other groups within the U.S. government, had been experimenting on thousands of American citizens without the latter's consent or even knowledge. Many people might wish to blame Timothy Leary for introducing college students to LSD, but, as it turns out, people at the CIA were serving as the wizard behind the curtain and were operating the levers that helped initiate the foregoing phenomenon.

Or, consider the fact that the Air Force Research Laboratory put out a call for research proposals that was to remain open until 2009. It was titled: "Research in Support of the Directed Energy Bioeffects Division of the Human Effectiveness Directorate"

The purpose of the foregoing call for research proposals was so that fully articulated theories and models involving the use of nonlethal forms of directed energy could be developed. The research being sought by the foregoing proposal was intended to generate technologies that were able to induce people to be compliant and behave in certain ways.

For instance, Extremely Low Frequencies or ELFs that involve non-ionizable forms of radiation require very little power. One can use directed forms of such energy that are only 1/50th of the strength of naturally occurring fields involving the Earth.

As such, those kinds of controlled, directed waves would tend to be considered as so much noise when engaged in connection with naturally occurring electromagnetic fields that are generated by the Earth. Yet, despite the relatively weak character of the pulsed signals that can be generated through ELFs, those kinds of signals still can have a substantial impact on what takes place within human beings.

The phenomenon of "cyclotron resonance" might be what enables the aforementioned low-power, pulsed ELFs to be able to penetrate biological processes within living organisms. Cyclotron resonance appears to be a means of transferring certain kinds of energies from one point (e.g., a transmitter) to another point (e.g., a human tissues and cells) without requiring any sort of mediating mechanism (e.g., membrane receptors) to assist such energies to gain access to, and, thereby, cause effects in, the biological terrain of human beings and other life forms.

All of the foregoing research is geared toward establishing what is known as a "frequency following response." This occurs when dynamics in the brain are entrained to follow, or be modified by, the presence of some sort of externally pulsed electromagnetic field that induces behaviors in the targeted individual or individuals which are being shaped by the incoming pattern of pulsed signal.

Moreover, the foregoing sort of research and events are not taking place just in the United States. The work and the real-world events which precipitate from that work are occurring all over the world.

For example, the Soviets were engaged in research concerning the impact that microwave radiation and extremely low frequency pulsed fields had on human beings. The United States discovered back in the 1970s that the Soviets had been directing microwave energy at individuals who worked at the U.S. embassy in Moscow ... directed energy that was capable of destabilizing emotional health as well as interfering with the process of thought.

In addition, the Soviets had not only developed a technology known as a LIDA machine which employed ELFs or Extremely Low Frequencies, but, as well, were researching other means of electromagnetic transmission involving those kinds of frequencies. The ELFs were often pulsed between 6 and 11 Hertz which is capable of resonating with, and, then, entraining, similar sorts of frequencies that normally occur in the human brain.

The research – wherever it is being conducted -- is being driven by the fear of, and desire to control, "the other." This latter category identifies those against whom it is supposedly "ethical" to use the weapons being alluded to in the foregoing Air Force documents, and, unfortunately, the process through which one becomes "other" tends to be fluid and flexible according to the needs of those who feel comfortable making unethical judgments as well as those who are more than willing to self-servingly employ those kinds of technologies to achieve some desired degree of control over the lives of "the other."

In a sense, the research of Dr. Makin serves as a proof of concept that many of the foregoing possibilities might already have been achieved, if not further refined and modified. Although her work has been directed toward attempting to improve the lives of people rather than being dedicated to the manipulation or enslavement of human beings, nevertheless, she has shown that: Emotions; mobility; attitudes; levels of substance P (associated with pain); endorphins (associated with relief from pain as well as a sense of dreamy well-being); and, cytokines (associated with bodily inflammatory conditions) are all capable of being manipulated.

In the latter part of his book: *Controlling the Human Mind: The Technologies of Political Control or Tools for Peak Performance*, Dr. Begich does explore constructive uses involving the phenomenon of "frequency following response" or behavior in which directed pulsed forms of energy are employed to enhance processes of human learning, memory, performance, and so on. Unfortunately, through no fault of Dr. Begich, a lot more government or corporate time, effort, and money seem to have become entangled in exploring the dark side of frequency following response than its constructive side.

Be that as it may, the research of Dr. McMakin concerning how to use directed frequencies to resolve, among other things, what allopathic medicine often tends to treat as intractable problems of ill-health, as well as the research of individuals such as Dr. Begich that is dedicated to discovering ways in which directed energy can improve various modalities of cognitive functioning, are both expressions of the frequency following response phenomena. Interestingly enough, both Dr. McMakin and Dr. Begich, each in her or his own way, have experienced push back from various segments of the allopathic medical industry.

Through sanctions, censuring activities, investigations, propaganda, and control of the CDC and FDA, many individuals representing the allopathic modality of technocracy have sought to impose their own form of frequency following response phenomena on individuals who are exploring the constructive uses of that phenomena. Apparently, many individuals who are wielding power within the allopathic establishment, along with many of their acolytes, seem to believe that constructive uses of frequency following responses threaten various aspects of their oftentimes fanatical-like medical theocracy.

In closing out the present chapter, one might also note that the manner in which somatids, endobionts, microzymas, or bions, impact the dynamics of cells, tissues, and organs might also give expression to the phenomenon of frequency following response. Indeed, epigenetic dynamics could be described as the study of frequency following responses in which the energies that are transduced by, for example, somatids help organize the epigenetic activities of the biological terrain so that a state of detoxified/stability is maintained or recovered in which the microbiome and the biological terrain are in a state of symbiosis with respect to one another.

Chapter 15 – Energies of Life

Dr. Jerry Tennant went through medical school and, eventually trained as an ophthalmologist. At a certain point in his adult life, while practicing as a doctor, he developed encephalitis.

His particular case was extremely serious. He started to experience significant memory problems, as well as had uncontrollable spastic movements, and, for a while, had a bleeding disorder.

In addition, he lost, for the most part, about seven years of his life (1995-2002) when he began to sleep for 16 hours a day. During the remaining eight hours of his day, he had difficulty focusing on much of anything, but he did have approximately a three hour window within the aforementioned 8-hour daily period when he had sufficient cognitive faculties at his command to be able to read a newspaper.

He sought the assistance of medical experts at Harvard and the National Institute of Health. However, they were baffled by his condition.

Dr. Tennant is of the opinion that he contracted encephalitis from one of his patients on whom he was performing Lasik surgery and who was also suffering from leukemia. He believes that a virus, of some sort, escaped from his patient's eye, made its way through his mask, and, then, entered his brain after travelling through the nasal canal.

There is no reliable way to confirm how Dr. Tenant actually became ill. His viral account is, in the absence of any supporting evidence, nothing more than a narrative.

Given that a number of medical experts were puzzled by his condition, one might entertain the possibility that, perhaps, the etiology of his illness could have been something other than what he supposed had been the cause of his condition. In fact, in certain ways, his illness had many of the earmarks of someone who had undergone an encounter with some form -- or forms – of EMF toxicity that either was (were) acute in nature or were chronic and had accumulated over a period of time.

At some point his biological terrain might have reached some sort of a tipping point with respect to the presence of such EMF toxicity. As a result, his body broke down, and he began to suffer an array of neurological and blood-related problems.

Whatever the etiology of his illness might have been and in the absence of any kind of medical expertise that might have helped him to deal with his difficulties, he started to reflect on how to escape from the pathology that had consumed so much of his life in such fundamental ways. Yet, as noted earlier, he only had about three hours a day in which his brain seemed to work well enough for him to be in a position to try to figure out what to do.

One of his first thoughts was that he believed that all cells of the body worked in a similar fashion. If he could find a way to heal one cell, then, he might have found a way to heal all of his cells.

With that possibility in mind, he purchased some 10-15 books on cellular biology. Apparently, Dr. Tenant was working on the assumption that the basic unit of life is the cell, but as Béchamp, Enderlein, Rife, Naessens and other proponents of the pleiomorphic/pleomorphic theory of microorganisms indicate, the cell is not necessarily the basic unit of life, and if this is the case, then, Dr. Tenant might have begun his inquiry based on a problematic assumption.

Notwithstanding the foregoing considerations, one of the principles that emerged from the research of Dr. Tenant into cell biology is that all cells appear to be designed to operate within a pH range of 7.35 to 7.45. In effect, he felt that pH describes a form of voltage in liquid form in which electrons had the opportunity, depending on circumstances, to either donate or receive electrons.

The movement of electrons gives expression to physics. From such physics, chemical transactions arose, and, so for Dr. Tenant, physics seemed to have a role to play in relation to resolving his physical problems.

According to Dr. Tennant, a pH reader really serves as a voltage meter. Thus, a pH of 7.35 translates into a voltage of -20 millivolts involving the movements of electrons that are being donated, whereas a pH of 7.45 gives expression to a voltage of -25 millivolts that are generated through the process of electrons moving as they are being donated to, or received by, one or another atom or molecule.

By convention, if a particular solution tends to receive electrons, a plus sign is placed before the voltage that is being generated. On the other hand, if such a solution tends to donate electrons, then, a minus sign is placed before the voltage.

Voltage can be converted via a logarithmic scale that will produce results ranging from 1-14. And, as indicated previously, cells operate optimally when the pH of those cells stays between a pH of 7.35 (-20 millivolts) and a pH of 7.45 (-25 millivolts).

In order to maintain the foregoing sorts of cell voltage, cells need energy. -25 millivolts are needed for cells to be able to operate properly, and -50 millivolts of energy are needed for the formation of new cells.

Different cells within the body tend to wear out at different rates. When such cells wear out, they have to be replaced.

For example, cells in the nervous system tend to turn over every 8 months. Liver cells need to be replaced every 8 weeks, while skin cells go through replacement cycles that take place every 6 weeks, or so.

Obviously, energy is needed in order for the foregoing sorts of replacement processes to be able go forward. Moreover, prior to their replacement, in order for cells to be able to last until they are replaced, energy is also required to keep the day-to-day functioning of those cells operational.

For Dr. Tennant, all chronic disease involves, in one way or another, the presence of an inadequate voltage to be able to underwrite or accommodate cellular energy needs. Consequently, whatever the ultimate cause of Dr. Tennant's disease might have been, the bottom line is that according to his perspective, his disease condition emerged as a result of – somehow -- inadequate voltage being present in certain cells, tissues, organs, and so on.

In addition to the energy that is required to maintain cells and to help subsidize the replacement process, energy is also needed to tend to the problems that are caused by environmental toxins such as the glyphosates that come from certain pesticides, or the heavy metals that are present in many products or which are by-products of different manufacturing or industrial processes (for example, the mercury that is given off as an emission when certain kinds of coal are burned).

Such toxins constitute constant sources of stress on biological systems. As a physician friend of mine pointed out to me with respect to a bout of illness that had befallen me nearly two years ago, most Americans suffer from adrenal insufficiency because their biological systems or terrains are constantly under stress from all the toxins that are being dumped into the environment – including EMF-based environmental toxins.

According to Dr. Tennant, the human body is a movable electronic module. Therefore, it needs access to battery packs that can supply it with the energy it needs to, among other things, move about in the world.

He identifies four such battery packs in the human body. To begin with, the muscles in our bodies serve as rechargeable battery packs.

The fascia -- or band of connective tissue (usually consisting of collagen) that surrounds muscles -- gives expression to an extensive wiring system that runs throughout the body. Piezoelectricity – which arises when mechanical stresses are placed on a given substance and generate a flow of electrons – plays a major role in the energy dynamics of the muscles.

Each organ has its own battery pack as a result of the system of muscles that run from our toes to our head. In effect the fascia that surround muscles form semi-conductors.

A semi-conductor is an arrangement of molecules which conduct a flow of electrons in only one direction at the speed of light. These semi-conductors are at the heart of the battery pack recharging system that helps serve the energy needs of the organs which those semi-conductors are associated.

There are six loops of circuitry involving the system of battery packs that are entailed by the networks of muscles, and surrounding fascia that are found throughout the body. The nature of such circuitry is fairly complex, and every stack of battery batteries can be associated with an acupuncture meridian.

For instance, the Stomach-Spleen battery pack supplies the energy that underwrites the activities of the endocrine system. In addition, the aforementioned battery pack supplies the energy for the reproductive systems in both females and males, as well as supplies energy for the macula of the eye and various kinds of cognitive processes in the brain.

Notwithstanding the complexity of the foregoing sorts of circuitry, there is a process akin to the sort of differential diagnosis process that a car mechanic might go through to figure out where voltage is not being maintained within a computerized vehicle. For instance, one might have to check the levels of the thyroid hormone T3 because this hormone plays a key role in regulating the voltage of every cell membrane in the body.

Or, maybe one will have to check the levels of the T2 thyroid hormone. This hormone has an intimate relationship with what transpires in the mitochondria, and there are many other such checks that can be performed.

According to Dr. Tenant, a second rechargeable battery pack system is located in cell membranes. These battery packs exist in the form of a network of capacitors. Capacitors are able to store energy.

According to some traditional theories, membranes of cells consist, among other things, of two opposing layers of fat cells or phospholipids. The phospholipids are made up from constituents that form two conductors separated by an insulator. By definition, this constitutes a capacitor which is capable of storing electrons.

At this point one might wish to keep in mind something that was touched upon early in the last chapter of the present book. More specifically, according to the research of Herbert Hillman, the traditional way of characterizing the cell membrane as a tri-laminar structure (consisting of two opposing layers of fat cells or phospholipids) might be an artifact of the methodological procedures used when trying to obtain a micrograph of a cell membrane rather than being a reflection of the actual structure of a cell membrane.

If the tri-laminar character of cell membranes turns out to be an artifact that is generated by the methods that are used to produce a micrograph of some kind, then, the cell membrane does not consist of two conductors separated by an insulator. Moreover, if the cell membrane does not consist of two conductors (the phospholipids) separated by an insulator, then, no capacitor exists for storing electrons.

A third battery pack system exists within the mitochondria that uses a complex process of electron transfer involving the dynamics of energy formation via ATP (adenosine triphosphate) and energy expenditure via ADP (adenosinediphosphate). When this battery is charged, reference is being made to the presence of ATP, and when the battery stands in need of recharging reference is being made to the fact that ADP has resulted from the donation of an electron to some cellular process and, therefore, needs to undertake a journey back to ATP (i.e., its recharged state).

The recharging process is known as the Citric-Acid or Krebs cycle. For the most part, this metabolic pathway involves taking fatty acids through a series of transitions that generate and transfer electrons in conjunction with the molecular components that make up the cycle, and if oxygen is present during the various steps of the cycle, then, for each unit of fatty acid that is processed by the Krebs cycle, 38 ADP batteries are recharged.

A fourth form of battery recharging comes through DNA. This involves the dynamics of scalar forces (which, in turn, seem to be connected to the golden mean -- 1.618 – as a function of distance between units that are make up the structure of the helix) that are used by DNA to complete its various tasks of replication, transport, and assembly.

According to Dr. Tennant, chronic disease arises when there is one, or more, failures in any of the foregoing systems of rechargeable battery packs. In other words, such systems cannot sustain an electric charge of the requisite sort (i.e., -20 to -25 millivolts) within the cells of those organ systems.

However, is there any reason to suppose that various kinds of acute diseases – and not just the sort of chronic diseases to which Dr. Tennat refers -- could also arise as a result of, for whatever reason, some sort of loss of voltage in one, or more, of the four battery pack systems within the human body. Both chronic and acute diseases might arise as a result of the presence of some kind of environmental toxin – such as tend to be generated through EMF-based forms of technology that spill dirty or jagged, pulsed forms of electricity into the environment on a constant basis.

Dr. Tennant notes that the energy recharging stations of the body are wired up like many circuit boards in computers. Many of the latter circuit boards make use of Tesla resonating circuits.

A Tesla resonating circuit consists of a capacitor (energy storage) and a coil (conductor), and each is wired in parallel. When the foregoing kind of an arrangement exists, the circuit has the capacity to communicate (in the language of electro-magnetic interactions) with other kinds of Tesla circuits – whether these are part of some sort of external form of circuitry or they are part of the circuitry involved in the energy recharging stations of the body.

Consequently, resonance interactions that occur between what is transpiring electronically outside the body and what is taking place electromagnetically within the body could be taking place. These sorts of resonance interactions might play a role in undermining the way the energy recharging systems in the body operate and could be part of the reason why voltage might be lost as such systems are engaged by environmentally toxic systems of EMF-based technology in problematic and destabilizing ways.

There is a great deal of quality work that has been done concerning the biological toxicity that is being generated through EMF-based forms of technology by, among others: Arthur Firstenberg (and all the many individuals about whom he writes in *The Invisible Rainbow* who have made fundamental contributions to this work); Elana Freeland (*Under and Ionized Sky* and *Geoengineered Transhumanism*); Robert Becker and Andrew Marino (e.g., *Electromagnetism and Life*); Daniel T. DeBaun and Ryan DeBaun (*Radiation Nation*); Samuel Milham (Dirty Electricity); Dr. Devra Davis (*Disconnect: The Truth About Cell Phone Radiation, What the Industry is Doing to Hide It*), as well as the work of Olle Johansson, Dr. Martin L. Pall (who has shown how EMF adversely affects human and animal biology by interfering with voltage gated calcium channels) and many, many others.

However, just as certain forms of electricity are harmful to, and destructive of, biological processes, there also are forms of electricity that can have constructive impacts on helping the body to repair whatever might be causing a loss in voltage within various battery packs (and the research of Dr. McMakin is just one example of how to go about restoring the health of someone's biological terrain). In this respect, Dr. Tennant has invented what is known as a BioModulator which is capable of recharging the ATP-ADP battery pack process. He also indicates that different muscle battery recharging packs can be treated by using various kinds of patches on the bio-terminals of what is known as a BioModulator.

When the cells in tissue are damaged by, for example, some form of EMF-based toxicity, the tissue goes to -50 millivolts which is well outside the parameters of optimal cell functioning. This in turn causes the arterials running through such tissues to dilate, which, in turn, gives rise to the symptoms of inflammation (such as temperature heat, swelling, redness, and pain).

If the battery charging system associated with adversely affected tissue cannot provide the necessary voltage which is capable of underwriting the energy costs of repairing damaged tissue, then a person might transition from some sort of acute condition of disease to a more chronic form of that disease as a result of a continued absence of the voltage that is necessary for healthy cell, tissue, and organ functioning.

As voltage is dropping, oxygen levels also will begin to lower. The efficiency with which metabolism takes place is, to a large extent, controlled by the relative presence or absence of oxygen, and the amount of oxygen that might be available is controlled by the degree of voltage that is present, and as a result, this can have problematic consequences for the amount of ATP that is available for subsidizing the biological activity that takes place with the cells of tissues and organs.

When the body is healthy, oxygen levels help to suppress the tendency of the bacteria within us to generate digestive enzymes that will dissolve cellular material in order for the bacteria to be able derive the nutrients that such bacteria need. As voltage and oxygen levels drop, bacteria tend to lose their cell membranes and become cell-wall deficient organisms – or stealth pathogens – which begin to generate various kinds of toxins that are capable of damaging the cells and tissues with which those toxins come in contact.

Such toxins can produce a variety of symptoms. These symptoms range from: Headaches, and a fever, to: Vomiting, diarrhea, as well as different kinds of joint pain, depending on the tissues being affected by the presence of such toxins.

If the voltage becomes sufficiently low –- say in the vicinity of +30 millivolts) other entities begin to show up. For instance, this might involve the emergence of cell-wall deficient fungi which present their own problems for a struggling biological terrain.

Consequently, what starts out, for instance, as some kind of EMF-based form of environmental toxicity, could, in time – as a function of the loss of voltage, along with the emergence of toxins that bacteria or fungi might produce -- lead to a whole host of other problems that are capable of affecting different systems within one's body -- neurological, respiratory, blood processes, metabolism, energy/voltage levels, and so on. All of the foregoing issues start – whether acutely or chronically – with a loss of voltage which EMF-based technologies (and other kinds of environmental toxins) are capable of bringing about under the right set of circumstances.

The foregoing seven or eight pages provide an overview of Dr. Tenant's perspective concerning the energy of life. It gives expression to a theoretical model that seeks to organize an array of data involving energy dynamics within the human body.

There are several alternative ways of engaging the data which Dr. Tenant is trying to organize that might resonate with certain facets of his perspective and, yet, go about the process of energy dynamics in a different manner. For example, one might try to account for the energy of life by looking at the dynamics of water within living organisms.

Pursuing the foregoing kind of critical reflection need not necessarily negate what Dr. Tenant is advancing. Instead, looking at the dynamics of water within living organisms – human or otherwise – might complement what Dr. Tenant is claiming as well as introduce some ideas concerning the energies of life that might even be more fundamental than the principles which were advanced during the foregoing overview involving the theoretical perspective of Dr. Tenant.

During the early part of his book: *The Fourth Phase of Water: Beyond Solid, Liquid, and Vapor*, Gerald Pollack mentions the name of Gilbert Ling a number of times. For example, on the book's dedication page Dr. Pollack acknowledges how Gilbert Ling introduced the author to the idea that the behavior of water within the biological terrain is quite unlike the way in which water behaves in a cup, and, then, a short while later in his book, Dr. Pollack notes how Gilbert Ling invented the glass microelectrode which was an invaluable tool in electrophysiological research because, among other things, it helped to generate evidence which indicated, contrary to existing models and theories concerning the cell, that water operated in accordance with various principles of structuring which conventional theory had not only missed but which, if accepted, would substantially alter how biologists might view what went on within a cell by shifting their focus from the dynamics of molecules within a liquid medium to the dynamics of water and how those dynamics affected molecular transactions that took place within that medium.

Gilbert Ling is mentioned for a third time within a few pages of the aforementioned book when Dr. Pollack points out how many, if not most, scientists of that time did not embrace the innovative research of Dr. Ling. Instead, they tended to reject him and sought to persuade people like Dr. Pollack that becoming associated with Dr. Ling or his research was not a good career move and was likely to sully one's professional reputation.

Thus, Dr. Ling inspired Dr. Pollack in two important ways. On the one hand, the focus of Dr. Ling's research substantially influenced various facets Dr. Pollack's own, subsequent, research, and, on the other hand, Dr. Pollack perspective was also shaped by the courage and integrity displayed by Dr. Ling while challenging some of the scientific theocracy of his day.

As a result of the foregoing sorts of inspiration, Dr. Pollack believes that like the notion of epicycles that was employed in an attempt to save the appearance of Ptolemaic theory when the latter offered explanations that were inconsistent with what was indicated through direct observation of the heavens, Dr. Pollack believes that theories of water have become too burdened by epicycle-like dynamics which have become bogged down in a collection of ad hoc beliefs that have been assembled into a theoretical edifice which is at odds with what can be observed when water is studied directly. Therefore, rather than merely becoming entangled in processes which did little but add ever more epicycle-like ideas which distort one's attempt to understand the nature of water, Dr. Pollack wanted to simplify the study of water by moving away from uncorroborated, ad hoc, theory-driven notions of water and, instead, move toward an empirically or observationally-driven investigation of water.

Although most everyone knows that the chemical formula for water is H_2O, the actual structure of water has been the subject of a considerable amount of debate. Dr. Pollack begins his foray into that debate by distinguishing between two kinds of water, namely: bulk water and structured water.

Bulk water is what one might encounter when one fills up a cup from the tap. Structured water, on the other hand, entails a variety of characteristics that tend to remain hidden in ordinary tap water.

For example, when water is juxtaposed next to some material that has hydrophilic properties – that is, the material is water-loving – then, an Exclusion Zone (the term was introduced by John Watterson, an Australian) emerges in such water. This zone – as the associated term indicates – excludes almost everything from that sector of water, and in the process of doing so, generates a separation of charge in which the exclusion zone is shaped by the presence of negatively charged electrons, while positive charges (to be discussed shortly) are pushed away or repelled from the place where the negatively charged exclusion zone is adjacent to the aforementioned hydrophilic surface.

Technically speaking, Exclusion Zones are never completely free of contaminants. However, experiments have been done by Dr. Pollack and others which indicate that there is an inverse relationship between the size of the Exclusion Zone and the extent to which contaminants are present, and, therefore, the fewer contaminants that are present, then, the larger the Exclusion Zone tends to be, while the greater the relative degree of contamination that is present, then the smaller the associated Exclusion Zone tends to be.

Another factor that affects the size or robustness of a given Exclusion Zone involves the character of the hydrophilic surface that serves as the nucleation site for the emergence of such an Exclusion

Zone. Hydrophilic templates that are robust tend to give rise to exclusion zones that reflect that robustness, but there are a number of factors such as structural character of that template or the extent to which contaminants are present which also can affect the properties of an Exclusion Zone.

In bulk water, exclusion zones do not form. Moreover, there is a relative absence of charge in bulk water, or, said in a slightly different way, the molecules in bulk water have a neutral charge in which the two atoms of hydrogen cancel out the charge of the single atom of oxygen.

When water becomes structured, then the protons within water tend to become organized in certain ways that are in response to the way in which the Exclusion Zone forms and becomes negatively charged. This results in the formation of positively-charged hydronium ions (H_3O^+).

Furthermore, just as negative charges have degrees of freedom that govern their movement within the Exclusion Zone, so too, hydronium ions (H_3O^+) have the capacity to move about to varying degrees within their own region of activity. The respective movements of the two kinds of charges can affect both the size of the Exclusion Zone as well various kinds of dynamics that might occur along the boundaries which demarcate the Exclusion Zone and the adjacent region of positively charged hydronium ions.

In effect, the hydrophilic surface, plus the negatively charged exclusion zone, plus the presence of hydronium ions creates a battery. The exclusion zone is populated with negatively charged electrons, and it is book-ended by a hydrophilic surface on one side and a zone of hydronium ions (H_3O^+) on the other side, and the foregoing separation of charge (the battery) can be maintained if it is suitably charged.

For instance, when radiant energy (e.g., from the sun or some other source) engages the foregoing battery, the battery becomes charged. Part of the foregoing radiant energy helps to maintain the separation of charge that constitutes the battery.

The negatively charged Exclusion Zone has the capacity to form a series of layers. Each of which consists of a repeating sequence of honeycombed-shaped structures made up of oxygen and hydrogen molecules that lend a crystal-like character to those layers.

The aforementioned honeycombed layers stack one on top of another in parallel fashion relative to the hydrophilic surface that served to nucleate the structuring process within water. The negative charge which characterizes the Exclusion Zone is a function of the way the honeycombed sequences come together as various layers of those sequences are formed.

More specifically the honeycombed, hexagonal character of the foregoing layers was due to a conclusion that was drawn on the basis of an array of different kinds of physiochemical data. This data consisted of measures involving freezing points, density considerations, diffraction patterns, boiling points, as well as spectral analysis of the frequency properties that are present in structured water. When considered as a whole, the foregoing data was consistent with, and seemed to point in the direction of, the idea that a latticework of hexagonal structures seemed to characterize the Exclusion Zone.

The lattice that is formed by the repeated hexagonal units which make up any given layer of the Exclusion Zone consists of a ratio of three molecules of hydrogen to two molecules of oxygen, and, therefore, every hexagonal unit carries a negative charge. This is why, collectively speaking, the Exclusion Zone as a whole is negatively charged.

Another one of the properties that is associated with the foregoing sort of hexagonal or honeycomb lattice structures is that those layers have the capacity to slide by one another in different circumstances. This means that the interactive dynamics between layers tends to entail a low degree of friction which could affect the sorts of dynamics that might occur within structured water.

For instance, when a given latticed layer within the Exclusion Zone interacts with the layers above and below it, there are a variety of ways in which those layers can be stacked one on top of the other. These variations are due to the way in which areas of negative and positive charge on one layer align with negative and positive regions of adjacent layers as they slide by one another, and such variations can lead to an array of different kinds of localized dynamics within such water depending on prevailing circumstances.

When the bond angles that are present in structured water have been examined, they have been shown to differ from the bond angles that are present in water when it is in a liquid, gaseous, or solid phase. This is one of the reasons why structured water is considered to be the fourth phase of water.

In addition, when electrons are able to move through a latticework fairly freely, they usually exhibit the property of being able to absorb ultraviolet wavelengths in the order of 270 nm. This property shows up in different kinds of materials that consist of hexagonal arrangements, and, consequently, when the Exclusion Zone in water was experimentally demonstrated to absorb ultraviolet wavelengths at 270 nm, this was another indication that the structure of the latticework appeared to be hexagonal in nature.

One might also note in passing that some individuals might question whether appreciable amounts of hexagonal-shaped layers of a crystalline-like latticework would be able to form given the existence of different kinds of thermal agitation which might be present within cells or tissue. Dr. Pollack points out that the more that such layers accumulate, then, the less likely will the dissipating force of thermal agitation tend to arise because such layers actually have a dampening down-like effect on the activity of those sorts of forces.

Before moving on, one might also note that the layers of hexagonal-shaped latticework that arise within structured water play a fundamental role in helping the Exclusion Zone to develop and expand. More specifically, on the one hand, the hexagonal-shaped structures which make up the latticework are quite narrow and, therefore, tend to exclude most solutes from entering into the Zone, and, on the other hand, the different layers tend to not be lined up with the layers to either side of them, and, as a result, this also tends to keep most solutes – including hydronium ions -- from being able to enter into the Exclusion Zone.

Although most of Dr. Pollack's book explores the Exclusion Zone as a region that is characterized by a negative charge, he also points out that positively charged Exclusion Zones are not only theoretically possible but have been empirically demonstrated to exist. Such zones were discovered to have occurred in conjunction with the presence of certain kinds of metals and polymers.

Although positively charged Exclusion Zones appear to be less common than negatively charged Exclusion Zones, nonetheless, the reality of such a possibility tends to induce one to ask certain kinds of questions. For example, is it possible (given the right nucleating surface within any given biological terrain – say, in conjunction with various metals which occur naturally or which have entered a given biological terrain via some sort of medical injection or environmental poisoning) that positively charged Exclusion Zones might form which could have various kinds of impact (either constructive or problematic) on that terrain?

The properties of positively-charged Exclusion Zones appear to be the inverse of what is observed in conjunction with negatively-charged Exclusion Zones. However, experiments also have demonstrated that due to the relative absence of oxygen in positive Exclusion Zones, those zones tend to be more susceptible to breaking down or dissipating than negatively charged Exclusion Zones.

Nevertheless, if, given the right set of circumstances, positively-charged Exclusion Zones were to occur in biological terrains, and if those zones were inclined to dissipate more readily than is true in relation to negatively-charged Exclusion Zones, one wonders about whether, or not, the presence of such fragile systems still might have the capacity to destabilize some facet of the biological terrain in which they form and, in the process, induce certain elements within the microbiome to transition away from a normal symbiotic relationship with that terrain and give rise to some kind of pathological condition.

The foregoing consideration seems especially relevant topics for critical reflection given the extent to which environmental pollution has been occurring for quite some time in different parts of the world. Increasingly, various kinds of heavy metals have been finding their way into the bodies of all manner of living organisms, and, consequently, asking whether the presence of those metals – along with an array of different synthetic polymer compounds that have been permitted to be dumped into the environment without any sort of adequate safety tests taking place – might be involved in potentially problematic positively-charged Exclusion Zones emerging (even for relatively short periods of time) within living organisms.

On the other hand, one might also reflect on the possibility that positively-charged Exclusion Zones could arise in conjunction with (that is, be nucleated by) naturally occurring metals that are in the body, or Exclusion Zones might arise in conjunction with molecules (for example, proteins) that contain some sort of metallic ionic component, such as zinc, which are known as metalloproteins, and these sorts of molecules occur fairly frequently in living organisms. The bioelectric and biomagnetic currents which occur in different aspects of the biological terrain might not just be generated through the formation of the batteries that are entailed by the sort of structured water which is characterized by a negatively charged Exclusion Zones, but, as well, such bioelectric and biomagnetic currents might be generated through the formation of batteries that arise in conjunction with positively-charged Exclusion Zones.

There could be a multiplicity of possibilities involving the kinds of constructive electrical circuitry that are possible within the context of any given cell, tissue, or organ. While the majority of the localized batteries that give expression to such circuitry might be a function of negatively-charged Exclusion Zones, and even though positively-charged Exclusion Zones might have a tendency to dissipate more easily than their negatively-charged counterpart, nevertheless, positively-charged Exclusion Zones could have a role to play within the dynamics of bioelectric and biomagnetic phenomena as a result of the batteries that come into play within the biological terrain.

At one point early on in his delineation of the properties of structured water, Dr. Pollack introduces terms such as "droplets" of water, "bubbles", as well as "vesicles" and, then, differentiates the use of those terms. Thus, whereas (1) a droplet consists of a positively charged interior surrounded by a negatively charged Exclusion Zone, (2) a bubble has, with one exception, the same structural properties as a droplet and that exception is that its interior consists of some sort of gas, usually in the form of water vapor, and (3) the term "vesicle" is a generic way of referring to both droplets and bubbles with the proviso that when a sufficient amount of energy is transferred to a droplet, the latter becomes a bubble because the interior is transformed into some sort of gas, usually in the form of water vapor.

Starting with hydrophilic surfaces to which water is adjacent, and proceeding on through: (a) The creation of negatively charged Exclusion Zones that become structured into crystalline-like layers of honeycombed sequences made up of two oxygen and three hydrogen molecules that preferentially absorb ultraviolet wavelengths of 270 nm and which can be stacked in a variety of ways involving forces of attraction and repulsion that can lead to different kinds of localized dynamics; (b) the simultaneous formation of a zone of hydronium ions (H_3O^+); (c) the separation of charge that exists between the Exclusion Zone and the zone of hydronium ions that possesses battery-like properties; (d) the maintaining of that separation of charge through the influx of some source of radiant charge; (e) the possibility of there being both negatively-charged and positively charged Exclusion Zone-based battery systems that occur in cells as well as tissues, and, finally, (f) the notions of droplets of water, bubbles, and vesicles, Dr. Pollack has introduced a network of ideas that can be used to explain an array of water-related phenomena which have mystified many observers. For example, the foregoing ideas can be used to account for why gelatin preparations, which consist mostly of water, don't leak water, or why tsunami waves are able to sustain themselves over long distances whereas ocean waves tend to dissipate within relatively short distances.

The foregoing ideas also can be organized to account for how warm water can be used to induce an ice cream mix to freeze more quickly than would be the case if one were to use cold water. Alternatively, when properly understood, the foregoing ideas are able to plausibly explain why some of the water in a person's body's rushes to a destabilized area of the biological terrain during the process of inflammation, as well as account for the forces that enable water to reach the top of a 300-foot Redwood tree without breaking the capillaries that transport that water, as well as enable to provide a possible explanation for how certain lizards are able to walk – or run – on water.

Different chapters of *The Fourth Phase of Water* by Gerald Pollack are devoted to not only generating answers to the foregoing issues, but, as well, various chapters of that book also explore other equally interesting phenomena involving water that some people might have thought were understood on the basis of previously developed theories concerning the nature of water but which, with the right kind of critical examination, can be seen to involve principles other than the ones which had been presumed to be true with respect to those kinds of phenomena. By critically reflecting on a series of problems such as those noted above and which can be understood through the appropriate use of the aforementioned itemized list of ideas or principles that are present in structured water, Dr. Pollack assists readers to develop a deeper insight into how water might be operating in the context of everyday life – including the biological events that give expression to that life.

While the foregoing comments allude to an array of interesting phenomena involving water, none of those topics will be pursued in what follows. Dr. Pollack addresses all of the those issues, as well as many more, in his aforementioned book, and there is a lot on which to reflect if one takes the conceptual journey that is being mapped out in his work.

Instead, the plan for this chapter has been to introduce enough information about the dynamics of structured water to lend plausibility to two principles that I believe are actively present in the biological terrain ... principles which are consistent with everything that has been said up to this point in my book. The two principles that are being alluded to are: (1) the dynamics of structured water constitute a primary source for the energy that either helps subsidize or takes the place of the different kinds of battery packs that were outlined when providing an overview of the work of Dr. Jerry Tennant in the first part of this chapter; (2) the dynamics of structured water within living organisms are organized by the epigenetic capacities that have been hypothesized to be present in microzymas, endobionts, or somatids. Or, said in another way, epigenetic processes (according to the blueprint of order that is inherent in, for example, somatids) are initiated or triggered by introducing various kinds of hydrophilic molecules (such as proteins) into different facets of cellular and tissue functioning in order to generate the energy-producing batteries that are present in structured water and which, thereby, enable metabolic transactions to take place in a manner that is directed toward engendering a condition of detoxified stability within any given biological terrain so that symbiotic relationships might be maintained by, or re-established through, that terrain and the microbiome which occupies it.

Part of the foregoing process of generating detoxified stability involves the manufacture and distribution of energy in a way that helps maintain the basic voltage necessary for cells to function properly that was stressed by the Jerry Tennant material. This voltage value – in humans – runs between -20 to -25 millivolts (and is associated with a pH of, respectively, 7.35 (-20 millivolts) and a pH of 7.45 (-25 millivolts).

The foregoing voltage and pH values are part of the blueprint through which the specialized somatids, endobionts, or microzymas which (according to Béchamp, Enderlein, Rife, and Naessens) populate the cells and tissues of different organs and which govern the dynamics that take place in those sectors of the biological terrain. Those dynamics give expression to an array of adaptive learning processes that are regulated by the epigenetic programs and algorithms which are present in the hypothesized blueprint with somatids, endobionts, or microzymas that set the voltage of life values which Jerry Tennat maintained were crucial to properly functioning cells.

Dr. Tennant also indicates that the electrical dynamics involved in the circuits of life could have semi-conductor like properties associated with some of those circuits. Interestingly, Dr. Pollack notes that the existence of various kinds of contaminants (which he believes can never be entirely removed) which are present in and around the Exclusion Zone could give expression to the activity of an n-type semiconductor under the right conditions.

A semiconductor exists when certain kinds of electrical conductivity are present within a crystalline-like structure. An n-type semiconductor is created when an impurity (contaminant) of some kind is added to a semiconductor which affects the manner in which that latter structure conducts electricity.

Earlier, mention had been made concerning the possibility that positively-charged Exclusion Zones might occur within the biological terrain and how both constructive and problematic properties could be associated with those sorts of Exclusion Zone-based batteries. During that discussion, the notion of metalloproteins was introduced in passing, and, conceivably, those sorts of metalloproteins, along with other kinds of metallic molecules, could form n-type semiconductor-like dynamics within cells.

In addition, while previously exploring some of the dynamics associated with the cell-membrane battery-packs that have been proposed by Dr. Tennant, I mentioned a possibility in which the tri-laminar character of cell membranes might not be correct and, instead, such a structure might actually constitute an artifact that is generated by the methods which are used to produce a micrograph of some kind. If this is true, then, contrary to what is claimed by Dr. Tennant concerning the issue of cell-membrane related battery packs, those membranes might not consist of two conductors separated by an insulator, and, consequently, if cell membranes do not consist of two conductors (the phospholipids) separated by an insulator, then, according to the model of Dr. Tennant, no capacitor would be available to store electrons.

However, Dr. Pollack's notion of a battery pack that is formed through the emergence of the separation of charge [between, say, a negatively charged Exclusion Zone and a zone populated largely by positively-charged hydronium ions (H_3O^+)] does exhibit properties which might entail a capacity to conduct currents as well as to store electrical charge. Therefore, there are elements present in structured water which might have capacitor-like qualities capable of conducting and storing electrical charges within cells and tissues that are quite independent of whatever dynamics might, or might not, occur in relation to cell membranes.

Dr. Thomas Cowan mentions something similar in his book: Cancer and the New Biology of Water, when he indicates how Gilbert Ling critiqued the traditional notion of a sodium-potassium pump. Dr. Ling claimed that such a pump was actually a function of the properties inherent in structured water rather than being a function of the dynamics of proteins that, supposedly, are located on, or which extend through (as transmembranes) any given cellular membrane.

When discussing the kind of sodium-potassium pump which has been proposed by Gilbert Ling, Dr. Cowan suggests that such a process does not require energy in order for the formation of structured water to be able to take place. If, by the foregoing suggestion, Dr. Cowan is indicating that no <u>extra</u> energy is required for those dynamics to occur, then, I would agree, but, perhaps, a certain clarification is needed.

For example, in order for an Exclusion Zone to be generated, some sort of hydrophilic surface must be present which one cannot assume just materializes ex nihilo but, presumably, that surface is present through the expenditure of some kind of energy. Furthermore, the force of attraction which is present in the phenomenon that makes something hydrophilic also gives expression to a form of energy which is being expended as water and that surface interact.

In addition, the forces of repulsion which come into play during the creation of the Exclusion Zone and which maintain a separation of charge also give expression to a process of energy transactions that are taking place. Moreover, the formation of the hexagonal latticework that characterizes the Exclusion Zone, together with the formation of hydronium ions along the periphery of that zone, also involves energy transactions.

If the foregoing arrangement of energy transactions is induced to dissipate, then the dynamics of structured water will disappear. Therefore, while no extra energy is needed to induce those dynamics to take place once the right set of conditions are present, nonetheless, those conditions and the dynamics to which they give rise are all different modalities of energy transactions.

According to Dr. Cowan, Gilbert Ling proposed that there are certain molecules known as "cardinal absorbents" which are capable of triggering or inducing phase changes in various aspects of cellular water. As noted previously in this chapter, such phase-changes tend to lead to the formation of negatively charged (usually) Exclusion Zones in which positive charges (i.e., hydronium ions), are relatively absent or separated (excluded) from the foregoing zones. This separation of charge establishes the conditions necessary for the emergence of a battery that can bring about the removal of sodium from a given cell while, simultaneously, potassium becomes concentrated in that cell.

Although Dr. Cowan discusses how trigger molecules can alter the phase properties of water within cells, he doesn't appear to indicate what regulates the presence or absence of those sorts of molecules. One might suppose, however, that the dynamics of those kinds of triggering molecules are regulated by the epigenetic instructions that are being issued through the presence of somatids, endobionts, or microzymas within cells and tissues, and, as a result, different facets of cells or tissues can be induced to change the localized phase character of water in a given region by introducing the appropriate triggering molecule at the right place and at right time which would set in motion whatever kind of structured water dynamics were needed to carry out a given biological operation or set of operations in that region or locale.

According to Dr. Tennant, there is an additional battery pack system that exists within the body that is associated with the mitochondria which populate the cytoplasm of cells. As previously noted, this battery pack utilizes a complex process of electron transfer, known as the Citric-Acid or Krebs cycle.

For the most part, the foregoing cyclical, metabolic pathway involves taking fatty acids through a series of transitions that generate and transfer electrons in conjunction with the molecular components that make up the cycle. If oxygen is present during the various steps of the cycle, then, for each unit of fatty acid that is processed by the Krebs cycle, 38 ADP (Adenosinediphosphate) batteries are recharged into Adenosine triphosphate (ATP), and, the latter molecule, is used to subsidize various kinds of energy requirements within cellular, tissue, and organ dynamics.

However, in the aforementioned book by Thomas Cowan – i.e., *Cancer and the New Biology of Water* – the author indicates how Gilbert Ling contends that the traditional understanding of the Krebs cycle as the power plant of a cell is misguided. According to Ling, and contrary to the opinion of many scientists, the Krebs cycle does not generate ATP (adenosine triphosphate) as a means of providing energy to run various metabolic pathways within the cell.

Instead, Ling proposes that the function of ATP is to help proteins to unfold in ways that enable those proteins to bind with, or interact with, different regions of structured water within the cell. The energy that actually makes biological processes possible is a function of the batteries that are generated when the appropriate sort of triggering mechanism induces Exclusion Zones to form, which, in turn, lead to a separation of charge (i.e., battery formation) between the negatively charged (usually) Exclusion Zone and the adjacent regions that have become populated with positively-charged hydronium ions.

In order to provide a sort of proof of concept notion concerning the idea that the role of ATP in the cell involves unfolding proteins rather than offering a source of energy that, supposedly, operates biological functions within the cell, Dr. Cowan refers to the way in which the making of Jell-O utilizes heat to unfold gelatin proteins so that the latter molecules will bind with water in order to help create a viscous gel-like condition which will form when that mixture is subsequently cooled. For Ling, and Dr. Cowan, ATP serves the same function in cells as heat does in the making of Jell-O, and, therefore, ATP helps proteins to unfold so that they can bind with water and help shape the dynamics that will occur in and around the gel-like conditions that emerge in conjunction with structured water.

Although Dr. Cowan does not directly address the following issue (however, he does speak of "the life force of the organism"), one might suppose that just as earlier the idea had been introduced which suggested that the epigenetic dynamics inherent in somatids, endobionts, or microzymas (which, Naessens, Enderlein, and Béchamp did consider to be the life force of organisms) are responsible for regulating the triggering dynamics involving what Ling referred to as cardinal absorbents, so too, the epigenetic dynamics that are inherent in somatids, endobionts, or microzymas, might also control how, where, and when the ATP that is produced by the Krebs cycle will be used within any given aspect of the biological terrain. Presumably, a certain degree of efficiency would be introduced if one were to suppose that the same center of command and control which is responsible for regulating the activities of triggering molecules also would be responsible for the dynamics of the ATP production that provide the mechanism through which different proteins are able to unfold so that they can interact in appropriate or necessary ways with the structured water that has been triggered to arise in different localized areas of cells, tissues, or organs.

Another proposal which formed part of Dr. Tennant's battery pack theories concerned sources of energy that might be available to the body for purposes of maintaining the voltage of life (outlined in the first part of the present chapter) has to do with the notion of scalar forces which Dr. Tennant indicates are generated in conjunction with DNA. Supposedly, these sorts of forces lead to, or, are somehow associated with, the emergence of battery packs that are used by DNA to complete various tasks of replication, transport, assembly, and so on.

One issue connected to the foregoing has to do with whether, or not, the foregoing kinds of scalar forces are actually capable of generating the requisite batteries, circuitry, and storage capacities that might be necessary be able to fully subsidize the genome's capacity to underwrite an array of tasks involving transcription, transportation, translation, as well as the epigenetic processes that shape the way in which the DNA code is to be parsed. Another issue present in the foregoing scenario involves asking the following question: Why not just suppose that structured water is able to occur in the regions where the genome resides and, if this were to occur, that water would be fully capable of providing the localized sorts of battery-generated currents, circuits, and electrical storage properties that are needed for whatever sorts of DNA-related activity takes place, and, therefore, if the foregoing were the case, there would be no need to posit a scalar-oriented set of forces that regulates various functions associated with the expression of genes?

The comments in the previous paragraph are not intended to indicate that such scalar forces do not exist in relation to molecules of DNA. Rather, the intent is to suggest that acknowledging the possible presence of those sorts of scalar forces is not the same thing as demonstrating how those forces would not only be able to generate or become associated with a system which would be capable of providing the energy that subsidizes genome-related activities but, as well, would take place within a system that was capable of regulating the use of such energy during processes of transcription, translation, transportation, assembly, and so on.

As noted earlier in the chapter, Dr. Tennant maintains that, in one way or another, all chronic disease involves the presence of an inadequate voltage (i.e., something other than being maintained between the -20 and -25 millivolts that are needed to underwrite or accommodate the sorts of cellular dynamics which generate health). Consequently, whatever the ultimate cause of a given form of chronic disease might be, nevertheless, according to Dr. Tennant, somewhere during the course of life that condition emerged as a result of the presence of an inadequate voltage in various cells, tissues, or organs.

The perspective being put forth by Dr. Pollack is not inconsistent with the foregoing general position that is being proposed by Dr. Tennant. However, Dr. Pollack – along with Gilbert Ling, Thomas Cowan, and others – are proposing that, among other things, the problems associated with the existence of an inadequate voltage might be a function of various kinds of pathological dynamics that are undermining conditions which are conducive to the formation of structured water within cells, tissues, or organs.

If one were to add some of the considerations that were advanced during the previous chapter on epigenetics to the foregoing perspective concerning structured water, then, one might suggest that both acute and chronic diseases occur when the process of forming regions of properly functioning structured water within cells, tissues, and organs becomes dysfunctional due to way in which the epigenetic communication between, on the one hand, somatids, endobionts, or microzymas and, on the other hand, water within the biological terrain is being interfered with or undermined in some fashion. In other words, in order for a condition of detoxified stability to exist in which the biological terrain of an organism is in symbiotic balance with the microbiome that occupies that terrain, then, a healthy form of communication must be maintained between the 70% of cells that consists of water and the epigenetic system that is present in somatids, endobionts, or microzymas that are being hypothesized to be responsible for regulating the formation of regions of structured water within cells through the process of "frequency following response" that was explored in the last chapter.

As noted previously in the present chapter – Dr. Tennant believes that the four proposed energy recharging stations of the body are wired together like many circuit boards in computers. He believes that those kinds of circuit boards establish conditions which constitute Tesla resonating circuits.

According to Dr. Tennant, a Tesla resonating circuit consists of a capacitor (energy storage) and a coil (conductor) being wired in parallel. Consequently, there appears to be nothing that is required to form a Tesla resonating circuit which, at least in principle, might also be found in the way in which different regions of structured water within a cell could be linked or "wired" together to form parallel circuits that involve both the property of conduction (i.e., a coil) and the property of energy storage (i.e., a capacitor) and, therefore, constitute a Tesla resonating circuit.

Dr. Tennant maintains that those resonating circuits have the capacity to communicate (via frequencies) with other kinds of Tesla circuits. These resonating circuits could be part of some sort of external form of electronic circuitry in, say, a weapon (which was seeking to induce "frequency following responses" in targeted individuals) or those Tesla resonating circuits might be part of the energy dynamics that exist within the body both in the form of linked regions of structured water, as well as in the form of the dynamics that might be taking place within somatids, endobionts, or microzymas and which epigenetically communicate with or regulate (via frequencies) the formation of regions of structured water within cells, tissues, and organs that carry out an array of biological functions or give expression to various kinds of metabolic pathways.

Finally, one might note that the Exclusion Zones of structured water have properties that are quite resonant with the notion of liquid crystals which were touched upon during the discussion of the work of Dr. Begich in the previous chapter. During the course of that discussion, some of the constructive and destructive potentials inherent in the notion of "frequency following responses" were explored.

The notion of structured water seems to be immersed in the dynamics of frequency following responses. For instance, this seems to be taking place when (through, for instance, the release of triggering molecules) the dynamics of phase changes that give rise to structured water are set in motion by means of the epigenetic processes (which, among other things, govern the activity of triggering molecules) that are organized by somatids, endobionts, or microzymas, thereby, creating conditions within the biological terrain which will entrain an array of biological molecules within cells, tissues, and organs to respond to the epigenetic programming that is regulating cell, tissue and organ dynamics at the behest of the basic unit of life – namely, somatids, endobionts, or microzymas.

Moreover, given Naessens' report (noted in Chapter 5) that the exterior portion of somatids could not be penetrated even when a diamond-tipped drill was employed, then, the shell or membrane which encloses such an entity is not likely to be characterized by various kinds of receptor or transmembrane dynamics. Instead, the means through which somatids, endobionts, or microzymas communicate with the world beyond the interior of those entities would seem to be in terms of frequencies and resonances.

All of the foregoing considerations are not meant to be definitive treatments concerning the dynamics of energy within the biological terrain, but, rather, they only are intended to provide an overview of possibilities. Dr. Pollack and others have explored the details of those kinds of dynamics much more intently than what is being presented here, but, nonetheless, the general perspective that is being advanced in the present book has been enriched by virtue of the ideas concerning energy sources that have been critically reflected upon in the present chapter.

Chapter 16: Fields, Quantum Dynamics, Transducers

Given the amazing properties (the so-called fourth phase) that are potentially present in water when the right sorts of conditions exist – conditions which, to some degree, have been delineated during the last chapter – the topic selected for transitioning in to the issues with which the current chapter are concerned also has to do with water. However, this present exploration will take us through some different realms of possibility.

In 2001, a book written by Masaru Emoto was published. It was entitled *The Hidden Messages in Water*, and it was a sequel to his earlier 1999 book: The Messages of Water.

Prior to exploring the phenomena which were the focus of the foregoing two books, Masaru Emoto had been engaged in research concerning the measurement of wave fluctuations that occur in conjunction with water. At some point, he became interested in the formation of crystals that took place when water was frozen, but, more to the point, he became fascinated by the way in which water seemed to be able to capture certain kinds of relationships that were transpiring prior to water being frozen and which, to varying degrees, were able to be fixed via the crystallized patterns of one kind or another that formed in water which had been frozen and, then, induced to melt.

The aforementioned book – namely, *The Messages of Water* – consisted mostly of photographs. Trying to communicate in words the possibilities that were being depicted in photographs would be a daunting task, however, during his second book: *The Hidden Messages in Water*, he sought to provide an hermeneutical perspective, of sorts, concerning some of the forces that might be at work and which led to different kinds of patterns becoming fixed in the crystals of frozen ice, and, therefore, most of the ensuing comments will be directed toward the aforementioned second book rather than toward his initial work.

Dr. Emoto begins by noting that, while the percentage tends to change as we age, human beings consist mostly of water, ranging from a high of 90% when we exist as fetuses, and dropping to, perhaps, somewhere slightly over 50% during old age. What happens to that water during the aging process has a lot to say about, among other things, our health and emotional state of mind.

While conducting research in America, Dr. Emoto discovered that water appeared to have the capacity to copy and store information. In support of the foregoing claim, he cites a 1988 experiment of Jacques Benveniste that was intended to lend credibility to the homeopathic principle which indicated that a diluted solution of a given substance could have the same efficacy or effect that an undiluted solution of that same substance had.

In his experiment, Benveniste took a medicine and diluted it to such a degree that the presence of the medicine could no longer be detected via clinical methods. Nevertheless, the diluted solution was demonstrated to have the same efficacy as an undiluted form of that same medicine, and, therefore, in some sense, the diluted solution appeared to have retained a memory of the properties of a medicine that had been diluted to a point where the latter's presence could no longer be detected.

In order to study the patterns in crystals that might arise in conjunction with frozen ice, Dr. Emoto developed a process that permitted him to take photographs of water during the 20 to 30 second period during which crystals form on the surface of ice as the latter begins to melt. One of the first things which he discovered was that the kind of crystal structures that might form -- if they formed at all -- depended on the nature of the water being studied.

For example, the water in Tokyo is chlorinated, and this interfered with and prevented the formation of crystal structures. If, on the other hand, water came from natural sources – such as springs – then crystalline structures would appear for a short period of time.

Presumably, the foregoing form of interference is a straightforward matter of chemistry. In other words, crystals did not form because, in some way, the presence of chlorine molecules prevented the formation of ice crystals.

Next, Dr. Emoto began to expose water to different kinds of stimuli prior to the time when the water was to be frozen but, subsequently, would be photographed during the critical timeframe during which crystal formation might occur. Initially, such stimuli involved music.

For example, when he played various compositions of classical music in the presence of the water that was to be frozen, different kinds of beautiful patterns and structures were subsequently captured during the brief period when crystals would form. Yet, when he exposed water to heavy metal music, whatever patterns appeared in the crystals seemed to be jagged and incomplete.

One question that might be raised at this juncture is the following one. Is the water responding to the music, per se, or, alternatively might it be responding to Dr. Emoto's obviously positive attitudes toward classical music as well as his apparent distaste for heavy metal music, or, perhaps, the crystalline patterns that form might be a function of both the kind of music that was played as well as the attitudes or emotions which someone like Dr. Emoto might feel concerning that music?

For instance, if someone who didn't like classical music was involved in the foregoing sorts of experiments, would the results be the same? Or, if someone who liked heavy metal music was participating in those experiments, would the patterns of crystallization still be incomplete and fragmented?

One also wonders about what impact other kinds of music might have on the formation of patterns within the crystals that emerged during the critical period in which they were photographed. For instance, what would happen if: Jazz, country, pop, Christian spirituals, rhythm and blues, atonal music, qawwali, Gregorian chants, or Chinese traditional music were used rather than either classical music or heavy metal music were played?

Would differences emerge in the nature of the crystalline patterns that might form in response to any of the foregoing kinds of music, and, if so, what would the nature of those differences be and what, if any, significance should be assigned to those differences. Alternatively, if there were no significant differences (whatever this might mean) in those patterns, what conclusions should be drawn concerning the foregoing sorts of outcomes?

Moreover, if there was some kind of fragmented or incomplete crystalline pattern that appeared in conjunction with water being exposed to other kinds of music, would those kinds of patterns be the same or would those patterns be different in some way? One might also wonder what the nature of the interference dynamics are that might result in such incomplete or fragmented patterns.

Being able to demonstrate that water appears to be able to differentially respond to the presence of various kinds of music is one thing. Being able to determine what the precise nature of the response dynamics are which leads to the formation of crystals of one kind rather than another is a different issue.

Part of the aforementioned sorts of dynamics has to do with the issue of storage or memory. In other words, there is a period of time that passes prior to the time when crystalline patterns form and, then, are photographed.

Therefore, during this period of time, some sort of dynamic must be present which is capable of storing, and, then, when the time comes, imprinting -- in the form of a pattern on a crystal -- whatever effect such music has had on the water. Even if the nature of such a dynamic involves nothing more than electromagnetic frequencies, one still would like to know how those frequencies are stored in water prior to being photographed, and, then, one would like to know what the nature of the transfer dynamic is that converts storage into a crystalline pattern.

If water were to crystallize in the same way irrespective of the attitudes of the people who were engaged in the experiment, then, one might ask another kind of question. Why was the water picking up on what was going on with the music and not at all picking up on the emotions, feelings, or attitudes of the individuals who were present during the time when water was being exposed to different kinds of music?

The foregoing question is actually quite relevant. This is because the next set of experiments pursued by Dr. Emoto involved words and their possible impact on the patterns that might appear in water as it was crystallizing following a period of freezing.

Various kinds of words (e.g., "Fool") and short phrases (e.g., "Thank You") were written on pieces of paper, and, then, wrapped around the containers of water that were to be frozen and later photographed during the period of crystallization. Once again, Dr. Emoto indicated that the crystals which formed in conjunction with the phrase "Thank You" exhibited complete hexagon shapes, whereas the crystals that emerged with respect to the word "Fool" were incomplete and malformed as had occurred when heavy metal music was played.

What would have happened if the individual who was wrapping the written words around the containers of water was insincere or intended to be sarcastic and, therefore, gave expression to an attitude which was inconsistent with the message "Thank You?" Alternatively, what if the thoughts associated with the written word "Fool" were not meant as a noun which was intended to convey a negative attitude toward someone else but was being used as a verb to describe what happens when a magician artfully performs a trick that fools the audience?

Moreover, if the thought processes, emotions, and attitudes of the individual who was wrapping the word or phrase around the water container made no difference to the character of the pattern that appeared in crystalline form, then, certain questions seem to bubble to the surface. More specifically, why does the water only appear to capture a certain kind of interpretation of the written message, of if the attitudes of the individuals engaged in the experiment proved to be irrelevant to the nature of the crystalline patterns that formed, then, why is the water apparently resonating with the written message rather than with what is transpiring in the person or people who are participating in the experiment?

If the attitudes, thoughts, and emotions of the people involved in the experiment are irrelevant to the sort of crystalline pattern which forms, then, another question emerges. Are we to suppose that water has some sort of linguistic capability which enables it to transduce the written message into some sort of storage/memory dynamic that can be imprinted on, or incorporated into, a crystalline pattern?

Irrespective of how the foregoing questions are answered, if there is a relationship between music and water, and/or between written words and water, and/or between people and water, then, what is the character of the dynamics that translate music, and/or words, and/or emotions into crystalline form? Should one suppose that the process is only a function of electromagnetically induced frequency phenomena, or, is it possible that some other kind of force, set of forces, or field is present which mediates the processes of storage/memory and pattern formation in the ice crystals?

Are there laws or principles governing that process? For instance, is there some sort of inverse square law which is operative which sensitizes water to some stimuli (e.g., most proximate) while ignoring other stimuli (e.g., less proximate)?

Are some phenomena to which water is exposed "experienced" as being more ordered (resonant) or less chaotic (resonance of a different kind) than are other kinds of stimuli to which water might be exposed? Perhaps, water is responding to the relationship between order and chaos that exists in any given stimuli or set of stimuli rather than responding through some aesthetic sense of beauty or moral sensibility.

Whatever the precise nature of the dynamics are which might be governing the formation of patterns and structures in water crystals, those dynamics appear to involve resonance phenomena of some kind. In other words, there appears to be a process of "frequency following response" that is taking place in which the pattern in the crystallized ice (the response) is following some sort of frequency associated with a given stimulus such as music, words, and so on.

Although the notion of "frequency" is most familiar in a context of electromagnetic phenomena, nonetheless, that concept might be applicable to other contexts as well. For instance, frequency has to do with the number of times something occurs within a given period of time, and, conceivably, if some sort of transducer phenomenon is taking place in the generation of crystalline patterns such that one kind of energy dynamic is translated into another kind of energy dynamic, then, presumably, an important aspect of that translation process involves the transformation of frequency in which the number of times that one kind of phenomenon occurs within a given period of time becomes the number of times that another kind of phenomenon occurs within a given period of time.

The precise of the foregoing sort of process in which one kind of frequency is transformed into another kind of frequency might not be known. However, the general character of such a process involves transduction of some kind in which one kind of energy is transformed into another kind of energy through, among other things, a change in the way in which the dynamics of the frequency phenomenon are manifested.

While the foregoing notion is somewhat hypothetical in character, there are concrete phenomena with which we are familiar – at least to a degree -- which seem to resonate with the aforementioned possibility. For example, when codons consisting of three DNA or RNA molecules are transcribed and give rise to any one of 22 specific kinds of amino acids that are possible from among the 500 amino acids that exist, a process of transduction is taking place in which one kind of energy dynamic (namely, that which takes place within DNA and RNA molecules) is transformed into another kind of energy dynamic (namely, that which takes place within amino acids).

We don't know how the frequencies that are present in DNA or RNA get transformed into the frequencies that are present in amino acids. However, our ignorance concerning that process of transformation does not alter the fact that a transduction of some kind has taken place.

The frequencies associated with a given set of codons -- consisting of DNA and RNA -- have become the frequencies associated with the dynamics of amino acids and the subsequent formation of peptide sequences. Nucleic acids are nothing like amino acids, and, yet, the frequency dynamics of the former have been transduced into the frequency dynamics of the latter.

A family that subscribed to a magazine published by Dr. Emoto made contact and informed him about an experiment which the members of that family had conducted. More specifically, rice from the same source was placed in two glass jars.

Each day, for a month, the family members took turns, at different times throughout the day, saying "Thank You" to one of the jars containing rice. The other jar, which also contained rice, was subjected to the words "You fool," and these words were directed toward the latter jar at various times during the day by different members of the family.

At the end of the month, the two jars were compared. The jar that repeatedly had been on the receiving end of the words "Thank You" began to ferment and exuded a sweet, malt-like aroma, while the rice in the other jar that had been repeatedly subjected to the words "You Fool" had turned black and was rotting.

Were the two jars responding to words – which were not necessarily sincere reflections of how any given family member might have been feeling at the time such words were spoken – or were the jars responding to certain kinds of preconceived ideas and/or emotions that might have been associated with those words? For instance, conceivably, the family conducting the experiment might have been taking part in a self-fulfilling prophecy in which the experiment was being engaged through a conceptual orientation that was framed by the ideas being expressed by Dr. Emoto through his magazine and, therefore, the members of the family might have fully expected that one of the two jars would turn out more favorably (fermented with sweet aroma) than the other one did (black and rotting).

Of course, even if the foregoing experiment were shaped by placebo and nocebo-like forces, this did not mean that nothing was transpiring. Indeed, the two jars of rice went in two, different developmental directions, and, therefore, no matter what the precise nature of the dynamics might have been, the differences that occurred seem both to be due to some kind of frequency following behavior in which each jar of rice responded to the sorts of frequencies that were being directed toward those two jars.

Dr. Emoto believes that words entail an array of powerful vibrations which give expression to the status of an individual's soul. In this regard, he mentions a Japanese word which, when transliterated, becomes "kotodama" and refers to the "spirit of words," and he believes that such a spirit – which reflects the condition of a person's soul – might have a considerable impact on the quality of the water that makes up the biological terrain through which we live our lives.

Furthermore, he maintains that illness, of whatever kind, has a sort of dimension of contagion embedded within it. In other words, to a certain degree, illness within any given individual is a reflection of -- or a frequency following response, of sorts, to -- the manner in which dysfunctional forces (both individually as well as collectively) are present in the world.

The condition of the souls of people can affect the health of individuals. Similarly, the condition of the soul of an individual can have an impact on the health of the collective.

Crimes that are committed by an individual impact the health of society. The dysfunctional condition of any given society impacts the character of the decisions that are made by individuals, and some of those decisions might lead to criminal acts.

Just as the stimuli to which water is exposed appear to become transduced in some fashion by means of the crystals that form in that water when it is frozen and, then, melted in an appropriate manner, so too, Dr. Emoto also believes that people who view the photographs of the foregoing crystals will be impacted or affected in some way. For instance, he says that the most beautiful crystals which form were in response to the words "love and gratitude" and people who view the photographs taken of the crystals that form in response to those word are also changed in some way.

Moreover, he claims that "love and gratitude" are principles which are at the heart of all of the world's religions. He maintains that if people were to incorporate or realize such principles in their everyday lives, then, there would be no need for laws.

As appealing as the foregoing perspective might be, the dynamics that take place within human beings might be a lot more complex than Dr. Emoto seems to suppose is the case. For example, various individuals might understand the nature of "love" and "gratitude" in ways that are different from one another, and, as a result, the behaviors associated with those terms might lead to forms of social dynamics that tend to run counter to each other.

Thus, if one person believes that the way to show love and gratitude involves submitting to whatever a husband, and/or a family, and/or a country, and/or a government, and/or a religious leader says should be done in a given set of circumstances, while another person believes that the way to show love and gratitude involves discovering one's essential identity and struggling to act in accordance with the natural law in which one's identity is rooted, then, there is likely to be some sort of conflict which tends to arise when the two foregoing perspectives encounter or engage one another. Or, stated in another way, while it might be true that each of those individuals could be affected or changed in some fashion by being exposed to photographs of crystalline patterns which form when the words "love and gratitude" are wrapped around a container of water that is subsequently frozen and, then, permitted to melt, nevertheless, there is no guarantee that they each will be affected or changed in the same way, or even that they both will understand the nature of the foregoing dynamic in the same fashion.

Later on during his second book, Dr. Emoto mentions in passing how quantum mechanics maintains that substance is nothing more than vibration. He, then, adds that the quantum view of existence consists of a strange combination of particles and wave.

If one were to recall that one of the architects of quantum theory – namely, Richard Feynman – once said that no one really understands quantum mechanics (even though the mathematical language through which it is expressed permits one to make very precise kinds of physical determinations), then, one might not be able to viably claim that substance is nothing more than vibration because, in a very fundamental sense, we don't necessarily actually understand either the nature of vibration or substance, or how the "stuff" or phenomena of the universe seem to be able to shape-shift and be manifested as what seem to be inherently irreconcilable phenomena involving particles or waves depending on the nature of a given set of circumstances.

Perhaps, the relationship between particles and waves is another kind of transduction process like that between DNA/RNA and amino acids. As noted previously, we don't know why or how frequencies of DNA/RNA came to signify frequencies of amino acids (i.e., the origins of the genetic code are shrouded in mystery), and, similarly, we don't know why or how the frequencies associated with particles get transformed into the frequencies associated with waves, or vice versa.

Particles and waves might be artifacts of an underlying field. Under the right set of transducer conditions, such a field might give expression to a form that has substance-like properties, while under other conditions of transduction, the field is induced to give expression to a vibratory or wave-like set of properties, but, as such, "reality" is neither wave nor particle and neither substance nor vibration.

The question, then becomes, what set or sets of forces is responsible for ordering or arranging field conditions in ways that will yield particles under one set of circumstances while ordering or arranging field conditions which exist in other circumstances that will be capable of giving expression to waves. Quantum mechanics is very good at figuring out what probabilities will be generated by different kinds of wave functions, but it has no clue as to why the probabilities that are manifested on any given occasion have the values which they do.

The foregoing comments allude to the problems of decoherence which have bedeviled quantum mechanics since the latter's inception. In other words, although the mathematic framework that is at the heart of quantum mechanics is capable of generating very precise solutions concerning the values that are likely when any given wave function collapses and, in the process, gives specific answers to specific questions, no one seems to know what causes the wave function to collapse in the way that it does and give the answers that it does. The mysteries which permeate attempts to reconcile the precise mathematical calculations of quantum mechanics with the unknown etiology of the realities which are being mathematically described has led to many of the controversies surrounding that discipline – from: Niels Bohr's probabilistic-based Copenhagen theory that seeks to compartmentalize, if not evade, questions concerning how the classical world and the quantum world are related to one another; to Schrödinger's Cat; to Hugh Everett's many-world's doctoral thesis; to Einstein's thought experiments that were intended to demonstrate that God does not play dice with the universe; to John Wheeler's notion that reality does not exist until a measurement is made when consciousness intervenes in a given experiment.

Notwithstanding decades of point-counterpoint involving those sorts of controversies, no one has been able to come up with a viable set of first principles in quantum mechanics which permits one to explain why: Photons, electrons, quarks, neutrinos, along with many other dimensions that make up the standard theory of quantum mechanics, have the properties that they do. String theories have been trying to provide answers to the foregoing issues for more than fifty years, and, like other physical theories of everything, those theories have come up empty.

Dr. Emoto goes on to mention a reported saying of the Buddha that appears in the Heart Sutra ... a saying which might actually be nearer to the truth of "things." More specifically, the Buddha is reported to have said: "That which can be seen has no form, and that which cannot be seen has form," and, therefore, one might understand the foregoing saying to mean that what is seen is illusory and, as such, does not actually have any substantial, enduring existential form of its own, while That which is responsible for the manifestation of all such illusory forms cannot be seen but is substantial in some mysterious manner – i.e., has an unknown and, perhaps, unknowable way of Being which makes illusory forms possible.

Shortly after making reference to the foregoing saying that is attributed to the Buddha, Dr. Emoto refers to a verse from the Old Testament of the Bible – namely, "In the beginning, there was the Word." What is the "Word?"

Some people interpret the notion of the "Word" as indicating that the universe was brought into being through the process of "vibration" or "frequency." Conceivably, however, while vibration or resonance might be one dimension of the way in which that Word is given a "visible" – if (according to the Buddha) illusory – form, the Word itself gives expression to an underlying, unknown impetus which is not itself necessarily a function of vibration or resonance but, rather, could be using vibration and resonance to communicate some of what is inherent in the unknown impetus that led to the Word becoming manifest.

If so, then, the Word is more than frequency, vibration, or resonance. The Word is the dynamic that makes frequency, vibration, and resonance possible even as it communicates an impetus or message that cannot be reduced to frequency, vibration, and resonance. The Word serves as a transducer which takes an intention which, initially, is not manifest and, consequently, is invisible – yet, nonetheless, real – and, then, transmogrifies that formless intention into what is manifest and visible, but which is not necessarily real in any essential way.

The Word is that which is both tangential and asymptotic at the same time. The Word is a sphere (Pascal), or a circle (Voltaire), or a form whose essence is everywhere but whose perimeter is nowhere.

Each of us has a unique relationship with the Word. The Word has a unique relationship with each of us.

Various kinds of frequencies (linguistic, conceptual, creative, social, moral, physical, and spiritual) are communicated to us through the Word, and, at the same time, we communicate with the Word through our thoughts, emotions, intentions, and acts. When an individual enters into a condition of symbiotic relationship with the Word, then, there is a resonance which is established between the Word and the individual that is similar to what transpires when the biological terrain and the microbiome become engaged in a symbiotic relationship with one another.

Both of the aforementioned modalities of symbiosis constitute conditions of health or well-being. Thus, when the capacity for epigenetic forms of adaptive learning are fully functional within somatids, endobionts, or microzymas so that a condition of detoxified stability exists in which the microbiome and the biological terrain engage one another in a symbiotic fashion, then, a condition of physical health or well-being exists, and, similarly, when the soul fully exercises its own capacity for epigenetic forms of adaptive learning by employing qualities of character, reason, insight, inspiration, and so on to engage, via symbiotic forms of resonance, the Word that has arisen through the Formless creator of forms, then, a state of spiritual health or well-being exists.

There seems to be a principle of: "As above, so below" sort of ambience involved in the foregoing dynamics. Thus, the energy dynamics of one level or dimension of Being are linked to modalities of energy dynamics that occur in other dimensions or realms of Being through processes of transduction.

Ultimately, or essentially, the notion of energy doesn't have to be tied to, or a function of, any particular kind of physical dynamic. Energy, like the closely connected notion of force, refers to a capacity to bring about an effect.

When the Unmanifested gives rise to the manifested, the latter is the effect of the former. We refer to the dynamics of that effect as involving some sort of causal energy or force even if we don't have any understanding of how the Unmanifested becomes manifested.

If the energy properties of the "effect" entail a different kind of dynamic than the energy properties of that which induced such an effect, then, the link that ties the two together involves a transduction of some kind. The underlying dynamics of those kinds of transduction processes might be cloaked in mystery and unanswered questions, but, nonetheless, the presence of those sorts of transduction processes would appear to be undeniable.

In other words, just as transduction phenomena seem to be involved as one moves from the unmanifested underpinnings of the "Word" to the manifest, but illusory forms of everyday phenomena, and just as transduction phenomena seem to be involved as one moves from particle to waves (or vice versa) within the context of the phenomena of quantum physics, and just as transduction phenomena seem to be involved as one moves from the frequencies of DNA/RNA to the frequencies of amino acids, so too, transduction phenomena of some kind appear to be involved as one moves from the epigenetic dynamics of somatids, endobionts, or microzymas –- and, therefore, the organizing and regulating processes which are inherent in the adaptive learning algorithms present in such entities -- to the frequency phenomena that give expression to the anabolic and catabolic dynamics of the biological terrain as it seeks to maintain or regain a condition of symbiotic relationships with the microbiome which resides in that terrain. In each of the foregoing cases, one kind of energy, frequency, or causal dynamic appears to be transduced into another kind of energy, frequency or causal dynamic. Indeed, there seems to be a clear-cut series of transducer dynamics which takes place as one transitions from the Unmanifested, to the manifested, and, then, to the realm of particles and waves, and, then, to the epigenetic domain of somatids, endobionts, or microzymas, and, then, to the metabolic pathways that are engendered by the epigenetically directed transducer processes involving DNA/RNA and amino acids.

The transition that takes place when water is exposed to various kinds of stimuli and, then, frozen and melted to yield crystalline forms might also involve a transduction phenomenon of some kind. However, irrespective of whether this is, or is not, the case, the patterns which form in crystals of water do seem to constitute a modality of frequency following response dynamics.

Dr. Emoto believes that we each have a God-given capacity to change the world. While the following saying -- namely: 'Be the change that you wish to see in the world' -- has been, apparently, falsely attributed to Gandhi, nonetheless, I believe that the idea has heuristic value which might be able to help answer questions concerning how one might become engaged with a process of changing the world.

Our God-given capacity to change the world begins with, and in many respects, ends with ourselves. We cannot force or even necessarily, induce other people to change, and, therefore, one might have to find a way to try to maintain a balance between the principles of: Neither control, nor be controlled.

However, by individually committing oneself to a process of seeking to acquire qualities of character such as honesty, humility, perseverance, courage, nobility, repentance, generosity, charitableness, forgiveness, gratitude, sincerity, piety, tolerance, friendship, love, and the like (and, therefore, more than love and gratitude are involved in such a process of change) we might be able to begin to establish relationships of resonance with others who are similarly engaged in their own process of struggling to acquire the aforementioned qualities of character, and, in the process, mutually work toward, and co-operatively attempt to develop more symbiotic relationships with one another that are conducive to the generation of social health and well-being.

For most people, including myself, individual change comes only through undergoing an array of existential difficulties of one kind or another. Nevertheless, there are instances which seem to be sprinkled in inexplicable ways across the sands of time that fall through the hourglass-like process which measures the temporal aspects of one's life and through which individuals are graced with a transitory and very fragile desire to engage in change and to become open to what the Word is, and what It has been busily broadcasting to all of creation, night and day, since that Word became manifest.

Unfortunately, such instances are easily missed. Indeed, regrettably, even when those instances come knocking on the doors of our existence, we often turn them away or turn away from them.

When we are inspired by others to truly become better versions of ourselves, such moments of inspiration involve being touched by a form of Grace that is being transmitted through a particular locus of manifestation – i.e., the person who inspires us. However, one must choose to actively embrace those fleeting, temporal portals of opportunity involving change, or they will disappear and, oftentimes, if those moments pass by unanswered, we tend to become entangled in the inertia entailed by dimensions of ourselves that are not open to change and which, therefore, become bogged down in an existential orientation which actively resists and flows counter to whatever desire might be present to try to struggle toward realizing one's essential potential as a human being.

Around the same time that I read Dr. Emoto's book on *The Hidden Messages in Water*, I also read Veda Austin's work: *The Secret Intelligence of Water*. Many of the same kinds of questions arose in conjunction with her book as occurred in relation to Dr. Emoto's research concerning water, but there also were a few additional issues that tended to bounce about in my consciousness with respect to her work.

For example, whereas Dr. Emoto was interested in exploring the messages which might be contained in water as evidenced by the crystalline patterns that occur in water which is first exposed to a stimuli, and, then, frozen, and, later, melted in order to generate crystals capable of conveying -- possibly – a message, Veda Austin believed that she had encountered the sort of evidence which indicated that some sort of intelligence might be present in water.

The notion of intelligence is conceptually slippery in and of itself. The problems surrounding that term are complicated when we either project intelligence onto some phenomenon when this is not warranted, or, alternatively, we try to withdraw some dimension of intelligence from a given context or phenomenon to which the term deservedly applies.

When a tape recorder responds to human consciousness by transposing the audio waves that emanate from such consciousness into electrical signals which are stored in such a device, we do not normally refer to such a dynamic as constituting evidence that the recording device possesses some form of intelligence. At the same time, the capacity of a tape recorder to do what it does clearly indicates that intelligence has something to do with the presence of such a capacity.

If conditions surrounding the process of recording an audio signal that is generated as a result of the vocal activities of human consciousness change the foregoing signal, then, although such changes are part of the recording and alter, in some way, what has been said, then, once again, we don't normally interpret the presence of those kinds of alterations as indications that some form of intelligence is present. Similarly, even if the recording device itself should alter some aspect of the audio signal, we tend to write this off as a chronic or acute glitch in the quality or performance of the recording device.

When water is able to capture some facet of intention generated by human consciousness, is this evidence of the water's intelligence. Or, alternatively, is it evidence, possibly, that water has the capacity – however it acquired such capacity (say through natural processes of physics and chemistry or through some other means) – to record, store, transmit, or reflect certain aspects of the kinds of frequencies to which it has been exposed?

In the opening chapter of her aforementioned book, Veda Austin begins with a quote from Rudolf Steiner which indicates that intelligence is present everywhere in nature but that such intelligence draws its properties from the universal intelligence to which the former modality of intelligence merely gives expression in its own characteristic manner. Human beings, like bodies of water, have capacities that offer evidence of intelligence, but like the aforementioned case of the tape recorder, such evidence might be more indicative of that which has made those capacities appear to be intelligent-like rather than actually being an indication that intelligence actually resides in either human beings or various bodies of water.

As was noted earlier, when the Unmanifested Word becomes manifest, then what is made manifest appears substantial and, therefore, seems to possess properties of its own, even though if the Buddha is correct – and I believe he is – that what has been made manifest has no actual form of its own but is a phenomena that has been generated through the Unmanifested Word which does have a substantial reality of Its own. Human beings and water might exhibit some sort of capacity for intelligence that has been built into them, or conferred upon them, but such intelligence actually might be evidence of the presence of something "other" than whatever kind of intelligence someone might wish to attribute to either human beings or to water or to some sort of artificially enhanced "intelligent" tape recorder.

Ms. Austin describes how she began to become interested in certain possibilities involving art, nature, and intelligence when she read an account that Dr. Thomas Hieronymus was reported to have observed in a Parisian meat market. According to Hieronymus, the frost which was forming on glass paneling beneath which various parts of refrigerated animal organs were being displayed was exhibiting patterns in crystallized form that appeared to be reflecting properties of the organs that were present below the display glass.

He believed the foregoing crystalline patterns formed as a result of subtle life forces which still were being generated by the body parts. One might recall at this point that Béchamp, Enderlein, and Naessens all subscribed to the idea that microzymas, endobionts, or somatids (whatever term one prefers) survived the death of the organisms in which they had been present during life, and, therefore, the 'subtle life force' to which Dr. Hieronymus referred could well have emanated from the microzymas, endobionts, or somatids (however one wishes to label them) which the foregoing three researchers all considered to give expression to the life force that helped make living organisms possible.

After reflecting on the ideas of Dr. Hieronymus, Veda Austin read and viewed the research of Dr. Emoto concerning the issue of messages in water. She also was inspired by the microscopic images of ice crystals that were taken – and, subsequently, published – by Laurent Costa.

As a result of the foregoing encounters, Veda Austin began to experiment with the dynamics of crystallography. During one of her first ventures into exploring those dynamics, she put water in a Petri dish and intended to freeze that water and, at some point, she wanted to take a photograph in order to see what pattern, if any, might be present in the crystalline structure that arose during the freezing process.

She indicates that prior to subjecting the Petri dish to a freezing process she noticed a piece of fluff of some kind which was present in the water and removed it with her hand. She remembers wondering if the movements of her hand might influence the water's memory in some way and, thereby, affect what might show up in the photograph which she planned to take, but she also notes that she had no preconceptions about what she might, or might not, see when she took a photograph of the crystalline patterns that might form once the water in the Petri dish was frozen.

When she looked at the photograph that she took, she was shocked to see a fairly clear impression of a hand in the photograph. Indeed, the photo which appears in her book is unmistakably the image of a hand.

While the foregoing scenario is quite intriguing, I'm not sure it indicates that water has intelligence. In her book, and as noted earlier, Veda Austin describes how she wondered if the presence of her hand taking away a piece of fluff might affect the memory of water, and, therefore, she already was framing the experiment in terms of water having memory (a notion that is often linked with the issue of intelligence) rather than merely indicating the presence of a certain capacity for storing data of some kind (like a tape recorder).

Furthermore, the hand depicted in the photograph which appears in her book shows a static hand – that is, a hand that is not doing anything. However, the hand that came closest to the water – perhaps even touching it – was engaged in taking away a piece of fluff and, therefore, one wonders why the image that was captured through the photograph that she took appears to exhibit a static rather than an active hand.

By the notion of "an active hand," I am not trying to suggest that the image should have been some sort of motion picture. Instead, although static, the image could have shown a hand which was formed in a shape that indicated it might have been trying to pick up something.

Is it possible that what was captured in the photograph was a function of the phenomenology she was experiencing as she was engaging in the experimental process rather than being a function of, say, the water's phenomenological orientation toward those same experimental conditions? In other words, what phenomenological perspective was being given expression in the photograph?

The foregoing question entails two entirely different possibilities. In one scenario – and this still would be quite intriguing – the water might have been affected by the frequencies that emanated from Veda's thoughts and actions and, part of that dynamic of being affected involved the storing of those frequencies, while in the other scenario – the one which Veda Austin came to accept – the water somehow intelligently "chose" to respond to her presence (including her thoughts) by generating the image of a hand that was based on, but not entirely controlled by, however Veda's presence might have been affecting the water.

She went on to conduct many other kinds of experiments. These experiments ranged from placing written words beneath a Petri dish, to playing music, to providing the water with degrees of freedom for responding to something that was sort of an open-ended kind of stimulus.

For instance, in one experiment she asked the water about her identity. More specifically, she asked: Who am I?

The image that appeared in the photograph consisted of the initials for her name "V" and "A" that were linked together in a specific manner in which the right side of the "V" shared the same line as the left side of "A". What was truly remarkable about this image is how the foregoing arrangement of letters reflected the special way that Vera Austin used to "brand" various items associated with her – a way to which the water that was being frozen supposedly had never been exposed.

Did the foregoing result indicate that the water was responding to her in an intelligent fashion? Are we to suppose that the water had the capacity to understand spoken words (unless the foregoing question was asked non-verbally), and, then, access Veda's consciousness and memories – all within a period of 30 seconds (the time allotted for stimulus exposure during her experiments) – while proceeding to select the foregoing arrangement of her initials as a sort of definitive response to her stated or unstated question?

Wouldn't it be simpler to suppose – and, yet, still be remarkable – that Veda was sending out frequencies of various kinds and that the frequencies which were captured in the crystalline pattern had to do with a way of identifying herself that were vibrating within her rather than being intuitively grasped, somehow, by the water? Given the foregoing possibility, one of course, still might ask why the pattern that appeared in crystalline form was what it was rather than some other kind of pattern, but such a question might have more to do with Veda Austin than with the water.

For years now, my wife and I have said things to one another that reflected what the other person was thinking as, or just prior to, whatever was voiced was voiced. We often have wondered who is sending and who is receiving or whether, perhaps, we take turns serving as "receivers" and "senders", but irrespective of what the answer to such wonderings might be, those experiences have taken place on a multiplicity of occasions in which whatever was said seemed to have little, if anything, to do with what might have been going on in our immediate environment at the time the foregoing phenomena took place.

Are the frequencies (whether of words, music, questions, thoughts, or emotions) to which water is exposed during the course of the experiments that are being conducted by Veda Austin somehow imposed on the water (received by it) or does the water somehow select from amongst the frequencies to which it is exposed and send back a 'chosen' response? Are the ideas that occur to my wife, or myself, being imposed by the "sender" as those ideas are voiced by one, or the other, of us, or does the "receiver" somehow select from amongst all the possible frequencies that are taking place in the sender and isolate one of those frequencies which just happens to be the one that is vocally mentioned by one or the other of us?

Does water possess intelligence, or is water constructed in a way that allows intelligent-like phenomena to become manifest within it?

Alternatively, is water something that connects all of us – both externally and internally – and, as such, might constitute a medium of communication through which an array of frequencies can be stored, transmitted, and reflected?

Irrespective of which of the foregoing possibilities toward which one might be inclined, there is one feature that appears to be held in common by each of those alternatives. More specifically, a form of 'frequency following response' seems to be present, and, if this is the case, then, the only questions which remain are what -- and where -- the nature of the locus of intelligence is that is shaping the crystalline patterns which emerge in the photographs?

During the Introduction to her book, Veda Austin quickly mentions a number of individuals who had, or have, ideas that are relevant to her experiments in crystallography. For instance, she briefly talks about the recently deceased French scientist, Luc Montagnier who performed an experiment – somewhat reminiscent of the homeopathic experiment (previously mentioned) conducted by Jacques Benveniste in 1988 -- which seemed to indicate that the structural properties of DNA could be imprinted on water and that such a pattern could be transferred to another container in which that kind of structure had not been present initially.

She also mentions the research of Dr. Gerald Pollack concerning the fourth phase of water, as well as the quantum electrodynamic investigations of Dr. Konstantin Korotkov involving water. In addition, she refers to the work of John Stuart Reid, an acoustics engineer, who invented an instrument known as a cymascope that enables one, among other things, to visualize and analyze various bands of audio signals.

While referring to the foregoing individuals, Veda Austin also indicates that water can have a crystal-like lattice structure (talked about in the last chapter of the present book). She goes on to add that under the right circumstances, crystals can exhibit a substantial capacity for storing information, and, therefore, once again – at least for me -- this tends to re-introduce the possibility that the crystallography experiments which she conducted might have more to do with such a storage capacity, along with water's special sensitivity to an array of frequency phenomena, than those experiments have to do with any sort of intelligent behavior that is being exhibited by water.

As I Muslim, I believe the Qur'an when it indicates that: "The seven heavens and the earth and all that is therein praise God, and there is nothing that does not glorify God in praise, but ye understand not their manner of praise" (17:44). Water praises God through its having the nature that it does since those properties have been given to water by God, but that nature does not have to be intelligent in order for praise to be offered.

Indeed, it is by water being water in all of its myriad capabilities that its form of praise is expressed. However, as the research and experiments of individuals such as Benveniste, Montagnier, Pollack, Korotkov, Reid, and others have been demonstrating again and again, there is much about the nature of water that we do not know and, therefore, to the extent that we are ignorant about the full nature of water, then, truly, to that extent, we do not understand its form of praise.

One of the facts that Veda Austin discovered about water is that not all water is the same. For instance, she found that so-called "informed" water freezes more quickly than does "uninformed" water.

She doesn't seem to specifically indicate in her book what she means by the terms of "informed" and "uninformed" water other than to say that most samples of water consist of a mixture of the two kinds of water. Moreover, the foregoing comments appear in the context of her talking about the research of people such as Gerald Pollack and others.

The notion of water being "informed" does tend to signify that some sort of intelligence might be present. On the other hand, what is meant by "informed" or "uninformed" water might have to do with the capacity of water to be structured or crystallized and, consequently, display a facility for storing information, and, as such, be informed or uninformed to the extent that such a facility is active or dormant.

Irrespective of whether, or not, "informed" water is more intelligent in some sense than "uninformed" water, Veda Austin discovered that informed water adheres to the bottom of a Petri dish. As a result, it begins to freeze much more quickly than uninformed water does, and, consequently, she was able to see patterns in the informed water much more quickly than had been possible in conjunction with uninformed water.

Techniques that Veda Austin developed in conjunction with informed water enabled her to photograph much sharper and clearer images than she had been able to do when she first began to take photographs of crystalline patterns. She refers to that process as 'Collective Molecular Photography' and maintains that as molecules of water begin to slow down while the Petri dish is frozen those molecules become more ordered and are able to rearrange themselves in a more coherent fashion that reflects the frequencies, stimuli, and information to which the water previously had been exposed.

She believes the manner in which water coheres and rearranges itself to give expression to various kinds of patterns that appear to reflect properties of different stimuli which are impinging on the water prior to being frozen seems to suggest that some sort of intelligent design is inherent in what is transpiring. She admits that she is not a scientist but someone who is engaged in research involving crystallography and water, and while acknowledging that the notion of Collective Molecular Photography is just a theory, she feels that whatever is taking place throughout that process, it is yielding interesting results.

I would agree with her about the interesting nature of what she is investigating. However, I'm not, yet, inclined to conclude that whatever is transpiring in her experiments indicates that water is – in and of itself -- intelligent, although I am quite willing to state, along with Rudolf Steiner, that the qualities of water being exhibited certainly are reflective of the Intelligence of That to which the participants in Nature (including human beings) are able to give expression through whatever intelligent-like properties might be manifested through their way of being in the world.

Toward the latter part of her book, Veda Austin explores the possible relationships among issues involving prayer, healing, and water. One of the differences entailed by these sorts of experiments had to do with the fact that participants were located in places which – at least in terms of geographical miles – appeared to be physically removed from the space where the water was being frozen and photographs were taken.

For example, in her book she places two photographs next to one another. One photo was taken using just filtered tap water, while the other image is the result of how that filtered tap water changed in response to a five-minute prayer that was directed toward the water sample by a friend of hers who was on a boat off an island near New Zealand.

There are marked differences between the two photographs. The image involving just filtered tap water appears fragmented, consisting of a series of lines without any sort of intricate structuring, whereas the image of the same kind of water toward which a prayer had been directed from some distance contained a hexagonal structure with internal markings.

Since the purpose of the foregoing experiment appeared to be intended to show the possible impact which a healing prayer from a distance might have on filtered tap water, then, presumably, the difference between the two images would be attributed to such a prayer being said. However, one should keep in mind that Veda Austin had arranged for her friend to do something at a certain time – that is, to say a prayer of some kind – and, in addition, one might suppose there would have been at least a theoretical expectation on her part that some sort of unspecified difference might emerge in relation to that prayer, and, consequently, one has to consider the possibility that the outcome of the foregoing experiment might have been influenced to some degree by thoughts, emotions, ideas, and so on which were coming from Veda rather than her friend or in addition to what might have been emanating from her friend.

The filtered tap water toward which the prayer had been directed did show a single hexagonal structure. Moreover, the presence of such a structure is often interpreted to mean that water is being enabled to give expression to its inherent nature – which involves hexagonal structures – and, therefore, the water toward which prayer was directed appeared to be more structured – and, therefore, presumably, healthier -- than just filtered tap water on its own.

The hexagonal structures that are present in ice and snowflakes are said to be unique in character. Irrespective of whether, or not, all such hexagonal structures are unique, one would like to know if the structure that appears in the photographic image is the imprinted result of the frequencies which are being sent via prayer or, alternatively, is the structure in that photographic image a function of how the water is intelligently responding to those frequencies.

Moreover, apparently, there were no double-blind editions of the experiments that were conducted in which neither Veda nor the water knew if a prayer would, or would not, be sent at a given time. In other words, the foregoing experiment should have been run on a number of occasions in which different kinds of contingencies would be controlled during each experiment.

On some of those occasions, no prayer should have been directed toward the water, while on other occasions, such a prayer could have been sent without Veda knowing which kind of event was taking place. On still other occasions, whatever thoughts were directed toward the water should have involved something other than a prayer.

A further kind of contingency that would need to be controlled in some fashion has to do with Veda Austin's presence. As indicated previously, she knew that a prayer of some kind was coming within a given time frame, and, therefore, how does one know that whatever image shows up in the photograph is due to the prayer being sent by her friend rather than being due to her presence or her thoughts while she is present overseeing the photographic process – especially given that the prayer she is requesting seemed to be designed to see if water could be "healed" in some sense and, therefore, her knowledge about the nature of the experiment might have been influencing the kind of structure that would appear just by her knowing what she was asking her friend to do within a given time frame.

The experiment that was conducted by Veda Austin and her friend did seem to indicate that some sort of 'frequency following response' was taking place. However, what the precise nature of that response is appears to be uncertain if not unknown.

Did the response involve intelligent behavior on the part of water? Did that response reflect the prayer, or did that response reflect, in some way, Veda's presence, or was that response a function of the combined frequencies being sent out by both Veda and her friend?

The fact that a hexagonal structure appeared in the second photograph is, in and of itself, intriguing because, at a minimum, the presence of the structure seems to indicate that some sort of 'frequency following response' might have been taking place. Nonetheless, we still really don't know what the significance is of the photograph which contains a hexagonal structure since there were no control methods that were employed which might have helped one to eliminate various kinds of contingencies from, possibly, affecting what was being photographed.

Veda incorporated variations on the foregoing experiment into her book which involved different people. These individuals used an array of techniques or processes in conjunction with filtered tap water in order to determine whether, or not, any, changes might show up in photographs that followed the initial photographs of just filtered tap water which had been frozen and, supposedly, not subjected to any sort of stimuli.

Nonetheless, the very fact of filtered tap water being taken through even a straightforward process of: Being placed in a Petri dish; frozen; and photographed – all while in the presence of Veda who might have been thinking or feeling who knows what – would seem to entail all manner of stimuli. Therefore, one can't help but wonder why none of those stimuli seemed to have any appreciable or structured effect on the water.

Maybe nothing appeared in the baseline comparison photographs of the filtered tap water because an expectation existed during such a process that nothing of a structured nature was likely to appear. If so, then the lack of structure in the baseline comparison photographs involving filtered tap water could have been exhibiting another kind of 'frequency following response' in which the water recorded and reflected what was being directed toward it which, seemingly, was nothing much at all except perhaps an array of seemingly unconnected, and, therefore, fragmented stimuli associated with the freezing and photographic process.

Veda Austin also indicates in her book that she conducted some experiments in which she asked people who lived in different locations – and she didn't know some of these individuals – to focus on something that was of relevance to them during the experiment but which would be kept hidden from her. The photographs that resulted from those experiments are quite interesting and intriguing, but I'm not sure those experiments indicate that anything other than some kind of "frequency following response' was taking place which did not necessarily entail any kind of intelligent behavior on the part of the water toward which various thoughts were being directed.

Independently of the issue of whether, or not, water has intelligence, what does seem to consistently emerge within the context of the various kinds of experiments conducted by Veda Austin is the phenomenon of 'frequency following response'. In other words, at the very least, her experiments appear to indicate that there are influences impinging on water which are capable of being captured, stored, and reflected in different ways, and if those kinds of influences can be manifested in water – even when those influences appear to originate in locations that are distant from such water – then, really, it is not all that much of a leap to suppose that human beings who (depending on the state of their stage of development) consist of anywhere from 50% to more approximately 90% water, might also be capable of receiving and responding to various kinds of frequency influences which could impinge on them from a variety of environmental sources – including distant ones.

The foregoing considerations resonate – in intriguing, unknown, and, possibly, non-existent ways -- with the idea of entanglement that has surfaced in conjunction with quantum phenomena. From the first forays into the periphery of the entanglement topic involving John Stewart Bell's statement concerning certain parameters of inequality involving various quantum phenomena, to the various experiments of individuals such as John Clauser, Alain Aspect, and Anton Zeilinger, evidence has arisen which indicates that, at least in conjunction with certain, specified, experimental conditions, there appears to be a connection of some kind between certain particles within the context of those kinds of experiments in which particles are separated from one another in a way that whatever is taking place between them seems to be of a non-local nature and, therefore, cannot be explained as being the result of some kind of electromagnetic signaling dynamic between them that is limited to, or governed by, the speed of light.

Discussions involving the foregoing issue of entanglement have gone back and forth between those individuals, on the one hand, who want to say that quantum physics has shown that everything in the universe is entangled in various ways and, on the other hand, those individuals who have wanted to introduce some degree of caution into the discussion. The latter individuals have suggested that, at the present time, the actual extent to which entanglement might be present in the universe is epistemologically constrained by, and, perhaps, limited to what has been established through the experiments of individuals such as Clauser, Aspect, and Zeilinger, and, therefore, beyond the sorts of conditions that were present in those experiments, we don't really know much about whether, or not, the phenomena of entanglement are pervasive throughout the universe, and even if those phenomena are fairly common, we don't really know what the implications of the presence of the entanglement phenomena might be for our everyday lives.

The experiments conducted by Veda Austin appear to indicate, at the very least, that there are resonance phenomena which, under certain conditions, can be shown to exist between people and water. Whether these resonance phenomena are local (e.g., electromagnetically based) or non-local and, therefore, are giving expression to some kind of entanglement dynamics has, yet, to be determined.

Notwithstanding the foregoing considerations, one might note that in the light of the evidence concerning the idea of 'frequency following response' which appears to be associated with various experiments conducted by Veda Austin, and given what Béchamp demonstrated more than 150 years ago and which, subsequently, was supported and developed in various ways by the research of Enderlein, Rife, Naessens and others at various points during the intervening century and a half, then one is not necessarily engaging in a flight of fantasy if one were to suppose that the internal dynamics of microzymas, endobionts, or somatids could have the capacity to generate an array of frequencies which might impinge on, and influence, what takes place within the context of the structured water that is present in the biological terrain which contains the physical entities (i.e., microzymas, endobionts, or somatids) that might be responsible for transmitting and epigenetically organizing life-force dynamics. Whether any of the foregoing sorts of resonance relationships are of a non-local nature is another matter.

The Presence of the Past: Morphic Resonance and the Habits of Nature by Rupert Sheldrake was published in 1989. This work was an updated sequel to his 1981 book: *A New Science of Life*.

In both of the aforementioned volumes, Sheldrake attempted to expound upon the nature of his hypothesis known as: "formative causation." This notion is evolutionary in nature and tends to challenge a variety of traditional views concerning the notion of evolution.

More specifically, he maintains that the term 'formative causation' gives expression to his belief that every dimension of nature operates in accordance with principles of collective memory which accumulate over time and result in specific patterns of behavior in particular species (i.e., such forms of behavior are caused by principles of memory formation) ... behaviors that become habitual in nature and on which the members of a species (both now and in the future) can draw as they go about their lives.

Sheldrake contends that if his hypothesis of formative causation is correct, then, one should be able to observe the presence of its dynamics in the formation of new behaviors that become dispersed or distributed across a given species. For example, if one were to observe a blue tit bird acquire a new behavior – like ripping off a cap from a bottle of milk in order to gain access to the milk contained in the bottle – then, if formative causation is true, Sheldrake believes one should be able to see evidence for the presence of a similar kind of behavior beginning to establish itself in other members of that same species even if the latter members are located at considerable distances (both geographically as well as temporally) from the precedent-setting bird or birds.

Let us assume that such a new behavior does occur. Let us also assume that either the same kind of behavior, or behaviors which are very similar to it, begin to emerge in other members of the species over a relatively short period of time. Given the foregoing assumptions, should one necessarily conclude that some sort of collective memory dynamic is transpiring across the species and, therefore, is enabling other members of the species to be able to draw on that collective memory and, consequently, the habit of ripping off the cap of a bottle of milk in order to access the contents of the bottle becomes established in the blue tit species of birds?

Has a collective memory and associated habit been instantiated in that species of birds? There are various considerations (some of which are presented in the following discussion) which suggest that such a conclusion might not necessarily follow from the premises stated by Sheldrake in which a new behavior arises and in which that sort of behavior begins to spread to other members of that species despite such a form of behavior being initially present only in an isolated case.

For instance, is there a difference between, on the one hand, some sort of 'frequency following response" and, on the other hand, instances of 'collective memory leading to the formation of a habit'? To begin to try to address such a question, one might want to know what enables a given organism – in this case a blue tit bird – to be able to have the capacity to exhibit a new behavior in the first place.

The emergence of a new kind of behavior would seem to indicate that some modality of epigenetic phenomenon is taking place in which a form of adaptive learning is transpiring. If one accepts the perspective of people such as Béchamp, Enderlein, Rife, and Naessens, then, the capacity for the foregoing sort of adaptive change resides in the entities – referred to interchangeably as microzymas, endobionts, or somatids – that are differentially present within every kind of cell, tissue, and organ and which are responsible for serving as the loci of the life forces that govern what transpires within the biological terrain of any given organism.

In addition, one might suppose that whether, or not, a given kind of new behavior would occur in a given species could depend on what degrees of freedom and degrees of constraint are present within the aforementioned epigenetic capabilities of the entities which might be responsible for giving expression to the 'life forces' that are inherent within any given species – namely, the microzymas, endobionts, or somatids. Presumably, the reason why blue tit birds might be known for their ability to rip off the cap of a bottle of milk but are not known for their capacity to build microscopes, telescopes, or other technological devices is because the latter sort of epigenetic capacity out of which that kind of new behavior might arise is not present, even as a potential, in blue tit birds.

Blue tit birds only do what their nature permits. If their nature permits certain kinds of new behavior to emerge, then, inherent within some unknown percentage of the birds of that species a certain kind of capacity exists that might – given the right set of conditions -- be able to manifest that sort of new behavior.

If the foregoing kind of new behavior appears, and, then, begins to spread, the phenomenon could be driven by the dynamics of a 'frequency following response' rather than through a process of formative causation in which a modality of collective memory leads to the establishment of some sort of habitual pattern of behavior. In other words, if a species has the inherent capacity to discover certain modalities of adaptive behavior – such as a new behavior of some kind – then, one also might suppose that there could be some sort of capacity associated with the foregoing kind of adaptive behavior in which different members of a given species are capable of being sensitized to the presence of the sorts of frequencies that might be generated through the foregoing sort of adaptive learning dynamic.

What Sheldrake is calling collective memory might just be the capacity that is inherent in a given species which entails the possibility, among other things, that certain kinds of adaptive learning are able to take place. Furthermore, what Shelldrake is calling habit might only refer to the sort of entrainment process that goes to the very heart of what is meant by 'frequency following response' in which a given organism responds to those frequencies to which its nature is innately sensitized.

The nature of the forces which trigger an inherent, but inactive, capacity for a certain kind of epigenetic form of adaptive learning to become active often tend to be unknown. However, once activated, one might anticipate that other members of the species will manifest sensitivity to, or be influenced by, the presence of the frequencies to which such adaptive learning gives expression, and, as the experiments of Veda Austin appear to demonstrate, those kinds of influences are, somehow, capable of being sent across, and/or received over, considerable distances.

Contrary to what Sheldrake claims, what might be inherited is not necessarily some sort of collective memory. Instead, what could be inherited is, within certain degrees of freedom and restraint, a capacity, on the one hand, that is able to engage in various modalities of adaptive learning together with, on the other hand, a related capacity which constitutes having some degree of sensitivity to the presence of the frequencies to which the activated forms of the first kind of capacity give expression.

If some members of a species in which a form of adaptive learning becomes activated are able to learn the new kind of behavior more readily than might have been the case with the initiators or discoverers of that mode of adaptive learning, this is not necessarily because a collective memory of some kind has been laid down from which other members of the species can draw. Rather, the rapidity with which such a new behavior might spread among subsequent members of the species relative to the originator or originators of that behavior could be because none of those subsequent members of the species had to deal with the difficulties surrounding the origin and development of a new kind of adaptive learning, and, in addition, subsequent members of the species might have been able to rely on an already existing innate capacity involving sensitivity to the presence of certain frequencies once the foregoing capacity had been activated.

Moreover, one might discover that not all members of a species are equally adept at picking up on, or resonating with, the frequencies associated with some new kind of adaptive learning. Conceivably, some members of a species might be more sensitive to the presence of certain kinds of frequencies than are other members of that species as one might anticipate with any sort statistical representation which describes the range of capabilities and properties that exist among the population of a given species by means of a normal curve.

Memory is not just a matter of information being stored. Memory is also a function of the dynamics that generates, shapes, or forms the properties, features, and characteristics of that information.

Memory which arises in conjunction with something of a novel sort involves observation. That kind of memory also involves a process in which what is observed is characterized and/or classified as being one kind of phenomenon rather than another sort of phenomenon.

Initiating the foregoing kind of novel memory might involve curiosity. That sort of memory also would appear to be caught up, to varying degrees, with experimentation, or trial and error, of one kind or another.

Moreover, the foregoing sort of memory concerning novel behaviors would seem to involve various kinds of awareness, perceptual orientation, interpretations, and insight or understanding. Such factors might enable an organism to distinguish between what could be of relevance and value, as well as what might not appear to be of relevance or value, with respect to adapting some kind of new behavior.

One might also suppose that the memories which arise in conjunction with the parsing of new experiences entail some sort of purpose, motivation, need, or inclination (other than, say, curiosity) ... forces which might be able to induce an organism to engage in different kinds of novel forms of experience. Furthermore, if various kinds of behavior are governed by habit, then, how does an organism overcome the inertial potential that is inherent in those habits and, thereby, be in a position to generate something that will lead to new behavior?

In some species – say, human beings – one might also want to factor in considerations involving identity and how a given kind of new behavior is related to one's identity. The extent to which some form of new behavior might enhance, challenge, or threaten one's sense of identity could determine whether, or not, that sort of behavior is pursued with any degree of persistence and irrespective of whether, or not, such behavior has to do with innovation or habit.

Is the memory that is being formed in conjunction with all of the foregoing influences episodic, procedural, and/or factual in nature? Are there separate fields for each kind of memory, and, if so, what is the nature of the storage dynamic and the nature of the process through which such memories are accessed?

Is the foregoing storage process electromagnetic, holographic, or is some other kind of dynamic (such as entanglement) involved? If there are different dynamics involved in the forming or maintaining of different kinds of memories, do those various kinds of dynamics resonate with one another in various ways, and if so, what is the nature of that resonance dynamic?

Let us assume that a repository for storing collective memories of a given species does exist. How do the members of a given species identify what is relevant in relation to that collected memory in conjunction with whatever is transpiring with respect to the on-going contingencies, needs, or interests in which a given member of the species might be currently immersed?

Are all memories collective, or are only some of them collective – for example, only those that have to do with procedures involving some kind of new behavior that has practical value for survival? Do different fields give expression to different kinds of memories like gluons, the weak force, photons, and the Higgs boson seem to give expression to different kinds of fields which might, or might not, be able to be shown to be different modalities of manifestation that are functions of some underlying unified field?

Is it possible that episodic or experientially-based memories could interfere with being able to access collective memories? Alternatively, is it possible that a given species' notion of what constitutes a 'fact --' or confusion about what differentiates fact from belief, or confusion about what differentiates reality from illusion -- might interfere with the formation and/or accessing of some modality of collective memory?

If a new kind of behavior arises within a given species and other members of that species subsequently exhibit a capacity to reduce the time that is needed to grasp and act in accordance with whatever the nature of the collective memory might be which is forming, or has formed, in relation to some new behavior, then, how are such improvements involving adaptive learning possible? In other words, how does some member of the species access, at a later time, the collective memory that has been laid down by the innovator of some behavior and, then, differentially respond to that collective field in a way that results in the kind of faster learning time or which leads to a more efficient -- and, therefore, speedier – performance of the sort to which Sheldrake is alluding in his book because the latter sort of adaptive behavior would appear to involve being able to change the nature of the underlying algorithm that governs, and is inherent in, the collective memory that is first laid down or generated by the innovator of some behavior?

How does any subsequent member of a species differentiate between, on the one hand, the original part of the collective memory that is laid down by the innovator of a certain behavior, and, on the other hand, those parts of the collective memory that have been added on by other members of the species that have been able to pick up on, or been able to grasp, the character of the original innovative behavior and, yet, at the same time, also have changed the habit-like or inertial properties of that initial edition of the collective memory as a result of having learned such behavior more quickly than had been the case with respect to the originator of the behavior? The existence of some sort of collective memory, in and of itself, does not appear to be sufficient to provide an account of how subsequent members of the species are able to engage that collective memory and, then, change it in order to be able to exhibit faster learning times.

Consequently, Sheldrake's idea that the formation of a collective memory leads to the emergence of new behaviors as well as habits doesn't appear to account for the capacity of those who subsequently engage the collective memory to be able to both be guided by that memory as well as to be able to change it. Furthermore, his hypothesis of formative causation doesn't appear to be able to account for how subsequent members of the species would be able to choose among various dimensions of the collective memory that give expression to differential learning times with respect to some given kind of new behavior and, thereby, be able to identify and, apparently, prefer those aspects of the collective memory that are able to lead to faster learning times.

About a third of the way through *The Presence of the Past: Morphic Resonance and the Habits of Nature*, Sheldrake begins to explore the idea of fields. He indicates that the notion of fields tends to be mysterious as a result of the way in which that idea is often described as being more fundamental than either matter or energy since the latter two ideas are often considered to be functions of one, or more, underlying fields which, to date, have not been able to be fully reconcilable with one another through some sort of unified field theory.

Although quantum electrodynamics was able to provide an account of how light and matter interacted with one another, and while, later on, the theory of the weak force became integrated with quantum electrodynamics in the form of a more comprehensive framework involving quantum fields (known as the electroweak theory), nevertheless, this is about as close as scientists have been able to come to developing some sort of unified theory of forces in which one would be able to show how various physical fields (e.g., electromagnetism, the weak force, the strong force and the gravitational force) were functions of some set of basic unifying mathematical equations. To date, no one has been able to show or demonstrate how the properties or values of fermions and bosons (the two basic modes of particles) could be derived naturally from first principles without scientists having to insert by hand the empirically determined values and properties of those fermions and bosons into the basic equations of physics because no one understands why fermions and bosons have the properties and values they do. In addition, no one has been able to show how quantum dynamics could be reconciled with a general theory of relativity that can, with considerable precision, describe what goes on within a gravitational field but cannot necessarily account for what makes a gravitational field possible nor account for how such a field interacts with other kinds of fields (e.g., electromagnetic, weak, strong, and the Higgs field) on a quantum level.

One might also note in passing that inherent in the theories of quantum field theory is the specter of ghostly infinities that have haunted those theories almost from their inception. Mathematical techniques such as renormalization have succeeded in providing a way of exorcising those demons in order to save theoretical appearances, but, nevertheless, being able to mathematically sweep infinities beneath an explanatory carpet does not really account for how actual existential infinities – and not just their mathematical counterparts – are able to disappear in finite time within any given quantum context, and, consequently, in a very real sense, renormalization is one of the many fictions that have been invented to make quantum mechanics work just as corporations are a fiction that have been invented by the courts to make someone's version of political theory work.

Furthermore, the four or five fields which are acknowledged as being present in the universe might, or might not, have anything to do with generating phenomena such as: Consciousness, intelligence, creativity, language, thought, choice, identity, and spirituality. While the assumption generally tends to be made in today's world that all of the foregoing qualities are, in some sense, functions or products of different modalities of physical dynamics of a kind (or kinds) that has (have) not, yet, been completely specified or worked out, scientists do not currently have any form of evidence that definitively proves and, therefore, can account for what makes any of the foregoing phenomena possible.

Sheldrake points out that beginning in the 1920s, there were a number of individuals (Hans Spemann, Alexander Gurwitsch, and Paul Weiss) who proposed the existence of various kinds of fields to account for the process of biological development. Morphogenetic fields was one of the terms that arose in the foregoing context and was used to try to allude to the possibility of having a scientific account that could explain the properties of embryogenesis (the process of cellular differentiation which leads to the formation of an array of cells, tissues, metabolic processes, and organs that give expression to any given species of organism) ... properties that were not, yet, understood.

During the 1930s and 1950s, C.H. Waddington tried to develop the foregoing notion of a morphogenetic field further. He introduced notions such as "chreodes" which he believed gave expression to individuated developmental pathways for various species within the context of an epigenetic landscape in which various facets of development seemed to give expression to "canalized" (channel-like) forms of dynamics that led toward the manifestation of certain endpoints (basins and attractors) which were a function of the particular character of the biological events that transpired in those landscapes.

The foregoing dynamics were often described as being a matter of self-organizing transactions. Whether those kinds of self-organizing transactions were somewhat autonomous and gave expression to emergent systems of self-organization that might randomly or sporadically occur as a result of conditions within a given epigenetic landscape, or whether those transactions were a function of underlying principles that were inherent in the morphogenetic fields that shaped development was often a point of contention.

One should note, however, that Béchamp, Enderlein, and Naessens believed, respectively, that microzymas, endobionts, and somatids possessed the principles which governed the life force. Consequently, for them, whatever the form of epigenetic dynamics that might be involved in embryogenesis or development was the result of what the internal dynamics of the aforementioned transducers of life force made possible.

Moreover, whereas, on the one hand, the theories of morphogenesis that were postulated in the 1920s, 1930s, and 1950s by individuals such as Hans Spemann, Alexander Gurwitsch, Paul Weiss, and C. H. Waddington were intended to be analogous, in some biological manner, to the fields being discussed in physics, on the other hand, the pleiomorphic/pleomorphic theories of Béchamp, Enderlein, and Naessens made biological events – including embryogenesis – a function of the life force principles that were believed to be present in microzymas, endobionts, or somatids and which were not reducible to a set of physical forces. As a result, there was no guarantee that those sorts of life forces were intended to be analogous to, or a function of, one or more of the fields of physics to which Waddington and others alluded in their theories of morphogenesis.

However, irrespective of whether the field dynamics of morphogenesis were approached through the theories of, say, Waddington, or were, alternatively, engaged through the theories of Béchamp, Enderlein, Rife, and Naessens, they all shared one feature in common. More specifically, all of those theories maintained that it was the field or biological terrain which was paramount and that development unfolded as a result of the principles inherent in the underlying dynamics of the biological field or terrain and, consequently, the process of development was not a strict function of genomics in which the germ plasm reigned supreme and dictated what transpired within any given organism.

According to Sheldrake, there are differences of opinion over, on the one hand, whether, or not, fields have any actual reality, or if they do actually exist, what the nature of that reality is, and, on the other hand, whether the notion of a field is just a convenient, practical way of speaking that helps one to organize various kinds of data and ideas. For example, some people have a Platonic-like orientation and consider fields to be giving expression to some sort of changeless set of Forms or Ideas which, ultimately, might, or might not, be mathematical in nature (ala Pythagoras), while other individuals believe that (like Aristotle) fields have certain kinds of causal properties which are able to materially affect what takes place within the context of those fields.

Sheldrake differentiates his notion of a morphogenetic field from field notions that are Platonic-like and/or Pythagorean-like. In other words, he believes that his hypothesis of formative causation entails a process of dynamics in which subsequent biological forms and processes are not a function of transcendent ideas or mathematical descriptions that are timeless in nature but, instead, his approach to biology involves field dynamics (morphogenetic events) that are causally dependent on what has taken place in the past (i.e., the formation of collective memory).

In addition, Sheldrake indicates that the notion of resonance which is present in his perspective is different from other theories involving the idea of resonance (e.g., electromagnetic theories and acoustic theories). More specifically, he maintains that for him resonance does not take place through the transference of energy but, instead, occurs due to a non-energetic transfer of information which he refers to as Morphic resonance.

While one might be prepared to acknowledge the possibility that not all forms of energy are necessarily physical in nature (for instance, consciousness, intelligence, creativity, and spirituality might involve forms of energy that are not necessarily physical in character), nonetheless, the idea of a non-energetic form of informational transference seems a little more -- if not a lot more – "iffy" in nature. This appears to be the case if for no reason other than that one has considerable difficulty understanding or visualizing how such a transfer would occur in the absence of any kind of energetics whatsoever.

Earlier in his book, Sheldrake did broach the idea that memory might not be stored in the brain. However, irrespective of whether, or not, memory resides in the brain, nonetheless, the whole process of memory formation (the process that occurs prior to it becoming collective memory) would seem to be steeped in energy-based dynamics of some kind and, indeed, for this and related reasons, many questions were raised in conjunction with the memory formation process previously in this chapter when some of the ideas of Rupert Sheldrake first began to be explored.

Just to reiterate some of the issues that were raised earlier one might ask: once a memory is formed, how is it stored? What is the nature of the dynamics which, according to Sheldrake, allows the dynamic formation of memories (whether done through physical or non-physical forms of dynamics) to be transferred into form of storage that is purely informational?

What enables such stored information to be changed over time as subsequent members of a species are able to learn a given behavior more and more quickly and, therefore, alter the character of the collective memory that previously existed as a result of the efforts of the individual organism that discovered a new way of doing something? What maintains stored information and where is it being stored?

What is the nature of a non-energetic form of resonance? How does a morphogenic field of information (i.e., the collective memory) resonate with the biological terrain of a living organism so that the latter (i.e., the terrain) is sensitive to the presence of, or has access to, the former (i.e., collective memory)?

Whatever the answer to the foregoing questions might be, Sheldrake's morphogenetic perspective appears to be somewhat Aristotelian in nature. In other words, he believes that fields exist in which causal dynamics take place within the context of those fields which are not dependent on any kind of transcendent set of Platonic Forms or Ideas. However, within the framework of those kinds of field dynamics, Sheldrake contends that rather than presuming that causality is a function of physical energies, he believes causality – at least in the context of learning new behaviors -- is rooted in a set of non-energetic informational changes that occur within a field of collective memory which gives expression to different forms of morphic, morphological, or morphogenetic resonance dynamics.

Notwithstanding the foregoing considerations, one does not have to suppose – along with Plato – that if there is a transcendent realm – relative to what transpires in relation to the physical world, then, this necessarily means that ideas and forms must, in and of themselves be transcendent rather than – for example -- being a manifested function of That which is transcendent. In other words, while the Source of all manifestation could be transcendent, manifestation, per se, comes and goes, and, as such, tends to be ephemeral and impermanent.

Moreover, instead of having to suppose that Ideas and Forms have to be perfect because they connected to a transcendent realm, what might be perfect about the foregoing sorts of manifested 'forms' and 'ideas' is the way in which they comply with, or serve, the character of the framework of Order through which those 'ideas' and 'forms' are made possible. For instance, if there are many flaws, imperfections, and the like which are present in the manifested world, the existence of those flaws does not necessarily reflect that some sort of imperfection must be present in That Which has made those sorts of difficulties and challenges possible but, instead, the existence of such problems merely might indicate that, in some unknown way, flaws and imperfections have a role to play in the way of the universe and, as such, are not necessarily due to either mistakes or some array of unanticipated random fluctuations.

Contrary to what Plato seemed to believe, Forms and Ideas do not necessarily have to be timeless, perfect, or transcendent. They could be expressions of a limited hangout of some kind which operates – despite whatever flaws and imperfections might be present -- on behalf of That Which lies beneath those appearances.

Furthermore, one might want to keep in mind how frameworks of statistical and quantum probabilities are often used for purposes of trying to describe events which take place in the universe. Consequently, one needs to distinguish between, on the one hand, a given modality of description and, on the other hand, That which such descriptions are intended to definitively circumscribe but which often do so only very problematically.

Plato and Aristotle could be reconciled to a certain extent if one were to call upon the metaphysics of something which might be referred to as an Order field. More specifically, whatever degree of order that exists in the physical universe could be due to the manner in which an Unmanifested realm (e.g., Rudolf Steiner's notion of Intelligence or an allusion to the previously noted saying of the Buddha in which "That which can be seen has no form, and that which cannot be seen has form," or the Hindu notion of "Brahman," or the Wakan Tanka – Great Mystery – of the Lakota Sioux, or the Dhat – Essence – noted by the Sufi mystics) which gives rise to the manifested realm of appearances – i.e., an Order field – such that what seems substantive in conjunction with the latter, manifested realm is a function of what has made those appearances possible rather than being a function of what is inherent in those appearances in a way that, supposedly, is independent of their Unmanifested Source. Furthermore, the properties of the Order field of appearances being manifested entail notions of causality in which different facets of such a field affect, change, or alter other dimensions of that same field.

On the one hand, by making reference to transcendent Forms and Ideas, Plato seeks to provide an explanation for why the world is the way it is, but he does so in a problematic way because the manifested and the Unmanifested have become conflated with, or confused for, one another. On the other hand, although Aristotle provides a framework for addressing issues of causation in the realm of appearances, he does so in a problematic way because he fails to offer anything that plausibly accounts for why causality works in the way that it does, or why there is something rather than nothing upon which causality operates.

However, if engaged in the right way, Plato and Aristotle actually complement one another. More specifically each perspective offers something that the other needs.

In the case of Aristotle, Plato offers something that is missing in the Aristotelian perspective – namely, the notion of a transcendent realm which makes possible all that goes on in the world of appearances. In the case of Plato, Aristotle offers something that is missing in the Platonic perspective – namely, a way of talking about causality which can be explored on the level of appearances without having to suppose that those appearances (or the dynamics which they entail) are transcendent, timeless, or perfect.

Sheldrake believes that the underlying Order field which governs the foregoing processes involves a form of collective memory that causally shapes what transpires in the realm of appearances. Those who believe that everything can be reduced to quantum phenomena (and some of this kind of thinking will be explored shortly) contend that the underlying Order field which governs what transpires in the realm of biology is a function of the dynamics of the zero point energy out of which all appearances emerge – including time, space, matter, energy, and life.

Béchamp, Enderlein, Rife, and Naessens respectively maintain that microzymas, endobionts, frequencies, or somatids give expression to a life force which epigenetically shapes what transpires in the biological terrain. As such, those entities serve as transducers which transform the energies (whether physical or non-physical in nature) of an underlying Order field into the biological dynamics that characterize the sort of metabolic processes which are responsible for maintaining or re-establishing a detoxified stability that, in the case of humans, requires a state of symbiosis between the terrain and the pleiomorphic/pleomorphic microorganisms that occupy that terrain.

Depending on how various issues are parsed, the internal dynamics of microzymas, endobionts, and somatids could be understood to be consistent with either quantum phenomena or morphic resonance phenomena. Or, alternatively, the foregoing internal dynamics of microzymas, endobionts, and somatids might operate in accordance with other kinds of non-physical.

Irrespective of how any of the foregoing kinds of dynamics might operate (via quantum processes, non-energetic modalities of formative causation, or non-physical forms of energetics), the foregoing entities would serve as transducers. In one scenario, microzymas, endobionts, or somatids would transduce zero-point energies of an Order field that gives expression to various kinds of quantum phenomena (both known and unknown) and would translate that energy into structured living systems. In another scenario, microzymas, endobionts, and somatids would transduce one, or more, of the forms of physical and non-physical energy to which the underlying Order field gives expression and that make those microzymas, endobionts, and somatids possible. Finally, in a third scenario, Sheldrake's morphogenetic field would transduce, among other things, collective memory (an evolutionary Order field) into various kinds of habits by means of information-based causal mechanisms.

There are unanswered questions and mysteries surrounding each of the foregoing scenarios. However, the intent here has not been to put forth a perspective that is definitive and devoid of epistemological challenges, but rather, the intent has been to introduce ideas and information that might help induce critical reflection and further discussion concerning those kinds of topics.

Toward the beginning of her book – *The Field: The Quest for the Secret Force of the Universe* – Lynne McTaggart proposes that human beings are on the edge of a revolution in which the focus is shifting away from a preoccupation with chemistry and biochemistry toward an exploration into the energetics of the fields that surround us as well as those that reside within us. To whatever extent the dynamics of chemical reactions are being replaced by the dynamics of other forms of energy, this is a transition which has been taking place for nearly two hundred years rather than something which only relatively recently has begun to take place.

Moreover, to reiterate a point made earlier in the current chapter, whether, or not, the forms of energies that underlie the capacity of microzymas, endobionts, or somatids to be able to epigenetically regulate the dynamics of the biological terrain of any given organism must necessarily be quantum-based, continues to be, in many ways, an open question. Indeed, the ensuing discussion will attempt to put forth some considerations that might challenge the idea that all forms of field energy necessarily lead, ultimately, to some form of quantum phenomena.

However, there is one premise concerning fields that is present in the aforementioned book of Lynne McTaggart's with which I am in agreement – at least, up to a certain point. More specifically, that the properties of a field (whatever it turns out to be) forms the woof and warp through which, or out of which, the tapestry of dynamic appearances is woven.

While the foregoing perspective does tend to reflect the conceptual orientation of Lynne McTaggart, the following claim does not reflect that orientation even though it is not inherently inconsistent with her general position either. More specifically, just as Béchamp indicated how the biological terrain is everything and, as a result, whatever transitions in the life cycles of pleiomorphic/pleomorphic microorganism which take place within a given terrain are a reflection of the conditions that characterize the terrain being occupied by such microorganisms, so too, the field or fields in which particular biological terrains are ensconced tend (tends) to determine how those terrains can be induced to operate or behave over time.

Said in another way, the modalities of energetics which transpire in such a field are of fundamental importance to what might, or might not, take place within any given biological terrain. Nonetheless, the character of those dynamics is not necessarily exclusively quantum or even physical in nature.

As noted earlier, energy – along with the associated notion of force -- is about a capacity to underwrite and, thereby, activate or give expression to the properties of a given set of dynamics. While some forms of energy -- such as electromagnetism – might, in some sense, be physical in nature, not all forms of dynamics are necessarily functions of physical systems or physical forces that are a function of quantum physics

While during the course of her book, Lynne McTaggart appears to indicate that spirituality might, somehow, be a function of quantum dynamics, sometimes it seems that she seems to forget that quantum mechanics is a methodological system for describing physical phenomena, and on the basis of those sorts of descriptions, that system provides a way to generate predictions concerning some of the properties which are likely to become manifest under specified conditions. For instance, at one point, early in her book, she contends that particles – such as electrons, photons, and so on – simultaneously exist in all possible states prior to some act of observation or measurement singling out which of those states will be realized in a given set of circumstances.

The foregoing notion of all possible states of any given particle allegedly being able to exist simultaneously supposedly gives expression to a condition that is referred to as being "superpositional" in character. A process of decoherence is said to occur when the foregoing condition of being superpositional is terminated (via observation or measurement), and, like a butterfly emerging from a chrysalid, a determinant event of one kind rather than another is manifested (in other words there is a transition to a particularized condition and away from a generalized condition involving the alleged multiplicity of states of a given particle which, supposedly, are simultaneously present).

Scientists -- including quantum physicists -- have not been able to demonstrate that the idea of being superpositional is anything more than a theoretical construct. The matrix equations of Heisenberg, the wave equations of Schrödinger, the relativistic wave equation of Paul Dirac, as well as the Sum-Over History technique of Feynman are all designed to enable a person to solve for particular outcomes within a given set of circumstances.

The idea of being superpositional might be the theoretical starting point from which the foregoing methods take flight. However, none of those four methods – or any of the other dimensions of quantum calculations – has the capacity to demonstrate that such a starting point was ever an existential reality.

While there is a sense in which observation or measurement triggers a cascade of events which leads to the determination of values that enable solutions for quantum equations to be discovered (and, one can't help but wonder if that which triggers observation is something other than quantum in nature), observation and measurement only find what can be particularized in a given context. Thus, when the underlying field is engaged in a certain way, certain kinds of particularized events are capable of being identified, and this realization of a particular, determinate result seems to be a function of field dynamics rather than the mysterious collapse of a given particle's superpositional state.

There is a tendency among many commentators concerning quantum phenomena to want to read all manner of possibilities into what is not known. However, what quantum mechanics can say with any degree of precision or reliability and what many people would like quantum mechanics to be able to say is not necessarily the same thing.

In her aforementioned book Lynne McTaggart goes on to indicate that the nature of the field out of which we all are manifested is what is known as a Zero Point Energy Field. Supposedly, this is a sea of vibrational dynamics through which all things are allegedly connected and out of which all phenomena emerge.

Technically speaking, Zero-Point Energy gives expression to the allegedly random fluctuations that characterize quantum phenomena (caused by so-called virtual particles that, supposedly, constantly pop in and out of existence) when the latter are in their lowest state of dynamics or energetics within, for example, the vacuum of space. The Zero-Point aspect of the foregoing notion has to do with the way in which calculations have been made (e.g., when the velocity of particles is set to zero and particles are presumed to have their lowest potential energy), and these sorts of calculations supposedly indicate that when the total amount of positive and negative fluctuations of quantum events in the vacuum of space are taken into consideration – and such negative and positive fluctuations are believed to be infinite in nature -- then, those sorts of calculations are believed to give rise to a value which is either very close to zero or actually zero (one needs to remember, however, that this is a calculation or prediction and not an empirically demonstrable result).

One also might wish to keep in mind that if one sets aside the issue of gravity, one can't actually measure absolute energies. Instead, one can only measure changes in energy or differences in energy that occur over a given period of time.

However, gravity really can't be set aside, and, therefore, measuring energy differences in a vacuum becomes problematic. All forms of physical energy, whatever their nature, have a gravitational pull which is associated with them, and when one is considering those kinds of dynamics, then, the absolute energy in which those dynamics take place is what matters and not various modalities of relative change in energy over time.

Given the foregoing framework, then, according to Dr. Sabine Hossenfelder, exploring the issue of absolute energies only makes sense in the context of general relativity – that is, Einstein's attempt to refine and expand upon Newtonian mechanics. The basic metric for trying to measure the absolute energy of the gravitational field would be a function of what transpires within a vacuum, and according to Einstein's field equations for general relativity, this would involve, among other things, two constants which, by definition, are supposed to exhibit the same value throughout space.

One of the two foregoing constants – G -- has to do with Newton's reference to the strength of gravity. The other constant which is present within Einstein's field equation is referred to as 'lambda' – Λ -- the so-called cosmological constant.

In addition to the foregoing constants, there are several variables which are present in Einstein's field equation for general relativity. One variable – R -- has to do with the curvature of space-time, and the other variable -- T -- has to do with all other forms of radiation and particles that exist in the universe.

If one gives 'T' a value of zero in the Einstein field equations, this would mean that space is devoid of all forms of particles and radiation. When this occurs, then, according to Sabine Hossenfelder, Λ (lambda) can be understood as constituting the energy density of the vacuum which is a measure of energy in a given volume of space.

Supposedly, energy density doesn't become diluted if space should expand as some cosmological theories require in their attempt to make sense of various kinds of red-shift observations that have been made by an array of astronomers and astrophysicists. Rather, Dr. Hossenfelder indicates that energy density is a property of space-time and, therefore, irrespective of whether, or not, space expands, the energy density should remain the same.

Thus, on the one hand, if space were to expand, then, the number of particles which are present in a given volume of space would become diluted. On the other hand, energy density remains the same because it is a function of space-time which, according to Einstein, does not change.

There is a scalability factor – 'a' – that can be factored into Einstein's field equations for general relativity. This has to do with the way in which the rate of expansion or acceleration of the universe has a contribution to make which is proportional to the cosmological constant.

If Λ (lambda) is positive, then, the expansion of the universe tends to speed up. However, Dr. Hossenfelder indicates that the foregoing considerations have nothing to do with the issue of quantum fluctuations.

The energy density constant which is present in general relativity cannot be measured. It is a property which is inferred on the basis of various kinds of observation.

According to many particle physicists, the energy density of the vacuum has been predicted to be some 120 orders of magnitude above zero. Unfortunately, there is no way to conduct an experiment which would be capable of proving or disproving such a prediction.

Particle physicists claim that the vacuum is replete with energy, although the predictions which have been made concerning just how much energy is present seem to be way out of line – by some considerable number of magnitudes – with what is actually observed. According to Dr. Hossenfelder, while the energy density of the vacuum can't actually be measured, nevertheless, its presence can be detected as a function of whether, or not, space is accelerating at one rate rather than another.

On the particle physics side of matters, the notion of virtual particles is a fiction. Virtual particles aren't actually seen, but, rather, they are a theoretical construct which seeks to make sense of flows of energy that can be detected on the quantum level.

On the general relativity side of the ledger, the notion of space-time is a mathematical/theoretical construct. It is a co-ordinate system or metric for measuring, among other things, the curvature which can be detected in a given volume of space that gives expression to the presence of a gravitational field during a given period of time.

One might also keep in mind that Einstein considered the presence of the Λ (lambda) constant is his field equations to constitute one of the biggest "blunders" in his career. When his field equations were first formulated, he was seeking to account for, among other things, the properties of a steady-state universe, but when evidence subsequently began to accumulate which suggested that the universe might have come into being through a Big-Bang and, as a result, involved expansion, then, the presence of Λ (lambda) seemed to be an embarrassment because it appeared to serve as a conservative force which helped to keep the universe in a steady state, and, therefore, that constant seemed to be inconsistent with the idea of a Big Bang and an expanding universe.

Eventually, proponents of the Big Bang did find ways of reconciling the Λ (lambda) constant in Einstein's field equations with the idea of an expanding universe. However, astronomers such as Halton Arp put forth data – for which he was ostracized from the so-called community of astronomical researchers – suggesting that the Doppler red-shift which was being interpreted by many astronomers and cosmologists as signifying an expanding universe actually constituted evidence of another phenomena entirely – an ejection phenomenon leading to the birth of new astronomical materials and systems -- because he had discovered that there were galactic phenomena (quasars) were associated with bodies that exhibited greater red-shifts than certain other astronomical entities despite the fact that independent ways of measuring the distance of those structures from Earth seemed to indicate that certain bodies nearer to Earth were exhibiting the greater red-shift values which, if true, would entirely contradict the interpretation of red-shift (the rate at which certain heavenly bodies were receding from Earth) that was favored by the proponents of an expanding universe.

Just as virtual particles are a way of trying to make sense of what is observed, so too, space-time and red-shifts are a way of trying to make sense of what is observed. However, all of the foregoing ways of trying to make sense of things are a function of constructs which might, or might not, accurately reflect the character of some aspect of nature.

Neither particle physics nor general relativity takes into account possible forms of dynamics or energetics that are not physical in nature. Particle physicists say that one kind of dynamic – namely, the random fluctuations of virtual particles at their lowest state of energy -

- is present in the vacuum, while those who subscribe to the theory of general relativity (and there are theories of gravity which are non-Newtonian and non-Einsteinian in character) propose that another kind of dynamic having to do with the energy density of space-time is taking place in the vacuum.

If one is not prepared to acknowledge that there might be other kinds of dynamics or energetics which are present in, or being expressed through, the vacuum of space, then, obviously, one will not likely be employing forms of metrics that are capable of detecting the presence of those kinds of possibilities. Indeed, neither the idea of virtual particles nor the idea of space-time is capable of detecting, measuring, or accounting for forms of energetics which are not – if they exist -- physical in nature.

Many individuals suppose that the Quantum Field which consists of Zero Point Energy is characterized by random fluctuations which, somehow, become ordered into the particularized events of decoherence. No one actually has shown that such a field, if it exists as described (i.e., as a set of infinite negative and positive values), is random in nature, and, indeed, one of the difficulties that has bedeviled quantum mechanics almost from the beginning is a consistent inability to explain how a given, determinate particular arises out of such a supposedly randomly fluctuating field ... there are probabilities which indicate what could happen or might happen or is likely to happen, but there is nothing which can be reliably said about why those probabilities – rather than some other set of probabilities – are showing up.

If one likes, one can assume that the latter particulars are giving expression to random fluctuations. However, this is all that one is doing – proceeding on the basis of an assumption which has not been empirically confirmed.

Is Lynne McTaggart correct when she indicates that human beings are nothing more, or less, than a collection of quantum packets of energy which are exchanging information with other quantum packets that exist within the universe? Is she right when she says that the ocean of vibrational energy that gives expression to the Zero-Point Energy of a quantum field is inexhaustible, and, therefore, in a sense without limit with respect to what might be able to be accomplished through it?

If the universe is random, then, from whence does order arise? Can one justifiably assume (and, therefore, empirically demonstrate) that order is nothing but a statistical artifact of random events?

The foregoing assumption might make sense within the realm of mathematics in which one can re-arrange possibilities in any one likes as long as one stays true to the underlying principles governing the mathematical representation of those possibilities. However, when one moves from the realm of mathematics to the realm of lived existence, do the principles governing existential possibility change and, therefore, transition away, to varying degrees, from the principles that govern the dynamics of mathematics?

If the universe is quintessentially quantum in nature, then, how do consciousness, intellect, reason, creativity, language, talent, and spirituality emerge from quantum phenomena? Moreover, while one might be prepared to acknowledge that quantum phenomena are, in various ways, associated with the biological terrain, can one necessarily suppose that the only field human beings have access to, or which they might be affected by, is quantum in nature?

In any number of ways, 'frequency following response' phenomena have been shown to exist. Some of these phenomena seem to be governed by electromagnetic dynamics which appear to comply with the principles of quantum physics, but there are other kinds of 'frequency following responses' that, conceivably, might be governed by non-quantum dynamics.

For example, what about the case in which a friend of Veda Austin said a prayer at some distance from water that is to be frozen, and, subsequently, after freezing, the water displays a certain kind of hexagonal pattern? Can one justifiably conclude beyond a reasonable doubt that the relationship between, on the one hand, the person who is saying a prayer and, on the other hand, the water toward which the prayer is being directed and which later seems to be exhibiting some sort of frequency following response in conjunction with that prayer consists only of quantum phenomena?

What is directing a certain kind of hexagonal pattern to become manifest? Can the foregoing sort of ordering process -- which results in a possibly unique hexagonal structure of one kind rather than of another kind -- be reduced to nothing more than (as remarkable as this might be) a set of quantum processes?

Having access to energy is not necessarily the same thing as having access to energy that has been incorporated into an ordered system that can make use of the potential which is present in a given form of energy. The water that flows down a steep incline does not automatically generate electrical power, and a moving magnetic does not automatically turn a light on, but, rather, in each of the foregoing cases, an infrastructure of some kind is required so that the potential within flowing water or the electrical potential which is associated with a moving magnet can be harnessed in order to be able to generate certain kinds of effects.

Even if one were to assume that all of space consists of Zero-Point Energy -- and, as noted earlier during the discussion of Einstein's field equations for general relativity, there are reasons for not making such an assumption -- Zero-Point Energy seems a lot like water flowing down a steep incline or a magnet being moved about. In other words, having a source of energy potential is one thing but being able to convert that potential into some kind of ordered, structured dynamics appears to be quite another proposition.

One cannot necessarily assume – at least with any sort of viable credibility -- that a prayer is communicated to a certain Petri dish of water via quantum events, nor can one assume – with any plausibility – that the force or forces which lead to a hexagonal structure of one kind rather than another being manifested in crystalline form is necessarily a function of quantum events. Furthermore, even if quantum phenomena of some kind are involved with those kinds of events, one cannot necessarily justifiably assume that such structures arose because the quantum field has the capacity to self-organize itself, for example, whenever prayers of a certain kind and whenever water of a certain kind engage one another.

To be sure, the property of emergent behavior can be, and has been, demonstrated to be a real phenomenon within the context of an array of different circumstances. More specifically, if one is able to establish the right set of conditions, then, sometimes a form of behavior can be empirically shown to be able to arise out of those conditions ... behavior which could not have been predicted based on what had been understood concerning the way that chemical and/or physical systems operate up to the point in which the foregoing sort of demonstration was conducted.

Nonetheless, quite frequently, the notion of emergent behavior is used as a rhetorical device for theoretically or presumptively alluding to an explanation that – in a vague sort of way – might account for how something is possible without actually being able to show that such a possibility can be empirically demonstrated. In a sense, the notion of emergent behavior is often used in ways that are similar to what happens in conjunction with chaos theory in which some individuals will attribute all manner of hidden forms of determinacy to conditions which, on the surface, seem chaotic or random, but, actually, are not all that well understood, and, as a result, ignorance is used to leverage possibility into something that might sound credible but has, yet, to be proven to be true.

Returning to the previously mentioned Veda Austin experiment involving prayers and water, do we know that prayer or thought are inherently functions of quantum dynamics? There are lots of theories floating around about those kinds of possibilities, but, at the present time we don't necessarily know what thought and prayer actually are let alone what makes them possible.

If prayer and thought are not functions of quantum dynamics, can those phenomena be transduced in some way, and, thereby, become transmogrified into a quantum-based modality? Is it possible to simulate thought or prayer by generating frequencies that have been empirically demonstrated to be associated with certain kinds of thoughts or cognitive behaviors?

In Chapter 14, certain aspects of the work of Dr. Nick Begich were explored (*Controlling the Human Mind*). Apparently, on the basis of a considerable amount of research, Dr. Begich came to the conclusion that frequency following responses can be generated in human beings so that certain kinds of experiences, emotions, and, even, thoughts can be induced to manifest themselves in people who have been subjected to, or exposed to, certain kinds of frequencies.

The foregoing does not prove that thoughts, emotions, and the like are quantum phenomena. However, at the very least, his research would seem to indicate that certain aspects of conscious behavior can be simulated within, or through, the brain.

What if one were to suppose that the brain is not necessarily the source of thoughts, ideas, insights, understanding, and so on, but has the capacity to receive such phenomena, then, this would seem to indicate that the brain could have the capacity to transduce ideas, thoughts, and so on which are coming to it from without. In other words, perhaps the brain might have the capacity to transform such received phenomena (whatever their ultimate nature might be) into an array of frequencies that can be processed into a usable set of biological dynamics.

When ideas or thoughts occur to us, we don't really know where they come from. They are just there.

Those phenomena could have come from without – as when my wife and I seem to exchange thoughts in a non-spoken manner, or as seems to have taken place in some of the experiments which Nick Begich discussed in his aforementioned book. Alternatively, as those with a fundamentalist-like materialist bent might be inclined to believe, such phenomena are, somehow, produced by the brain even though, currently, they have no idea how the brain accomplishes that sort of production.

In the previously mentioned experiment of Veda Austin in which a friend thinks of, or says, a prayer that is intended for, or being directed toward, water that is situated in another location, do the intention and prayer come from within her friend or is the friend merely a locus of manifestation through which the prayer emerges? What is the nature of the relationship, if any, between, on the one hand, the intended prayer, and, on the other hand, quantum dynamics?

Do intention and prayer somehow organize, or draw upon, Zero-Point Energy so that the structural character of the intention and prayer is able to impact the targeted water? If so, what is the nature of this organizing or drawing process?

Is some sort of entanglement phenomenon taking place? If entanglement of some kind is present, is it necessarily a function of quantum dynamics, and if it is not a function of quantum dynamics, then, wouldn't the existence, or non-existence, of Zero-Point Energy be irrelevant?

In what manner does the targeted water that is in Veda Austin's lab receive the prayer which has been intended for it by her friend? Is the form of that intended prayer non-quantum in nature or is it quantum in character?

How does the water transduce that phenomenon? How does the water store what has been transduced, and how does a hexagonal structure of a, presumably, unique kind become manifest when the water is frozen?

Are the foregoing transactions functions of quantum dynamics? Or, are they non-quantum in nature and involve some other kind of energetics? Or, are they some combination of quantum and non-quantum dynamics?

If the information that is derived from the intended prayer is quantum-based, then, how does that set of quantum activities become ordered into one kind of hexagonal structure rather than another? If the intended prayer impacts the water in Veda Austin's lab (and this is an interpretation concerning the nature of what is transpiring) but is non-quantum in nature, then, how does one kind of hexagonal structure rather than another modality of hexagonal structure arise in conjunction with such an (assumed) impact?

How much of the foregoing structure is a function of what is intended due to the giving of a prayer that is of one kind rather than another? To what extent, if any, did the water contribute to the formation of the hexagonal structure that is manifested upon freezing in a way that is to some degree, independent of what was intended by Veda Austin's friend?

One can talk about quantum dynamics and Zero-Point Energy as much as one likes. However, none of that talk is able to provide a plausible, step-by-step account of how intention, prayer, transmission, the capacities of water, and the formation of a hexagonal structure interact with one another.

The entire infrastructure is missing that is necessary to connect intended prayer and a hexagonal structure and, then, show how everything that links one to the other is made possible through, as well as derivable from, Zero-Point Energy. The same fundamental problem that befuddled the architects of quantum theory is disclosing its resonating presence in the foregoing set of unanswered questions – namely, how do quantum events get transformed into the dynamics of classical phenomena with which we deal in everyday life? And, of course, the foregoing problem presumes that no form of non-physical energetics is involved in such events in ways that are complementary to, and/or are independent of, quantum dynamics.

In Chapter One of her book – *The Field* – Lynne McTaggart talks about an experience undergone by astronaut Ed Mitchell during the 1971 Apollo 14 mission. At some point during the mission, he was staring out one of the craft's windows and had an overwhelming sense of being connected not only with the rest of the universe beyond the window, but, as well, with all human beings throughout time.

During the experience, he felt that time was a construct. He sensed that individual intentions did not exist but, instead, there was only the presence of a universal 'intelligence' of some kind.

The experience was not primarily conceptual in character. It was visceral in a way such that his entire body and being experienced the connectedness which seemed to be present.

Apparently, the experience did not seem to be religious in character. Instead, the experience appeared to be a realization of the way that existence or Being is in and of Itself, and Ed had been connected to the omnipresence of Being through the experience of realization to which he had been opened up while looking out one of the Apollo 14's windows.

Without wishing to denigrate or deny the felt reality of the foregoing experience, nevertheless, certain questions do tend to bubble to the surface. Lynne McTaggart indicates that Mitchell had been in touch with 'the Force' or 'the Field,' but such a conclusion seems a little premature, or, said in another way, if he was in touch with some sort of 'Force' or 'Field,' neither he nor Lynn McTaggart necessarily understand what the nature of that Field was or entailed – although much of what follows in the various chapters of her book attempts to tie those kinds of experiences to quantum dynamics and Zero-Point Energy.

Had he actually been in touch with the entire universe? Had he actually been connected with all people, both present and past?

Is there actually no such thing as individual intention? Is the sort of Intelligence being alluded to in the foregoing experience all that is or which exists, and, if so, what is one to make of the personalized sort of experience that Ed Mitchell believed had enveloped his awareness? Who was the one experiencing and what was being experienced?

Is time really a construct? Or, possibly, was his experience some sort of phenomenological invention in which time appeared to be a construct?

Ed Mitchell was a strange combination of fundamentalist Baptist and scientific rigor. He had earned a doctorate in astrophysics from MIT and, in addition, was a test-pilot colleague of Chuck Yeager who, like Yeager, was made of 'The Right Stuff.'

Prior to the Apollo 14 mission, he had arranged to perform a number of off-book telepathy experiments during the mission in conjunction with several Earth-based scientists who were interested in exploring the nature of consciousness. The experiments involved copying various numbers that represented the Zener symbols (circle, star, square, a set of wavy lines, and cross) that were used by Dr. Joseph Rhine at Duke University as part of the latter's method for testing human beings to try to determine if telepathic capabilities might be present.

Although six sessions of the foregoing sort of number recording had been planned, only four were able to be completed. His confederates on Earth were tasked with the challenge of trying to discern what numbers were being recorded by Ed Mitchell during a given experimental session.

Later, after the Apollo mission had been completed, the results of the foregoing four experiments were analyzed. Those results achieved statistical significance and indicated that such scores would have been due to chance in only 1 in 3,000 cases.

Nassim Nicholas Taleb has written a number of books (e.g., *Fooled by Randomness* and *The Black Swan*) which indicate that the way we engage, and reflect on, the events of our lives often become entangled in a kind of delusional modality of thinking. For example, in *The Black*

Swan, he indicates, among many other issues, that life is filled with what are referred to as "black swan" events in which possibilities that are considered to be highly improbable, nonetheless, can, and do, take place, and, yet, many people go about their lives as if such black swan events don't exist or are so rare that they don't need to be taken into consideration when making decisions about how to proceed in life.

Statistics doesn't eliminate "chance" from being treated or understood as constituting a possible causal-like influence in an experimental process. In fact, the notion of chance is an interpretation of events which colors those events in shades of conceptually-driven (and not necessarily existentially driven) notions of randomness without necessarily correctly understanding what might actually underlay the occurrence of such events, yet, nevertheless, the likelihood that chance events are responsible for a given outcome can be statistically framed within, or restricted to, the somewhat arbitrary statistical notion of "significance" which creates a context of diminished possibility -- in which one can trust, or not, as one chooses -- that chance events (whatever this might mean) are responsible for what took place in a given experiment.

A little later in the first chapter of her book, Lynne McTaggart maintains that the phenomena of cause and effect no longer seem to be present when dealing with events on the sub-atomic or quantum level. Instead, according to her, cause and effect appear to be replaced by indeterminacy and random events.

Once again, however, a certain amount of caution needs to be exercised when engaging such issues. One should try to keep in mind that quantum dynamics is a methodology for describing, framing, and interpreting empirical data, and, consequently, one cannot be sure whether, on the one hand, any given answer that is generated through quantum methodology constitutes a way of framing reality which distorts, to varying degrees, the actual nature of reality, or whether, on the other hand, such an answer accurately reflects, within certain limits, the way that nature is.

To whatever extent telepathic phenomena are real – and the evidence in favor of such a possibility appears to be considerable – are those events caused by determinate events of one kind or another, or are they the result of some sort of indeterminacy phenomenon which is devoid of causal considerations? Are the turtles of indeterminacy really indeterminate turtles all the way down to the essence of Being, or -- as Einstein believed and Niels Bohr denied -- is indeterminacy, at some point, a function of hidden variables which preserve cause and effect?

Lynne McTaggart introduces the notion of "nonlocality" at this point. She indicates that the term refers to empirical discoveries which demonstrate, on a quantum level, how some particles are linked in a way that seems to be independent of spatial distance and, therefore, is not something that is a function of dynamics which are restricted by what can be communicated between such particles via the speed of light.

One might want to keep in mind that entanglement experiments usually use the metric of spin to measure whether, or not, the phenomenon of entanglement is present in a given set of circumstances. Spin is a property of particles which can be mathematically described or represented and that certain particles appear to possess but which no one really understands.

One might be able to show that the property of spin connects particles despite the fact that conditions of locality do not hold with respect to those particles (locality involves circumstances in which communication between particles is restrained by what can be transmitted by the speed of light within a given time frame). Nevertheless, such a demonstration doesn't really say anything at all about whether, or not, other properties of those separated particles might, or might, not be entangled as well, nor does it indicate what the possible significance of such connections might have, if any, for the macro-world or classical world in which we tend to live our lives.

In addition, even though scientists have been able to prove that entanglement phenomena exist, nonetheless, to date, their research has not shown that those kinds of phenomena only can be a function of quantum dynamics. Indeed, conceivably, non-quantum forms of entanglement might play a far more significant role than do quantum versions of entanglement, and such non-quantum forms of entanglement might be a consideration when quantum editions of entanglement do not seem to be sufficiently robust to account for what might be going on a given phenomenon – such as in conjunction with the phenomenon of telepathy or when a prayer is said that is intended to – and appears to -- affect water that is not geographically proximate to the individual through whom the prayer is being sent.

Contrary to the claims of Lynne McTaggart, being able to prove that some phenomena are linked via non-local entanglement dynamics doesn't necessarily disprove Einstein's contention that nothing is capable of exceeding the speed of light. Possibly, all that is being shown is that there are forms of entanglement which do not entail communication across, or signaling across, spatial distances in accordance with the restraints that the speed of light places on communication or signaling.

Although the notion of dimensionality is often tied to geometric forms of representation (e.g., Kaluza-Klein theory of gravity, string theory) which are inherently spatial, nevertheless, dimensionality need not be restricted in such a spatial manner. Dimensionality might involve qualitative differences that are independent of spatial distances and, if so, then, the manner in which particles or other entities become entangled with one another might have nothing to do with communication across spatial distances.

For instance, let's accept the Apollo-14 experience of Edgar Mitchell at face value. Given that premise, if he really were connected to the entire universe at the instant he was looking out the craft's window and if during that encounter he really were connected to all people both present and past, then, this would be an example of a form of dimensionality that appears to be non-local and, therefore, non-space in character.

One of the mistakes which string theory might have made is to suppose that the dimensions which are proposed by different versions of that theory must necessarily be spatial in character rather than being able to be qualitatively differentiated from one another. String theory requires that its extra dimensions must undergo a process of compactification into, say, Calabi-Yau spaces in order for the multidimensional character of string theory to be reconciled with our classical, four dimensional experience of the world.

To be sure, making dimensionality qualitative rather than quantitative would likely require one to develop, or discover, different modalities of metrics for gauging what transpires in those dimensions.

However, at the same time, one might begin to critically reflect on the fact that just as sight, sound, smell, proprioception, and tactile sensation constitute different dimensions of experience and, yet, manage to comingle with one another within a unified sense of consciousness, so too, the notion of dimensionality within physics might benefit from a certain amount of critical reflection concerning how the "stuff" or vibrational energetics that populate the universe might give expression to the 'dynamics of comingling' among a number of qualitatively different dimensions, some of which are physical and some of which are not physical in nature, but all of which contribute to the character or properties of such "stuff" or vibrational energetics.

In Chapter Four of her book – *The Field* – Lynne McTaggart explores, in some detail, various kinds of biological phenomena that shed a certain kind of light on the topic of cellular communication. For example, she discusses an experiment in which a group of French researchers were studying the effect that various kinds of physical interventions had on the heart of a guinea pig.

More specifically, they were measuring the effect that different vasodilators (tend to increase blood flow), which were histamine-like and acetylcholine-like, might have on the heart, as well as seeking to determine what impact adding mepyramine-like and atropine-like components – which are agonists (suppressors) of vasodilators – would have on the heart that was being observed. However, the influencers that were being added to the heart in question were not molecular in nature.

Instead, what were being introduced into the experimental heart were low-frequency renditions of electromagnetic signals that previously had been recorded (by using a certain kind of transducer and a sound-card equipped computer) as those signals emanated from the aforementioned molecules. In other words, the experiment was about whether, or not, the properties of molecular substances could be transduced into frequencies that would have the same impact on the heart as actual molecules would have had.

When the frequencies for acetylcholine and histamine were introduced into their experimental heart, those frequencies induced the heart to exhibit increased blood flow as if actual molecular vasodilators were being used. Similarly, when the frequencies for mepyramine and atropine were introduced to the heart, blood flow was restricted.

Nearly a hundred years ago, Royal Rife was using frequencies to cure cancer and other diseases. Moreover, earlier in the present book (Chapter 14 – Resonance) the work of Carolyn McMakin and Nick Begich indicated that frequencies were capable of having profound effects on what might transpire within various aspects of the biological terrain.

In the 1970s, Fritz-Albert Popp was doing research involving the idea that each substance seemed to have its own particular frequency or resonance ... a signature which differentiates one substance from another. His research had begun with trying to determine what, if any, effect ultraviolet light might have on carcinogenic compounds.

The particular compound he was investigating was a substance that was considered to be profoundly carcinogenic. It was known as benzo(a)pyrene which was a polycyclic hydrocarbon molecule.

Polycyclic compounds contain a number of aromatic rings. Initially, those sorts of compounds were differentiated on the basis of smell (i.e., aroma) before their actual molecular composition was, subsequently, determined.

Popp had discovered that when benzo(a)pyrene is exposed to ultraviolet light of a certain frequency (380 nanometers) the compound altered the UV frequency that was being transmitted through the molecule. However, when he performed the same kind of experiment with benzo(e)pyrene – which is almost, but not quite, identical to benzo(a)pyrene – then, the UV frequency passed through unaltered.

When Popp performed the same kind of experiment with a number of other compounds – some of which were carcinogenic and some which were not – he discovered that only the compounds that had carcinogenic properties possessed the capacity to scramble 380 nanometer UV light . While he was critically reflecting on the results of his experiments, he came across research concerning a phenomenon known as "photo-repair".

Considerable research had established that if one were to expose a cell to ultraviolet radiation to the point where 99% of that cell and its DNA were destroyed, nonetheless, the cell could re-acquire its full functionality if one were to subsequently expose that cell to the same UV wavelength which had been destroying the cell but did so at a much lower intensity. During the course of his investigation into the phenomenon of photo-repair, he discovered that the process operates most efficiently when the ultraviolet light is at 380 nanometers – the same wavelength at which carcinogenic compounds, like benzo(a)pyrene, exhibited the capacity to alter the frequency of UV light.

On the basis of his experimental work and the foregoing research into the photo-repair phenomenon he began to entertain a startling possibility. Perhaps, carcinogenic materials were carcinogenic because they were capable of interfering with the wavelength at which the process of photo-repair took place most efficiently.

Popp wrote up the results and conclusions entailed by his explorations into ultraviolet light, carcinogenic compounds, and photo-repair. His work was challenged on one point – namely, there was no evidence that the body produced a form of weakly intense ultraviolet light of 380 nanometers.

Later on, he took on a doctoral student by the name of Bernhard Ruth. The collaboration began with a challenge -- namely, Popp wanted Ruth to demonstrate that the body was not capable of generating light.

After several years of laboring, Ruth built a device that was capable of detecting whether, or not, photons of extremely weak intensities might be emanating from the body. After running through various experiments in order to eliminate whether, or not, different possible sources (such as photosynthesis) might be leading to the production of light that was being observed during their experiments, Ruth and Popp discovered that organisms did, indeed, give off what came to be termed biophoton emissions.

The two research scientists also discovered that the biophoton emissions were highly coherent. In other words, whatever was going on involved some form of cooperation or resonance among the photons that were being given off.

One of the next questions that he addressed was directed toward discovering what the source of the light might be that was emanating from different organisms. To determine this, he began to work with ethidium bromide and DNA samples.

Ethidium bromide has an effect on DNA. The latter molecule will unwind when exposed to ethidium bromide.

He discovered that the more of the compound which he added to a given sample of DNA, the more the latter molecule would unwind. He also discovered that the more the DNA unwound, the more light would be released, and, moreover, the less ethidium bromide that was added, the less DNA would unwind, but, as well, less light would be released.

On the basis of the foregoing experiments, Popp came to the conclusion that DNA was a storehouse of biophotons. He came to believe that when DNA became unwound within the cell, then, photons of various frequencies would be released by the DNA and this would lead to biophotons of various frequencies having a differential impact on biological dynamics.

The mainstream view of biological functioning is that the genome, via various modalities of RNA, leads to the production of amino acids which are assembled into proteins that regulate the bodies network of anabolic (building up) and catabolic (tearing down) forms of self-regulation. Popp was proposing that the biophotons consisted of an array of frequencies that were being released as DNA became unwound and that this release of coherent-like light might be playing a crucial role in orchestrating what transpired with any given organism.

Estimates have been made that each cell carries out more than one hundred thousand operations per second. If one considers the billions of cells that are present in the body, then, an almost unimaginable number of biological operations are taking place simultaneously within the body every single second of the day.

All of the foregoing activity gives rise to a very important question, and this is a question with which a developmental biology that, traditionally, has been tied to just the molecular dynamics of DNA/RNA processes has struggled to plausibly answer. More specifically, given all of the cellular activities that are taking place within an organism, how do organisms – especially multi-cellular organisms -- manage to operate in such a synchronized fashion, especially during the processes of embryology and subsequent biological development?

Popp proposed that the dynamics of biophotons might be able to provide an answer to the foregoing issue of morphogenesis. He maintained that the coherent activities of biophotons were responsible for successfully orchestrating the many intricate and fast-paced complexities that were involved in the synchronized activities of cellular life.

There were others before Popp – such as: Alexander Gurwitsch or Elmer Lund in the 1920s; Harold Burr in the 1940s; and H.W. Beams and G. Marsh in the 1950s – who had put forth theoretical ideas and experimental data indicating that different facets of biological activity seemed to be tied to changes in the electrical fields associated with those kinds of biological activity. In addition, Herbert Fröhlich had been an early proponent of the idea that, perhaps, proteins were induced to cooperate with one another through some modality of communication within and among cells that involved frequency or resonance dynamics.

Popp later conducted a series of experiments in which he recorded biophoton emissions from the hand and head of a 27-year old, healthy woman who, for a period of time each day, sat in a completely darkened room. The foregoing measurements were taken daily over a period of nine months.

He discovered that the biophoton readings he was recording appeared to follow, along with other kinds of activity, patterns of biological rhythms for different periods of time (e.g., a week, two weeks, 32 days, 80 days and so on). Moreover, when there were increases in biophoton activity in conjunction with one hand of the 27-year old woman, a similar increase would be measured in the other hand of that same woman.

When Popp performed the same kind of experiments with people who were ill, he found that there were characteristic differences in biophoton activity between healthy and ill people. In addition, he discovered that there appeared to be characteristic differences in the nature of their photon activity which surfaced in individuals with different kinds of illness.

According to Lynne McTaggart, Popp interpreted the foregoing results through the framework of a Zero Point Energy Field. Apparently, he believed that the closer an organism was to a zero-like condition of equanimity in conjunction with the surrounding Zero Point Energy Field, then, the healthier a person would be and, as such, different patterns of biophoton emission gave expression to the body's attempt to make whatever corrections were necessary to help the body work toward that state of equilibrium.

For instance, among other things, Popp had observed that when people are stressed, their rate of biophoton emission increases. He saw this as the body's attempt to regain a form of dynamic stability or equilibrium.

Although Popp framed his understanding of biology in terms of an organism's biophoton interactional relationship with the existence of an alleged Zero Point Energy Field in which, all organisms, supposedly, are immersed, there is another way of looking at his research. More specifically, earlier in the discussion of the development of Popp's perspective, the notion of photon-repair was mentioned which, as previously was noted, had to do with the body's ability to be able to repair extensive damage caused by exposure to ultraviolet light.

No one seems to know what makes the phenomenon of photo-repair possible. Furthermore, during the discussion of Popp's ideas, Lynne McTaggart indicated that Popp found that biophotons exhibit a property of coherence. However, other than some allusions to the way in which organisms might interact with the alleged Zero Point Energy Field, there didn't appear to be an explanation for the presence or nature of such coherence – although indications were given that DNA might, in some way, be responsible for releasing biophotons and that those quantum entities were somehow responsible for orchestrating the complexities of cellular and multi-cellular life.

Conceivably, however, rather than being a function of the way in which the body interacts with the alleged surrounding Zero Point Energy Field during a proposed quest to achieve some sort of equilibrium with respect to such a field, the dynamics of biophoton phenomena might be a function of what previously was proposed in the present book to be the result of the epigenetic activity of the microzymas, endobionts, or somatids that are differentially present in every kind of cell in any given organism. In other words, rather than trying to argue that living organisms seek to establish some sort of equilibrium in conjunction with a notion – i.e., a Zero Point Energy Field – which is entirely theoretical in nature and about which many questions can be raised (and, previously, were raised) for which quantum physicists appear to have no demonstrable answer – why not suppose that the coherent dynamics of biophoton activity is a function of entities – namely, microzymas, endobionts, or somatids – which not only have been proven to exist but -- as individuals such as, among others, Béchamp, Enderlein, Rife, and Naessens have shown – appear to have a potential to serve as mediators of life forces which are independent of organisms and, yet, are integral to phenomena such as pleiomorphism/pleomorphism, and, in addition -- as Naessens has demonstrated – seem to have the capacity to make the process of transplantation be rejection free.

Perhaps the reason why the phenomenon of photo-repair is not understood is because most mainstream scientists have not taken the time to investigate, grasp, and develop the research of individuals such as Béchamp, Enderlein, Rife, and Naessens concerning the dynamics of microzymas, endobionts, or somatids. As previously indicated, photo-repair is a process in which cells, including their DNA, have been destroyed and, yet, 'something' present in those cells is capable of bringing life functions back to them when that 'something' is treated with low-intensity editions of the very same wavelengths of ultraviolet radiation that originally had put such cells at death's doorstep.

Somatids have been shown to be able to survive exposures to various temperatures, doses of radiation, and other toxic conditions that are normally lethal to life forms and, yet, despite those kinds of exposure, continue to be functional. Somatids cannot be penetrated with diamond-tipped drills, and, yet, they are able to continue to interact with cellular life.

A plausible candidate for the interaction or communication between, say, somatids (or microzymas and endobionts) and cellular activities could involve some form of frequency following responses that are generated by, or transduced through, the internal dynamics of somatids, endobionts, or microzymas. Such frequencies might induce biophoton activities to emerge in cells, tissues, and organs and could be epigenetically orchestrating various activities of the genome.

Rather than suppose that the unwinding of DNA causes biophoton activity to increase, why not suppose that it is the epigenetic activity of microzymas, endobionts, or somatids which is generating such biophoton activity. The unwinding of the DNA occurs not because ethidium bromide is present but because part of the epigenetic activity of the biophotons is to direct which aspects of DNA will unwind, and when, and with what modifications in order to be able to establish the sort of adaptive learning processes that will enable detoxified stability to be maintained or recovered so that the biological terrain can be in symbiotic relationship with the pleiomorphic/pleomorphic microorganisms that populate that terrain.

On the one hand, the coherent activity that is given expression through the aforementioned spectrum of biophoton frequencies might be generated through the inner dynamics of microzymas, endobionts, or somatids. On the other hand, microzymas, endobionts, or somatids might serve as transducers in which non-energetic communications, signals, or directives from some underlying Order Field (which need not be either quantum or Zero Point Energy-like in character) are transformed into coherent packages of biophoton activity that epigenetically organizes the activities of the genome.

The foregoing considerations are theoretical or hypothetical in nature. However, a theory or hypothesis is being advanced during the course of the present book which, nonetheless -- despite addressing a multitude of topics involving evolution, microbiology, virology, immunology, epigenetics, junk or non-coding DNA, vaccine-related issues, notions of resonance, the properties of water, as well as quantum dynamics – that hypothesis or theory has demonstrated itself to be consistent, heuristically valuable, and capable of providing plausible answers to, or ways of thinking about, an array of questions and issues which are fundamental to both biology and medicine but for which much of what is considered to be mainstream biology and medicine does not appear to have a great deal to offer that is either viable or plausible.

Chapter 17: Interfering with Following the Science

The methodological principle that supposedly informs how the FDA (Food and Drug Administration) goes about its business of trying to both safeguard and assist Americans to navigate their way through the labyrinth of issues in which pharmaceuticals, medical devices, injectables, cosmetics, and food stuffs are entangled is, on the surface, quite straightforward. More specifically, the FDA is supposed to operate with the sort of due diligence which would be able to ensure that harmful and ineffective products do not reach consumers, while, simultaneously, doing whatever it can to make sure that beneficial products are being made available to the citizens of the United States in a timely fashion. There are a variety of obstacles that stand in the way of such a straightforward purpose being realized.

For example, to varying degrees, the FDA has been, and continues to be, suffering from what is known as regulatory capture. This means that in all too many instances, FDA policy is not set by individuals who are serving as objective, independent, moral, fiduciary agents who are working for the benefit of Americans on behalf of the United States government, but, instead, in all too many cases, public policy concerning pharmaceuticals, injectables, food stuffs, cosmetics, and medical devices is being set, or heavily influenced, by the very industries that are supposed to be regulated by the FDA.

Regulatory capture is possible because some of the human beings who work for the federal government are all too human and, as a result, they have proven to be susceptible to the many kinds of incentives that can be dangled before them in exchange for a little consideration here or a little consideration there that will enable companies to get their products to market quickly, but if employees of, or consultants to, the FDA were actually doing their jobs in a rigorous, objective, competent, moral, and uncompromised fashion, such products might never be approved or passed through without appropriate warnings attached to them.

For instance, when Curtis Wright IV worked for the FDA, he played an instrumental role in helping Purdue Pharmacy get approval for OxyContin without proper warning labels being attached to the product indicating that the drug was highly addictive. As a result, he helped to trigger a drug epidemic that: (1) has cost tens of thousands of people their lives, (2) led to a rampant increase in crime as the desperation of people who, suddenly, found themselves needing to subsidize an extremely powerful drug habit that had taken over their lives was leveraged by an array of unsavory suppliers; (3) precipitated a onslaught of cases involving newborn babies suffering from neonatal opioid withdrawal syndrome, (4) tore apart, if not destroyed the lives of hundreds, if not thousands, of individuals, families, and communities across America, as well as (5) induced a lot of doctors (in private practice, clinics, and hospitals) to put aside the idea of "first do no harm" and replace that code with the sort of cash-based ethics which came from writing prescriptions that never should have been written and ordering forms of treatment that never should have been given.

The reward received by Curtis Wright IV for serving the interests of Purdue Pharma was a $400,000/year job offer from that company. However, Curtis Wright IV is not the only federal official to have been caught up in what is known as the revolving-door dynamic during which federal agents are induced to compromise various official responsibilities in exchange for subsequent lucrative payoffs of one kind or another from this or that corporation which are given in reciprocation for favors that were rendered by a government official who was supposed to be serving the American public but ended up serving other interests instead.

The foregoing assessment is not a subjective, ill-conceived opinion that cannot be substantiated. Various decisions in different courts across America, as well as different government bodies (including the CDC, various legislative bodies, as well as the President's Commission on Combating Drug Addiction and the Opioid Crisis,) have indicated that dangerous, false, and misleading statements have been made by pharmaceutical companies and many of their representatives concerning the safety, addictiveness, and effectiveness of various kinds of opioid drugs, and the agency that enabled those companies and representatives to not only get away with, but profit from, such grossly manipulative forms of advertising was none other than the FDA, with special assistance from people like Curtis Wright IV.

In 2002, the FDA established a group of ten allegedly independent experts to assess whether, or not, the warning labels attached to opioids ought to be changed. For quite some time (nearly ten years), evidence had been accumulating which indicated that not only was the problem of addiction entailed by opioid use growing but, in addition, the number of prescriptions being written for opioids seemed wildly inconsistent with the actual clinical need for those drugs. Supposedly, the committee which was being put together by the FDA was to determine whether, or not, limitations ought to be imposed on clinical uses of opioids so that they would be prohibited from being prescribed for, and being used in conjunction with, common run-of-the-mill sorts of pain issues (relatively minor sorts of aches) and, instead be authorized for use in only much more serious clinical conditions.

Eight of the ten experts that were installed on the foregoing committee which was being convened by the FDA had financial links to pharmaceutical companies – including Purdue Pharma – that were producing opioid products of one kind or another. Surprise, surprise, those "outside experts" advised the FDA that there should be no changes to the warning labels attached to opioid products despite the existence of overwhelming evidence indicating that America was being devastated by the problems that were being generated through the dangerously addictive, if not lethal, properties of opioids.

One might, or might not, be inclined to give the foregoing ten experts a pass for voting in a manner that served their individual financial and professional interests. However, what manner of stupidity, if not corruption, was involved in the manner through which the FDA selected the individuals who were to become members of its opioid committee given that if the FDA had exercised anything remotely like due diligence with respect to the foregoing selection process, then they would have discovered that eight of the ten people appointed to its committee had conflicts of interest because of their financial ties to the pharmaceutical industry and, therefore, were not suitable candidates for engaging in a supposedly objective and fair process that might determine what kind of future uses concerning opioids should be approved by the FDA.

The Food, Drug, and Cosmetics Act specifies that companies and businesses which manufacture, sell, and/or distribute products that fall under the purview of the aforementioned Act must be able to show how their products are not only safe and effective, but, as well, organizations must be able to demonstrate that the benefits promised by such companies, businesses, and manufacturers outweigh any risks that might be entailed by the use of their products. While companies which produce products that fall under the jurisdiction of the FDA are responsible for ensuring that they are acting in accordance with the provisions of the Food, Drug, and Cosmetic Act, nonetheless, the FDA is also responsible for checking the extent to which companies or businesses actually comply with that Act.

Both the pharmaceutical companies and the FDA failed in their respective responsibilities with respect to observing and enforcing The Food, Drug, and Cosmetics Act. The result is a tragedy that has been spreading across America for 28 years with tentacles of corruption and destruction that have been whipping about – and continue to do so -- in predictable and unpredictable directions.

The foregoing, nearly 30-year opioid epidemic that was caused by acts of omission and commission on the part of the FDA is not an isolated incident. There have been many "mistakes" – and not necessarily innocent mistakes – that have been committed by different individuals and groups of individuals at the FDA over the years, and, in fact, the mistakes which have been, and are being committed, by the FDA are often inimical to the possibility of going about their activities in an objective, unbiased, and fair manner.

For example, I have followed the research of Dr. Peter Breggin, a psychiatrist, for more than three decades who has written a number of books, as well as offered testimony in a variety of court cases, which have presented evidence – and not just conjecture – that many of the drugs being manufactured and, subsequently, prescribed for different kinds of difficulties involving mood, anxiety, sleep, attention deficits, and so on, have a dark side to them which often leads individuals who are taking those drugs to commit acts of violence against others and/or themselves (i.e., suicide). One of the anti-depressant drugs which he was critical of was Prozac which began to come into prominence in 1989, and despite a growing literature – journalistic, scientific, and clinical – that the drug could induce people with no history of violence to commit acts of murder or self-harm, nonetheless, the FDA did nothing for fifteen years notwithstanding the fact that many of the foregoing documented cases of violence involving both murder and suicide had been sent to the FDA.

Neither the manufacturers of anti-depressants nor the FDA can put forth evidence capable of proving that depression or mood disorders are the result of a chemical imbalance in the brain – which is how depression and anti-depressants are often advertised to work. Therefore, in effect, those manufacturers who engage in such advertising are promoting false, misleading, and, possibly, fraudulent information concerning both the condition of depression and the nature of antidepressants, and, yet, the FDA continues to permit those who manufacture antidepressants to engage in such problematic forms of advertising.

In 2001, a product liability suit was brought to trial in Wyoming against GlaxoSmithKline and its antidepressant drug Paxil. The lawsuit revolved about an individual who had no history of violence and, yet, after taking two doses of Paxil, proceeded to kill his wife, daughter, granddaughter, and himself.

On the basis of expert, scientific testimony and evidence that was presented to the court during the aforementioned trial concerning problems surrounding the use of Paxil, the judge ruled in favor of the plaintiff. Although GSK did end up paying nearly 6 and half million dollars in compensation for the liability entailed by its product, the drug company did not make any changes to the way it manufactured, distributed, and promoted Paxil, and, in fact, proceeded to lose a number of other court cases involving product liability concerning its antidepressant and, apparently, seemed to be treating the sums paid out in such cases as merely the cost of doing billions of dollars worth of business in its sales of antidepressants.

Finally, in 2004, the FDA held hearings on the issue of antidepressants such as Prozac and Paxil. Nonetheless, despite a mountain of evidence indicating that anti-depressant medications were neither necessarily safe nor effective, the FDA continued to move, if at all, quite slowly and cautiously when it came to controlling the epidemic of violence that could be traced to the use of the foregoing sorts of pharmaceuticals, and, instead, appeared to engage in a process of willful blindness concerning the legal, scientific, clinical, and journalistic evidence indicating that antidepressants were often found to be neither safe nor effective.

Dr. Breggin indicates that antidepressants can often have a destabilizing impact on those who are taking those kinds of drugs. Such effects can lead to bouts of euphoric mania, sleeplessness, uncontrollable jitteriness, aggressiveness, and anxiety.

Richard Kapit, who was the individual who conducted the internal review of Prozac on behalf of the FDA, indicated in his final report that the packaging label for that drug should contain information about the unsettling and destabilizing effect which Prozac could have on some individuals and how this effect could significantly worsen their condition of depression and mental problems. The FDA, in collusion with the drug company Eli Lilly, ignored Dr. Kapit's warnings concerning the potential adverse effects that were associated with the consumption of Prozac.

The foregoing warning was made known to the FDA in the middle of the 1980's. Twenty years (when the FDA began to hold hearings on the possible adverse effects of antidepressants in 2004) were required for the FDA to acknowledge – without necessarily committing itself to taking any precautionary or protective actions – that there might be serious adverse effects associated with many, if not all, antidepressant pharmaceuticals

45% of the budget for the FDA comes from the pharmaceutical industry. This money is paid in the form of so-called "user fees" which, supposedly, are intended to speed up the process of granting approval to any given drug, but one might as well refer to those fees as hush money, or 'conflict of interest' fees which are paid to induce the FDA to engage in less than a robust form of due diligence when it comes to regulating the pharmaceutical industry.

A research project had been conducted by a University of Connecticut group led by Irving Kirsch and was published in 2002. The project focused on the alleged efficacy data that -- over a period of 12 years, or so -- was supplied to the FDA by various pharmaceutical companies with respect to six major antidepressants – namely, Zoloft, Celexa, Paxil, Effexor, Prozac, and Serzone.

The foregoing drugs all had been approved on the basis of two studies each which had shown some sort of positive evidence. However, what might be meant by the idea of a positive result and how significant such a result might actually be is often not a straightforward issue and, frequently, is subject to various ways of arranging data that enables one to point to this or that positive aspect of the conclusions that are being framed through one's way of presenting such data.

One needs to understand that the pharmaceutical companies did not just conduct two trials and they were both positive. Those companies conducted many trials and merely selected the two that seemed positive and, therefore, appeared to best serve their purposes of getting their drug approved.

The University of Connecticut research group wanted to examine all of the studies that were done by the pharmaceutical companies in relation to the FDA approval process and not just the two studies per antidepressant product that were submitted to the FDA by those companies.

After examining some 47 drug trials – constituting approximately 8 trials per product – the University of Connecticut researchers came to the conclusion that when the results of those trials were compared with placebo outcomes, none of the drugs studied showed anything more than negligible sorts of positive effects.

Four years later, Irving Kirsch worked with Joanna Moncrieff, a British psychiatrist, and produced another research study which focused on drugs that were based on SSRIs (Selective Serotonin Reuptake Inhibitors) such as Zoloft, Prozac, and Paxil. They concluded that none of the drugs which they studied have any kind of increased clinical benefit relative to placebos.

The FDA is aware that other clinical trials have been conducted by drug companies concerning the efficacy of their products. Unfortunately, the policy of the FDA is to not release such data.

Surely, the people who work at the FDA have the capacity to perform the same kind of analyses as were conducted by Irving Kirsch at the University of Connecticut and, later on, which he conducted with Joanna Moncrieff, and, as well, the FDA also has access to the data on which the foregoing reviews were based, but, once again, one has difficulty avoiding the conclusion that the FDA sits on information that has implications for the health and well-being of Americans but hides important information from the American people in order to serve the interests of the pharmaceutical industry.

Given the foregoing research, evidence exists indicating that antidepressants are not any more effective than are placebos. What about the safety facet of antidepressants?

In 2003, Dr. Breggin wrote a paper entitled: "Suicidality, Violence and Mania Caused by Selective Serotonin Reuptake Inhibitors (SSRIs). During the course of the foregoing paper, he indicated that a variety of antidepressants had the effect of destabilizing and over-stimulating psychological and physical functioning and, as a result, frequently led to conditions of extreme aggressiveness and violence towards other individuals as well as obsessive thoughts concerning the issue of suicide.

At the insistence of Dr. Breggin, a copy of the foregoing paper was given to every member of the advisory committee that was associated with the 2004 FDA hearings on antidepressants. Such "advisors" are chosen by the FDA, and most of them have discernible financial ties to the pharmaceutical industry as a result of grant money, speaker's fees, or consultancy payments.

The FDA is aware of such potential conflicts of interest because prior to public hearings, the FDA publishes letters which itemize those kinds of conflicts. Yet, inexplicably, instead of ensuring that its advisors have absolutely no ties to pharmaceutical companies and, therefore, will be able to arrive at objective and independent judgments concerning the safety and efficacy of various products, the FDA merely absolves committee members from any sort of legal liability they might have in relation to their on-going ties with the pharmaceutical companies which could substantially bias their advisory activities concerning the products being manufactured by the very companies to whom they have financial ties.

Two hearings were held by the FDA advisory committee in 2004 investigating the use of antidepressants in conjunction with children and young people under the age of 18. The committee eventually released a report indicating that during the hearings they had been exposed to evidence indicating that just three of 15 studies had shown any kind of positive effect involving the use of antidepressants in children and youth under the age of 18, and what, exactly, the nature of those "positive" effects might have been were not indicated.

In addition, in February 2004, the advisory committee published a statement on its website acknowledging that evidence existed indicating that use of antidepressants not only were associated with suicidal obsessions, but, as well, were linked to conditions of confusion, anxiety, aggressiveness, and violence toward others. However, individuals such as Dr. Breggin and Dr. Kapit had been issuing such warnings and backing those concerns up with evidence, for more than twenty years.

In early 2005, a new black box warning label was proposed to be added to the packaging insert accompanying antidepressant products that addressed the issue of children and young people under 18. While the black box warning label did indicate that antidepressants have been shown to increase the risk of suicidal thoughts and behavior in children and adolescents, nevertheless, the black box warning which was eventually agreed upon did not contain an even more forceful statement that originally had been proposed to be included in the aforementioned black box label concerning the causal role that antidepressants might have with respect to inducing violent and suicidal thoughts and behavior in adolescents and children because the FDA, while negotiating with various manufacturers of antidepressants, had decided to remove any mention of the issue of causality from the black box label that appeared in the packaging insert accompanying the container of antidepressants.

What is there to negotiate about? The FDA, via its advisory committee, was aware that only three of 15 studies provided any indication that antidepressants might have some sort of "positive" effect (whatever that might mean) and, consequently, antidepressants have been shown, in 80% of the studies conducted, to be neither safe nor effective when used by children or adolescents. Furthermore, the FDA, via that same advisory committee, was aware that consumption of antidepressants by children and adolescents was associated with the appearance of violent thoughts and behaviors concerning other people or themselves – something about which the FDA had actually known for twenty years.

How does one conclude that although given products (i.e., antidepressants) increase the likelihood of violent thoughts and behaviors in those individuals who consume those products, nonetheless, such products play no causal role in the emergence of violent thoughts and behaviors? If causality plays no role in the dynamics of an antidepressant's impact on a person's body, then, exactly how do antidepressants increase the risk that someone will experience an increase in suicidal thoughts and/or behaviors?

In 2008, Dr. Breggin published *Brain Disabling Treatments in Psychiatry.* He put forth evidence in that publication which indicated how the American Psychiatric Association, along with academics and others who were card-carrying members of the pharmaceutical cartel, were busily engaged in criticizing the FDA for even issuing the aforementioned black box label that it did in relation to antidepressants. In addition, the foregoing surrogates for the pharmaceutical industry also had been seeking to induce medical doctors to disregard those sorts of warnings and not treat those concerns with the consideration that they deserved.

In 1994, Dr. Breggin released the book: *Talking Back to Prozac.* During the course of that book, he noted how Prozac had been approved during the administration of Bush I and that not only had Bush Senior been a board member of the company which produced Prozac – namely, Eli Lily – but, as well, Bush's Vice President, Dan Quayle had a number of individuals on his staff who were former employees of Eli Lily and, in addition, the international headquarters for that company were located in Quayle's home state of Indiana.

Legislators supposedly have powers of oversight concerning the conduct of the FDA, yet, many of those legislators receive campaign contributions from pharmaceutical companies and most of those legislators are consistently lobbied by pharmaceutical companies. So, one can't help but wonder just how unbiased the oversight might be which Congress supposedly exercises over the FDA when it comes to the way in which the FDA "negotiates" with the pharmaceutical industry concerning the safety and health of the American public?

When Presidents, Vice Presidents, legislators, academics, the media (which is heavily subsidized by the pharmaceutical industry), an array of consultants, and professional organizations like the American Psychiatric Association are all working from the same operational page out of self-interest and conflicts of interests rather than through any sense of commitment to the fiduciary responsibility which they should have toward the general public, then, can one really be surprised when people effectively lose sight of the actual nature of science? Science is not a matter of learning – via school, politics, commerce, or the media -- how to follow some sort of consensus that has been arbitrarily – and, frequently, corruptly -- established in conjunction with issues like antidepressants.

Science requires one to pay attention to empirical observation and be prepared to engage in a thorough and rigorous evaluation of that observation in order to try to sift through an array of experiential data in an attempt to discover underlying patterns which are capable of accurately characterizing what is being observed. However, just as importantly, science requires objectivity, character, and morality, because if one is not prepared to take evidence and use an abundance of unbiased, critical reflection to follow that evidence to wherever it might be able to viably transport one (through hypotheses, experimental demonstration, and replication), then, one is not actually following science in any reputable sense of the term.

Very early on during the OxyContin affair, Purdue Pharma had come out with the claim – via its resident pain specialist, Dr. J. David Haddox -- that the risk of becoming addicted when taking its product was less than 1%. Subsequently, *Scientific American*, along with other media outlets, helped promote that claim by mentioning the foregoing factoid without, unfortunately, verifying its degree, if any, of legitimacy.

The source on which the foregoing factoid was based did not come from a scientific study of any kind. Instead, the idea that less than 1% of the population might be vulnerable to the risk of becoming addicted when taking various kinds of opioids was based on a one paragraph letter that was sent to the editor of the *New England Journal of Medicine* in 1980. The individuals who wrote the letter were basing their claim on observations which they had made in conjunction with the experiences of a very small group of people, and, as one of the authors of the letter later stated their observations had never been intended to indicate that there were not significant risks and dangers associated with long-term use of opioids.

The 'less than 1% meme' was passed around by physicians, hospital personnel, medical clinic staff members, and an array of journalists. Yet, apparently, none of those individuals ever bothered to check whether, or not, such a claim would able to be substantiated if it were challenged through scientific methods rather than merely being accepted at face value.

As a result, the medical system itself helped to create an opioid pandemic which is still unfolding. To date, the pandemic has cost hundreds of thousands of people their lives as well as led to well over a trillion dollars being consumed through such things as lost productivity, criminal activity, and the costs that have been associated with trying to deal with an opioid problem that had been set in motion by people who should have done their due diligence with respect to the vetting of opioids – i.e., should have been committed to following the methods of science -- but failed to do so.

The foregoing scenario resonates with many aspects of the "HIV-causes-AIDS" fiasco. For example, in the early 1990s, Kary Mullis (the scientist who won a Nobel Prize for inventing the methodology which makes possible the process of PCR -- polymerase chain reaction) was tasked with writing an article about HIV and AIDS.

He wanted to start the article by saying that HIV causes AIDS, but he also wanted to be able to cite a source which could substantiate that claim. He began to research the topic and could find nothing in the scientific literature which was capable of substantiating such a claim.

Consequently, he began to ask a variety of scientists who presumably would be informed about, and knowledgeable concerning, what the possible identity of the source might be for making the claim that HIV-causes-AIDS. None of the experts he asked could resolve his dilemma by offering words like: "Oh, take a look at such and such an article in such and such a journal."

Finally, at a party he attended, Kary Mullis cornered Luc Montagnier -- winner of the Nobel Prize for, supposedly, helping to discover HIV – and began asking a number of pointed questions concerning the issue. Luc Montagnier became perturbed with the questions being asked of him, abruptly walked away, and, therefore, was unable to provide Kary Mullis with a source that was capable of substantiating the claim that HIV-causes-AIDS.

At some point following the aforementioned meeting, Montagnier began championing the idea that HIV does not cause AIDS on its own but operates in conjunction with some other unknown co-factor to induce AIDS to arise. In passing, let it be noted that such a co-factor, if it even exists, is still unknown.

In 2021, Robert Kennedy Jr. came out with the book: *The Real Anthony Fauci*, which, among other things, tells the story of how Anthony Fauci had played a key role in the deeply disturbing facets – and there were, and are, many such facets – entailed by the so-called science surrounding HIV and AIDS.

Kennedy's book was widely acclaimed and has sold well over a million copies. The fact of the matter is, however -- and the foregoing Kary Mullis anecdote is only one of those facts -- all the startling revelations that were contained in the Kennedy book concerning the HIV and AIDS issue are nothing more than very old news ... indeed, his commentary concerning the HIV and AIDS issue is more than thirty years behind the times.

In the late 1980s, I was a grad school student at the University of Toronto. To try to make ends meet (not always successfully), I had a job as a supervisor for a photoduplication service that was housed in the U. of T.'s Science and Medicine Library. That service not only attended to the machines that were used by students to duplicate various materials but, as well, that service copied materials on behalf of faculty members who were doing research into this or that aspect of science and/or medicine (and there were some copyright issues that arose in conjunction with those services).

There were a number of part-time workers who fell under the purview of my supervisory responsibilities. These part-time employees were all students at the University of Toronto.

When time permitted, one of the foregoing students and I used to talk about a variety of issues. One day, we began talking about HIV and AIDS, and he offered to loan me a book he had on the topic.

I seem to recall – but I might be wrong -- that the book was entitled: *AIDS*, Inc. I believe the book was written by Jon Rappoport, an investigative journalist, and it had been released in 1988.

I was going through that book circa 1989. To make a long story short, the book – whatever its actual provenance -- provided an array of empirical evidence indicating, among other things, that not only was there no evidence to demonstrate that HIV caused AIDS, but, as well, there was no evidence capable of supporting the idea that viruses – and, therefore, HIV – existed.

In the 1980s and 1990s, a renowned molecular biologist working at the University of California, Berkeley -- Dr. Peter Duesberg -- had conducted studies and written some articles which indicated that AIDS was not caused by HIV. Among other things, he was a proponent of the idea that a bevy of recreational drugs, including poppers (alkyl nitrates), along with a lifestyle of promiscuity, sexually transmitted diseases (thus, a constant need for antibiotics), poor nutritional habits, and a tendency to burn both ends of life's candle were all contributory factors in the emergence of AIDS within certain populations that, as a result of their behaviors, seemed to be vulnerable to the on-set of opportunistic diseases such as Kaposi Sarcoma as well as various forms of bacterial pneumonia (e.g., toxoplasma pneumonia) – all of which, collectively speaking, eventually led to the onset of AIDS. Peter Duesberg's reward for offering a scientific narrative that ran counter to the one favored by Anthony Fauci -- the relatively newly appointed head (1984) of the National Institute of Allergy and Infectious Diseases (NIAID) that is situated within the National Institute of Health of the federal government – came in the form of the destruction of what had been, up to that time, a very successful professional career.

Almost from the very inception of the controversy, a group of researchers in Australia who became known as the Perth Group took issue with the idea that HIV-causes-AIDS. The foregoing group was led by the research of Dr. Eleni Papadopulos-Eleopulos (now passed on) and Dr. Val Turner.

The members of the group argued (and offered evidence to support their claims) that there was no proof HIV existed, let alone that it caused AIDS. In addition, they maintained that the Western blot antibody test as well as the ELISA test that were used to detect the presence – allegedly -- of HIV were deeply flawed.

Finally, they were of the opinion there was no evidence to demonstrate that the use of AZT (azidothymidine) served to ameliorate the condition of either HIV or AIDS. In fact, rather ironically, they believed that using AZT to combat HIV and AIDS actually was counterproductive because it was instrumental in bringing about the very condition (AIDS) that it was supposed to inhibit or counter.

For some thirty years, or so, individuals such as: Dr. Eleni Papadopulos-Eleopulos, Dr. Val Turner, Dr. Kary Mullis, Dr. Peter Duesberg, Jon Rappoport, and the student with whom I worked at the University of Toronto, were aware of evidence indicating that the notion that HIV-caused-AIDS was deeply problematic. Even I was aware of that material some thirty years before Robert Kennedy Jr. decided to write about the issue, and, consequently, one can't help but wonder why he is getting so much traction with material about which others knew some three decades before he began putting his book together.

Furthermore, not only is Robert Kennedy, Jr. late to the "rescue," so to speak, with his aforementioned book, but in a very important sense, he doesn't seem to understand some of the issues that are at the heart of the topic about which he decided to write. For example, toward the beginning of Chapter 5 ('The HIV Heresies'), he states that he wants there to be no doubt about where he stands concerning the relationship between HIV and AIDS – namely, he is agnostic concerning the issue, and, therefore, is a proponent of maintaining a neutral position concerning that alleged relationship.

He follows up the foregoing clarification with comments about how real science often tends to be iconoclastic or unsettling, and, therefore, it invariably serves a role which is the enemy of all appeals to authority and consensus politics. He even cites a quote of Dr. Michael Crichton which stipulates how science is the antithesis of social processes that are governed by consensus politics.

Fifteen or sixteen pages later, Kennedy indicates that as far as the public record is concerned, he is a proponent or advocate of the view that HIV causes AIDS. Within the span of a relatively few pages, his earlier position concerning a perspective of alleged neutrality toward the relationship between HIV and AIDS has, apparently, been abandoned.

Irrespective of which of the foregoing two positions of Robert Kennedy Jr. one considers, they both are problematic. More specifically, his first statement concerning neutrality appears to ignore the considerable research – noted earlier -- by Dr. Eleni Papadopulos-Eleopulos, Dr. Val Turner, Dr. Kary Mullis, Dr. Peter Duesberg, Jon Rappoport, and many others which indicates that there is absolutely no credible evidence to support the idea that HIV causes AIDS, and, therefore, one wonders what the nature of Kennedy's scientific reasoning is for claiming neutrality on the matter.

Moreover, despite previously endorsing the words of Dr. Michael Crichton which gave expression to the idea that consensus decision making and science are antithetical to one another, nonetheless, within just a relatively few short pages, Robert Kennedy Jr. changed his opinion and has adopted what is nothing more than a consensus view. In other words, he wants to go on record and state that he believes – as the other members of the mainstream consensus do – that HIV causes AIDS.

Notwithstanding the foregoing sorts of inconsistencies, whether Kennedy is neutral concerning the relationship between HIV and AIDS or, instead, he is an advocate for the idea that HIV causes AIDS, he is missing the real science. There is no credible evidence which is capable of substantiating or confirming the proposition that HIV or any other virus actually exists.

Robert Kennedy Jr. has made a least one video in which he claims that he is not against vaccinations in general but, rather, he is only against those instances which, in his opinion, provide evidence that the process of vaccination is being abused in some fashion. For example, he believes such abuses are present in conjunction with, say, Paul Offit's rotavirus vaccine.

Kennedy clearly indicates such opposition in his own book -- *The Real Anthony Fauci*. He states, in fairly strong terms, that the aforementioned Offit rotavirus vaccine is likely to have been responsible for more deaths and injuries than can be attributed to the disease that – allegedly – is cause by the rotavirus itself.

Most – but not all vaccines – are directed against viral infections. Yet, compelling evidence appears to exist indicating that no one has been able to show that viruses actually exist.

Virologists hide behind the ludicrous claim that they have isolated, purified, and sequenced an array of viruses. Unfortunately, what virologists mean by the notions of isolation and purification is a function of consensus science which refuses to undertake the scientific steps that are necessary to actually be able to prove that viruses can be isolated and purified. Furthermore, their laughable notions concerning the idea of genetic sequencing viruses is all a matter of computer programs that algorithmically extrapolate and interpolate alleged viral DNA or RNA sequences into an invented, fictional existence without ever actually obtaining a virus that has been properly isolated and, then, demonstrating how the internal properties of such a virus entail a DNA or RNA sequence that can be established independently of a computer program.

If viruses do not exist, then, every vaccine that purports to provide protection against this or that kind of viral infection is a fraud. Consequently, if Robert Kennedy Jr. is not against vaccinations in general, one would like to know which, if any, of the anti-viral vaccinations that presently are being imposed on children might be worthy of his support, and if there are such anti-viral vaccines which he advocates, why he does not consider them to be every bit as fraudulent and dangerous to society as he clearly believes is the case with respect to the rotavirus vaccine which Paul Offit helped to develop.

Please don't misinterpret what is being said here. There is a lot of evidence (but far from all) that is presented in the aforementioned book by Robert Kennedy Jr. which is important, but, perhaps, one also ought to keep in mind that all of the HIV-AIDS material which he put forth has been known for a long time and, yet, people like Fauci and others have been able to maintain and enforce a false narrative for more than three decades (and I do mean enforce, just ask people like Peter Duesberg).

However welcome the work of a Bobby-come-lately might be in some respects (e.g., being able to drive another empirical stake through the heart of a Michael Myers-like vampire that just won't die), nevertheless, the foregoing collusional delusion set in motion by various virologists, as well as by Anthony Fauci and others, has come with a huge, tragic price tag. More specifically, the HIV-AIDS fictional delusion has been responsible for not only the unnecessary deaths of thousands of people but has run up billions of dollars in costs that should have been directed toward programs of research and treatment that were actually rooted in a science based on rigorous empirical observation, careful forms of testing, and defensible forms of ethics rather than being wasted on forms of activity that, euphemistically, are referred to as science but tend to be governed by the idea that because a bunch of people have decided to come together in agreement concerning a given narrative, then, therefore the focus of such a story must be true, and no actual science is needed.

In 2010 – eleven years prior to the work of Robert Kennedy Jr. -- Dr. Nancy Turner Banks (a Harvard Medical School graduate and a practitioner of obstetrics and gynecological oncology for 25 years) released a book entitled: *Aids, Opium, Diamonds, and Empire: The Deadly Virus of International Greed*. She explored many complicated issues in considerable detail during the course of the aforementioned book – including hardcore data concerning the assassination of Robert Kennedy Jr.'s uncle, John Kennedy -- and followed up her initial publication with a more technical work six years later titled: *The Slow Death of the AIDS/Cancer Paradigm and the Apocrypha of the Eukaryotic Cell*). She was very clear in both of the foregoing books that, for very good and demonstrable reasons, she rejected the official HIV-causes-AIDS story which had been cooked up by the likes of Anthony Fauci, Robert Gallo, Luc Montagnier, and others with whom they colluded (officially or unofficially) and that such a narrative was rooted in an array of decisions that were inherently committed to not following the protocols of real science. The aforementioned official narrative was, then, unquestioningly accepted by thousands of other scientists, academics, journalists, and government officials who also all seemed to be equally unconcerned with the need to try to actually follow the rigors of real science rather than becoming shamefully compliant with the all too flaccid (but very lucrative) nature of pretend science.

As pointed out earlier, for more than thirty years, tens of thousands of lives and billions of dollars have been lost to an opioid pandemic which has an etiology that can be traced to people who talked the language of science but practiced something that is entirely alien to the discipline to which such language alludes. Moreover, for more than thirty years additional tens of thousands of lives and additional billions of dollars have been lost to an HIV-causes-AIDS narrative which has arisen through the dynamics of social engineering rather than through a process that is actually interested in seeking the truth concerning such matters. Furthermore, for over thirty years still additional thousands of lives and still more billions of dollars have been destroyed due to the scientific sins of commission and omission that were perpetrated by those who have tried to sell the idea – based on questionable if not non-existent evidence -- that problems such as mania, depression, anxiety, attention deficit disorder, insomnia, and any number of other cognitive difficulties are due to a chemical imbalance in the brain despite the fact that none of the proponents of such an idea can plausibly and credibly show how the absence or surplus of certain kinds of – for example -- neurotransmitters is able to generate the phenomenology of any of the aforementioned psychological or emotional difficulties or account for the fact that numerous studies have shown that not only are the drugs that are used to resolve the foregoing sorts of problems unable to outperform placebos, but, as well, those drugs have been shown to be able to induce many people to become lethally violent toward themselves and/or others.

At one point in time – during the early 1950s -- my mother was a den mother for a Cub Scout group. She had the dubious distinction of having me as one of her wards.

She was very talented with respect to writing plays for her denizens to perform, making costumes for us to wear, and dreaming up projects for us to do. One of those projects had to do with the March of Dimes, an organization initiated by Franklyn Roosevelt in 1938.

The task she assigned to us was to walk about the downtown section of the city in which we lived (Rumford, Maine) in order to ask for dimes from people on the street as a co-operative enterprise – our asking and their giving – in order to try to combat infantile paralysis. She supervised the foregoing collection process from a near-by office command post of some sort, but other than the foregoing facts and the vivid memory that it was very, very cold during that occasion, all I seem to recall (I was 7 or 8 at the time) it that we were not very financially successful in our drive ... where was John D. Rockefeller and his self-serving, image-enhancing, propagandistic extravaganza of dime-giving when you needed him.

A few years later, I got a polio shot. With the exception of a smallpox vaccination that took place somewhere around the same time, those two vaccinations were the only ones I received until I was forced to take a few shots in order to be allowed to travel overseas when I was in my thirties.

On one of the latter occasions involving vaccines, I had an adverse reaction. I got up, started to walk and, then, collapsed following the procedure.

Back then, much less attention was paid to the issue of adverse reactions than is currently the case. Even now, however, there are a lot of medical practitioners who either still don't know about the adverse reaction to vaccinations reporting system or who do know about that system but, nonetheless, are unwilling to take the time (although doing so is really part of their job) to fill out the required information and forward it to the appropriate authorities.

Earlier in the present book an overview was provided outlining how the smallpox vaccine did not eradicate the associated disease but, rather, evidence was presented which showed how decreases in the incidence of smallpox often took place quite independently of vaccination programs, and, as well, there is considerable evidence to indicate that the latter sorts of programs often actually helped spread the disease rather than curtail it. In what follows, something of an overview will be offered concerning different facets of the polio issue in order to show, in, yet, another way, that science – at least good science -- is not what has been, or is being, followed in the matter of polio research.

One might begin the current process of critical reflection by pointing out that in the book *Murder by Injection* -- which Eustace Mullins wrote -- the author notes that between 1950 and 1964, Morris Beale, who edited a influential publication called *Capsule News Digest*, had issued a standing offer concerning his willingness to give $30,000 to anyone who could offer proof that the polio vaccine was not a fraud and that it had not been responsible for a variety of deaths. No one ever took him up on the offer which, presumably, would have been easy enough to do if what he was alleging was not true.

Poliomyelitis is a disease that refers to an inflammation of portions of the brainstem or the gray marrow matter that is found in the spinal cord. The impact of such inflammation can lead to the atrophying of muscles as well as, in more serious cases, interfere with respiratory functioning.

The question, of course, which emerges in the foregoing context, is what causes the sort of inflammation that is being referred to as giving expression to the form of pathology known as poliomyelitis. Although the media – for purposes best known to them – had been hyping the idea that the disease was manifesting itself everywhere (and which led to projects like those of my mother and her den of kids that were mentioned earlier), the empirical reality was quite different because the disease actually was not all that common,

There was reported to be a wild type of the poliomyelitis virus that, supposedly, had been studied in various indigenous tribes in South America, and, then, that data was compared with the incidence of the alleged virus in white populations. The terms "supposedly" and "alleged" are being used here because as three earlier chapters of the present book attempted to show, the so-called evidence concerning the existence of any kind of virus at all – and not just the one which was being attributed as the cause of poliomyelitis – is both questionable and dubious.

Notwithstanding the foregoing considerations, the polio-oriented studies being alluded to in the previous paragraphs indicated that both white groups and native groups showed evidence of having the wild version of the poliomyelitis virus in their system, Yet, native peoples – despite, supposedly, being highly infected with that wild type – were rarely troubled by the disease, whereas white people seemed much more susceptible to the disorder.

The considerable disparity between the two groups pointed to an obvious question. Why did such a disparity exist?

One response to the above question is fairly straightforward. There is no actual disparity because what some people are treating as evidence in support of the idea that the given virus exists in both groups is based on a misunderstanding of the data.

For example, antibody tests were run which were being used to serve as surrogate indicators that the virus is present in both the indigenous and white groups being studied. However, as pointed out in a previous chapter, there are many questions surrounding whether, or not, antibodies -- in the sense meant by immunologists -- actually exist, and even if antibodies do exist, there are a variety of questions which can be raised about whether, or not, their presence means what immunologists believe that presence means – in other words, that the presence of such alleged antibodies is an indication that individuals who had such an immune response had come in contact, at some point, with the poliomyelitis wild-type virus.

In short, there are legitimate doubts that can be raised concerning the existence of the poliomyelitis wild-type virus. In addition, there are legitimate doubts that can be voiced as to whether antibodies exist or, if they exist, whether that presence actually means what many immunologists and medical doctors interpret such a presence to mean.

Over the centuries, scientists and medical practitioners have believed many things which aren't true. The notions of viruses and antibodies might just be two more things that they believe which are not true, and the fact that a lot of scientists and medical practitioners might be saying that something is the case (a consensus view) is not enough to justify accepting what they are claiming as being necessarily true.

In 1947, some years prior to his invention of an oral vaccine for poliomyelitis, Albert Sabin had made observations concerning the foregoing sort of anomaly (i.e., the disparity in incidence of the disease in with respect to native and white groups). He noted that although native individuals supposedly had tested positive for the presence of the poliomyelitis virus prior to the age of five, nonetheless, there were no subsequent cases of paralysis in that population, while, on the other hand, white servicemen who lived in the same general area as the native individuals that had been tested were experiencing cases of paralysis at a fairly significant rate.

In different parts of the world, geographical areas that were implementing programs of hygiene, sanitation, and public health were, to varying degrees, bedeviled by the presence of poliomyelitis. Yet, geographical regions in which the foregoing sorts of public health programs were relatively, or completely, non-existent tended to be devoid of the disease.

White people were, by and large, exposed to vaccines, DDT, processed flour, arsenic, mercury, refined sugar, antibiotics and many other chemical pollutants, whereas, relatively speaking, native populations in different parts of the world were not being exposed to those same pollutants – at least not to the same degree as white people had been exposed. Few researchers seemed to be asking whether it might be possible that one, or more, of the foregoing chemical pollutants could be responsible for the fact that white people were succumbing to poliomyelitis at a far greater rate than were native peoples.

Instead, apparently, framing experience through a set of theories concerning viruses and antibodies was far easier to set in motion. This was the case despite the fact that neither of those theories could account for the disparities which existed between white and native communities in the matter of the incidence of poliomyelitis.

Prior to 1958, there were all manner of paralytic diseases that might have been diagnosed as cases of poliomyelitis. Therefore, there was considerable confusion about what might be causing a given case of paralysis.

For example, DDT and arsenic toxicity could cause the sort of paralysis that was associated with the supposedly viral-induced cases of poliomyelitis. Guillain-Barré syndrome, transverse myelitus, lead poisoning, and undiagnosed congenital syphilis also could produce symptoms that might be diagnosed by some doctors as indicating the presence what was being referred to as "poliomyelitis".

Before the advent of the Salk vaccine, the ways in which medical practitioners diagnosed poliomyelitis were very subjective, loose, and iffy. As a result, various forms of paralysis were often confused for, and conflated with, the paralyses associated with poliomyelitis.

After the vaccine was introduced, distinctions were made between those who had been vaccinated for polio and those who had not been so vaccinated. One ramification of the foregoing distinction is that when diagnoses concerning the presence of paralysis were made in conjunction with those who had been vaccinated for polio, every effort was made to come up with a cause for the paralysis being observed that was something other than poliomyelitis even though no such evasive, diagnostic efforts were made prior to the process of vaccination.

By narrowing the definition of poliomyelitis, medical practitioners could make it seem like polio vaccines were responsible for decreasing the incidence of the disease. However, those kinds of decreases were a function of changing the way in which poliomyelitis was diagnosed rather than being a function of what was being accomplished via the polio vaccine.

For example, before the Salk vaccine was released in 1955, many medical practitioners would diagnosis even very short cases of paralysis – lasting only 24 hours – as constituting evidence for the presence of polio. After the Salk vaccine came out, the criteria for diagnosis changed and, as a result, unless a given case of paralysis lasted for more than 60 days, it was not considered to be poliolytic in character.

Consequently, the incidence of poliomyelitis dropped drastically. This was interpreted by some people as constituting evidence that the vaccine was effective, but such data actually only reflected changes in the criteria being used to diagnosis the pathology.

Even in the cases of paralysis that lasted longer than 60 days, this was not necessarily proof that poliomyelitis was present. Instead, the length of time issue might have been because irrespective of what might have been causing a given instance of paralysis, nonetheless, the problem of duration could have had more to do with how patients were being therapeutically treated rather than being an indication that poliomyelitis was present.

During the first half of the twentieth century, the vast majority of the rehabilitation treatments for individuals who had suffered some sort of paralysis due to one, or another, kind of disease process were relatively barbaric, crude, and ineffective. Surgical forms of trying to 'normalize' the curvature of bones and tendons, or various kinds of electrical procedures, or prolonged bouts with splinting techniques had all proven to be highly ineffective, painful (for the patient, not the practitioners), destructive, and counter-productive.

The very means that were being used to treat paralysis – for example, splinting; placing people in body casts for six months, and, sometimes, for as long as two years, or surgically cutting tendons -- were actually leading to the atrophying and destruction of muscle tissue, as well as causing nerve damage. As a result, the condition of becoming immobile in conjunction with some paralytic disease was often was a reflection of the form of treatment being used and not necessarily an indication that the individual being treated actually was continuing to suffer from some form of paralysis.

Sister Kenny was a woman from Australia who began treating cases of paralysis in 1912. She was successfully able to reverse many, if not most, cases of paralysis she treated without any of the painful, ineffective techniques of surgery, splinting, casting, and electrical stimulation that were in vogue within the mainstream orthopedic medical community of the time.

Instead, she used a combination of hot packs and various forms of physical therapy to help rid individuals of their paralysis. The treatments were relatively quick, very successful, and involved only a small-to-moderate degree of occasional discomfort.

Of course, from the perspective of medical orthodoxy, what Sister Kenny was accomplishing was heretical. This judgment was not because she failed at what she was doing, but, rather she was resisted, fought, and opposed by the mainstream medical community precisely because she was able to do what the members of that community could not do – namely, actually help people rather than make their conditions worse, and, consequently, Sister Kenny had to fight a sort of rearguard action for more than thirty years before, grudgingly, the effectiveness of her work slowly came to be acknowledged ... at least to a degree.

Unfortunately, during the time in which her work went unacknowledged, many hundreds, if not thousands, of patients had to endure the pain and ineffectiveness of the standard of care treatment that was being offered by the medical community. That standard of care was the result of not paying attention to, if not actively ignoring, evidence rather than working in co-operation with such evidence.

For instance, flies were often blamed as being carriers of the alleged poliomyelitis virus. As a result, DDT was used in an attempt to eradicate fly populations.

Parents were induced to spray their houses with products containing DDT. DDT-related products were used to soak – and, supposedly, free – bedding and clothes from the dangers of viral-infested flies.

Kids would be encouraged to run about in the clouds of DDT that, from time to time – especially in the summer -- were being sprayed by community health workers. Lunch boxes were cleansed with DDT-based products.

Just as AZT was later shown to be capable of causing the very disease – namely, AIDS – that it was supposed to cure, so too, DDT was later discovered to be capable of causing a variety of diseases – including paralysis – that it was supposed to be helping to protect against. Paralytic conditions, extreme fatigue, joint pains, and muscle weakness were all symptomatic conditions that were held in common by both poliomyelitis and DDT poisoning.

Due to its extreme toxicity, the sale and use of DDT in America and Canada were phased out in the early 1960s. This phasing out process took place at roughly the same time as poliomyelitis was beginning to disappear in those two countries.

The decline in cases of poliomyelitis was being attributed to the effectiveness of both the Salk polio injections and the Sabin oral vaccine. Unfortunately, few, if any, researchers were investigating the possible ties between the symptoms of poliomyelitis and the similar symptoms of toxicity which could be generated by exposure to DDT, and, therefore, most people never considered the possibility that the disappearance of poliomyelitis in both America and Canada in the early 1960s might have something to do with the fact that the use of

DDT also had been discontinued in those two countries during that same period of time.

Interestingly, but tragically, although the sale and use of DDT disappeared in America and Canada, its presence surfaced again in places such as China and India. Perhaps no one should be surprised that both of the latter two countries experienced outbreaks of diseases that have been diagnosed as polio but could just as easily have been diagnosed as being due to the effects of DDT-poisoning.

The symptoms associated with poliomyelitis have also been linked to lead and arsenic poisoning as well. According to Suzanne Humphries and Roman Bystrianyk in their book *Dissolving Illusions*, Sister Kenny discussed an incident in her autobiography concerning some children on a farm who had become semi-paralyzed or lame at about the same time as cows on the farm were exhibiting similar symptoms of lameness and bouts of paralysis.

The disease that had stricken the children was known as "cow disease." Cows don't suffer from poliomyelitis, but, from time to time, they are run through arsenic-containing solutions in an attempt to protect them against ticks. Paralysis is one of the symptoms which arsenic-poisoning – when it occurs -- has been known to induce in such mammals.

Furthermore, some of the earlier treatments for syphilis involved medications that were produced using arsenic-based compounds. From time to time, there might be increases in the incidence of pathologies involving paralysis that were diagnosed as being poliolytic in nature, but such outbreaks often occurred at the same time that arsenic-derived medications were in abundant use in an attempt to stem the tide of an epidemic-like spread of syphilis that might also be taking place in a given location.

During the 30s and 40s, syphilis was actually a lot more common than was polio. Therefore, what actually might be causing the foregoing cases of paralysis was not always clear even if medical practitioners treating those cases of paralysis operated in accordance with a form of certainty that was more a function of trending consensus-generated beliefs concerning polio rather than being based on scientific methods which might have been able to rule out – or rule in -- arsenic poisoning as being the cause of a given case of paralysis.

Suzanne Humphries and Roman Bystrianyk also point out in their aforementioned book how the CDC has indicated that less than 1% of the people who, supposedly, have been infected with poliomyelitis ever go on to develop some form of paralysis. Moreover, she, along with her co-author, point out that the CDC further stipulates that only 5-10% of that 1% actually die from the respiratory failure.

Thus, according to the CDC's way of looking at things, 99% of the people who allegedly have tested positive for the presence of the so-called poliomyelitis-causing virus do not experience or exhibit any symptoms of the disease. Yet, according to the guidelines drawn up, initially, by Robert Koch and, later, updated by Thomas Rivers (specifically to take into account viruses), if a given entity cannot be shown to cause a given disease in every instance in which the latter is present, then, one cannot necessarily attribute any given occurrence of such a disease to that cause.

Lead, arsenic, DDT, and other chemicals are all capable of causing forms of pathologies that are poliolytic-like in nature. Consequently, given that 99% of the people who test positive for the poliomyelitis virus never exhibit any symptoms (assuming that such a test is valid and that viruses actually exist), then just because someone tests positive for a given virus and, subsequently, exhibits a certain constellation of symptoms, one cannot necessarily conclude that those symptoms are caused by a given virus without also looking at other possible causal factors for such a condition, and, unfortunately, throughout much of the history of polio, rigorous processes of diagnostic confirmation were rarely employed and, instead, medical practitioners often proceeded on the basis of assumptions and consensus rather than conclusive forms of evidence.

An interesting consideration pertaining to the incidence of poliomyelitis is that children who have undergone tonsillectomies are anywhere from 2.5 times to 6 times more likely to be diagnosed with poliomyelitis than are children who have not undergone such a procedure. Furthermore, children who have lost their tonsils are 16 times more likely than their tonsil-possessing counterparts to experience the most serious form of poliomyelitis – namely, bulbar poliomyelitis (which can lead to respiratory failure and death).

The foregoing item is of interest to me because I was one of those children who, not necessarily for any discernibly good reasons, was induced to have a tonsillectomy. Subsequently, I was never diagnosed with poliomyelitis or its more serious bulbar modality, and, the reason which many individuals might be likely to offer for my good fortune is that I had been vaccinated against polio.

Apparently, the reasoning which is being used to frame the foregoing statistics and conclusion is that when one is going about life without tonsils, then, there is likely to have been some sort of peripheral nerve damage which occurred in conjunction with one's tonsillectomy, and it is precisely these sorts of damaged nerves that the alleged poliomyelitis virus likes to use to gain access to one's spinal column and/or brainstem (although I doubt that doctors have ever actually witnessed this route-taking phenomenon) and, thereby, be in a position to cause symptoms of polio. One might just as easily argue that by removing someone's tonsils, one has deactivated one more means through which the body seeks to protect itself against any sort of toxin or toxic substance from being able to gain access to the body's interior and, as a result, the absence of tonsils potentially puts one at risk for developing symptoms that could be poliolytic-like in nature but, actually, might only be indications that some form of poisoning or toxicity is present.

Individuals without their tonsils are 2.5 to 6 times more likely to be diagnosed with poliomyelitis than are those with their tonsils, and, as well, the former individuals are 16 times more likely to exhibit the respiratory problems associated with bulbar poliomyelitis than are their tonsil-toting counterparts. However, given the foregoing data, one also might like to know – for purposes of comparison -- how much more likely are those without tonsils than are those with tonsils to be diagnosed with some form of toxicity or poisoning upon being exposed that is capable of causing the sort of neurological conditions that could involve symptoms of paralysis and/or respiratory distress.

Being without tonsils might cause one to be a lot more susceptible to a variety of diseases and pathological conditions and not just susceptible to the possibility of polio. To mention only polio with respect to the foregoing statistics seems to slant one's understanding in potentially misleading and problematic ways.

In 1916 – two, or so, years before the alleged great influenza epidemic of 1918-1919 – the largest outbreak of poliomyelitis in American history took place. There were more than 5,000 deaths and 23,000 cases that occurred throughout New England and New York as well as a number of Mid-Atlantic States (including Maryland and Delaware).

Around the same time there had been smaller outbreaks of a disease which had been diagnosed as poliomyelitis in places such as Wisconsin, Minnesota, and Michigan. However, none of these latter locations experienced anything that, even remotely, resembled what took place in New England, New York, and several Mid-Atlantic locations within the same sort of time-frame.

The number of people affected in the eastern outbreak was, relatively speaking, quite extensive compared to the ones that took place toward the interior of the country. Moreover, not only was the death rate associated with the eastern epidemic very high (more than 25%) when compared with what happened in more westerly states, but, as well, for whatever reason, the eastern outbreak seemed to involve more children who were around two years of age ... something that had never been recorded in conjunction with other, previous outbreaks of poliomyelitis.

In their book – Dissolving Illusions -- Suzanne Humphries and Roman Bystrianyk refer to a theory put forth by Dr. H. V. Wyatt in 2011 which suggests that the foregoing epidemic might have been the result of a highly virulent engineered strain of the alleged polio virus that had 'escaped' – accidentally or on purpose – from a Rockefeller lab. However, in 1916, the electron microscope had not, yet, been invented (1930s), and, therefore, scientists could not even see viruses (if they existed), let alone adequately isolate, purify, and sequence those alleged entities.

Watson and Crick wouldn't come up with the double helix idea for another thirty-five years or so, and, for the most part, sequencing technology wouldn't be available for more than 60 years (Sanger sequencing began in 1977). Consequently, one wonders how anyone in 1916 would be able to go about engineering a virus even if such entities did exist.

Apparently, one of the features of the 1916 outbreak that induced the aforementioned Dr. Wyatt do wonder if that epidemic might have been the result of an engineered virus was based on the kind of biological destruction that had been observed in the 1916 cases. The individuals who were afflicted by the 1916 form of pathology – whatever it was – suffered from extensive neurological damage, and that kind of damage was reminiscent of the biological effects in experimental animals which were associated with an "MV" strain that had been developed at a Rockefeller lab.

Another factor that seemed to lend credibility to the idea that an engineered virus might, somehow, have been let loose on the world was the cover story that began to circulate in order to explain the epidemic. According to the narrative that was fed to the public, the outbreak of polio cases had begun as a result of some Italian immigrant children who had just arrived in America, but, when someone decided to check the timelines for the two events (i.e., epidemic and immigration), evidence was discovered which proved that the epidemic had begun before the arrival of the Italian children who were being scapegoated by the media (and by whomever might have provided the media with that kind of a narrative).

The existence of a fabricated storyline doesn't prove that the 1916 epidemic was the result of an engineered virus that escaped from a lab. On the other hand, the fact such a false narrative was introduced does suggest the possibility that a person or persons unknown might have been trying to cover up something or other.

One possibility for releasing the foregoing sort of story might have been in an attempt to avoid any sort of public panic concerning the unknown. In other words, conceivably, rather than admit ignorance and, thereby, stoke fears concerning the unknown origins for an outbreak that was highly lethal – especially among two-year olds -- someone might have thought it would be better to provide the semblance of an explanation by blaming some immigrant children who – given the anti-Italian sentiments that existed in many places at the time – were easy targets of opportunity.

A second possibility is that although no viral strain actually was engineered in 1916 which, somehow, was able to escape into civilized society, nonetheless, this didn't preclude the possibility that other kinds of things might have been inadvertently released into the environment. There were hundreds, if not thousands, of chemicals that have toxic properties which were being manufactured in 1916 that, somehow, might have escaped into the 'wilds' of the eastern United States.

For example, although America had not, yet, entered World War I, nonetheless, it was heading in that direction (April, 1917). Poison chemicals and gases were being employed during combat by all sides, and, therefore, it is possible that the military-industrial complex which was becoming established in the United States at that time might have been responsible for any number of leaks or spills during processes of being developed, manufactured, delivered, (perhaps while various toxins were being transported by trucks and/or trains), or while disposing of toxins related to the manufacture of those products.

A third possibility is that although the destructive MV-strain that was present in a Rockefeller lab was not engineered, nevertheless, it was a concoction that contained toxic components. In fact, when America entered the First World War, one of the ways in which troops were prepared for combat was to be given an array of serums and injections that were alleged to be able to protect them from all manner of diseases, and more than one commentator concerning those times has indicated that many of the people who died during the so-called influenza epidemic of 1918-1919 died from the destructive impact that such serums and injections had rather than from a virulent strain of influenza.

Therefore, conceivably, at some point during the development, manufacture, distribution, and/or disposal of the foregoing serums and vaccines, toxic materials were released into the environment and various people who, subsequently, were exposed, in some way, to those toxins also succumbed, in various ways (illness, paralysis, or death), to their presence. Or, perhaps, the hazardous wastes that were generated during the process of development and production of the foregoing sorts of materials needed to be disposed of but, unfortunately, the waste materials were haphazardly dumped in places that contaminated water, dairy farms, animals, fruits, and/or vegetables, and, as a result, what looked like the phenomenon of contagion actually might have been giving expression to the phenomenon of clustering that is present in the dynamics of large-scale forms of poisoning.

According to the aforementioned theory of Dr. Wyatt concerning the possibility of an engineered virus, the location of ground zero for the outbreak that was being diagnosed as poliomyelitis was just three miles from the Rockefeller Institute where Simon Flexner and his colleagues were experimenting with Rhesus monkeys. A train line ran by the Institute which ran throughout metropolitan New York, and, therefore, in one way or another, poisons might have been transported to different parts of New York City and beyond.

There are a variety of questions that might be asked concerning the tissue cultures being used in the foregoing experiment. More specifically, tissue cultures allegedly containing poliomyelitis viruses were being transferred from monkey to monkey.

How were those cultures introduced into any given monkey? Were those processes of introduction likely to lead to the emergence of forms of pathology that were due to the method of introduction rather than being a function the contents of the cultures being introduced?

For example, suppose those cultures were injected directly into the brains or spinal columns of Rhesus monkeys. Would a person be unreasonable if she or he were to entertain the possibility that having such materials injected into a brain or spinal column might be enough -- in and of itself and quite independently of what might be in such cultures – to cause illness, paralysis, or neurological problems of one kind or another?

Moreover, what if those cultures contained an array of toxic ingredients which had been used during the culturing process? What was actually in those cultures that were being transferred from monkey to monkey?

The researchers were sure that the cultures contained poliomyelitis viruses. Yet, how could they be sure of such a claim when – as previously noted -- they had no scientific way to see those entities, let alone isolate, purify, or sequence them?

Would one be unreasonable for entertaining the possibility that the reason why Rhesus monkeys became ill, debilitated, paralyzed, or died during various experimental procedures at the Rockefeller

Institute was because of the ingredients in the culture that were being injected into them? What evidence would compel one to conclude that viruses were necessarily present in those cultures?

According to Dr. Eckhard Wimmer, who was a member of a research team that was being funded by the Defense Advanced Research Project Agency (DARPA) many decades after the 1916 Rockefeller experiments had been conducted, the more modern research team had discovered that the toxicity associated with the poliovirus could be freed from the need to be attached to any sort of underlying genetic sequence that had to be translated by cellular machinery.

He said the empirical formula for the dynamics of the toxicity associated with poliomyelitis was: C332, 652H492, 388N98,-2450131, 196P7, 501S2, 340 .... He said – as previously intimated -- that the foregoing empirical formula could be generated in a test tube without genetic machinery needing to be present for the production of such a molecular substance.

In effect, what Dr. Wimmer seemed to be confessing is that a technology had been developed through which toxic formulae (capable of causing the same kind of damage that is being attributed to the poliomyelitis virus) can be translated into molecular poisons without requiring the presence of the genomic sequence for an entire virus that, normally, would be considered to be necessary to bring about a case of poliomyelitis. If so, then, apparently, gain of function research might have nothing to do with manipulating the genetic sequences of a virus in order to try to produce a viral variant that is more transmissible or more lethal than the original strain, but, rather, gain of function could be all about finding empirical formulas for toxins that can be turned into poisons (like a spike protein) which, subsequently, can be mass-produced by cellular machinery.

In conjunction with the foregoing considerations, the Cutter Laboratories affair during the 1950s – in which a poliomyelitis epidemic was caused by the manufacture of an improperly attenuated version of the Salk vaccine – becomes an interesting topic for a variety of reasons. One point of interest revolves about the issue of whether, or not, viruses actually exist.

If viruses don't exist, then, whatever is being manufactured in the form of a vaccine has nothing to do with viral content, whether attenuated or not. In fact, aside from the foolishness of talking about live and attenuated viruses, when, even if viruses did exist, they are not living organisms, one might wonder just what it is that is being attenuated or adjusted in a vaccine if viruses don't actually exist.

Before exploring the foregoing sort of wondering a little further, let's back track somewhat in order to introduce some of the narrative that surrounds and permeates the Cutter tragedy. To begin with, the Salk vaccine underwent a rapid process of experimental development and an even more rapid process of licensure.

The U.S. Department of Health, Education and Welfare sullied every theme in its department title by ramming through approval of the Salk vaccine in just two hours. The Department of Health, Education, and Welfare committee that had been given the responsibility for generating an informed decision concerning the foregoing issue of vaccine licensure was denied an opportunity to have access to, as well as be able to thoroughly study and critically reflect on, the research that had been conducted in conjunction with the theory underlying the Salk vaccine.

The relevant information concerning the research on the Salk vaccine was contained in a report that was being written by Thomas Francis. The committee members were being pressured into making a quick decision concerning licensure without being able to read, digest or comment on the contents of that report.

Someone told the committee members that speed was essential. Apparently, there was no time for reading, reflecting on, or discussing the Francis report, yet, no one on that committee was being given a clear indication as to why such speed was essential to the decision-making process.

In addition, when some members of the committee said they did want to engage in an extended discussion concerning the polio research, there was push back from someone of influence indicating that if further time were devoted to discussing the issue, then all the members of the committee would be required to travel to Washington or Bethesda, Maryland. Since traveling to Washington or Bethesda would have created difficulties for some of the members of the committee, the group was pressured into making a decision based on woefully incomplete information that could not be properly explored or discussed.

Field trials involving the Salk vaccine had taken place in 1954. The Francis report concerning those trials was not released until 1957 -- some two years after the aforementioned committee members were pressured into approving licensure for the Salk vaccine.

One can, of course, be critical of whomever it was that had been placing pressure on the committee members to make a quick decision on licensure. However, one also can be critical of the committee members for allowing themselves to be pressured into a decision because, among other things, traveling to Washington or Bethesda, Maryland presented them with some difficulties. To accommodate such an inconvenience, people later died or became paralyzed for life as a direct result of a rapid-paced licensure decision.

From the very start of the program that led to the Salk vaccine being "realized," there were people associated with its development who had been aware of some of the problems that were inherent in the whole process. Salk claimed that there was no live virus present in the vaccine and that the alleged virus had been completely deactivated through the presence of, among other things, formaldehyde.

Given that even if viruses exist, nonetheless, they are not live organisms, then, what does it mean to say that a virus has been deactivated? What exactly has been deactivated, and if deactivated, then, what remains of the alleged virus so that it could be able to induce the so-called immune system to generate certain kinds of antibodies which, supposedly, are keys to generating an appropriate sort of immunological response? ... although, at the same time, one might keep in mind the existence of evidence – previously noted -- which indicates that antibodies might not actually exist, or, if they do exist, they might not function in the way in which immunologists have theorized that they are supposed to.

Apparently, many scientists who were associated with the Salk vaccine project indicated there was something wrong with the deactivation process. However, every time someone would voice an objection to what was taking place during the process of vaccine development, those people's voices would either be suppressed in some way or they would be removed altogether.

Consequently, during the developmental phase of the Salk vaccine, the protocols of scientific methodology were ignored, suppressed, or countermanded. Furthermore, during the Department of Health, Education and Welfare committee meetings concerning licensure of the vaccine, the protocols of scientific methodology were once again ignored, suppressed, or countermanded.

As a result, children died, and individuals became paralyzed. Apparently, people in the household of those who had been vaccinated sometimes became infected as well.

If viruses exist, then, one might attribute the Cutter Laboratories fiasco to a flawed design and production process in which, apparently, the formaldehyde that was present in the vaccine did not properly deactivate the virus (whatever this actually means) and this, in turn, led to individuals becoming exposed to a fully functional virus against which their systems had not been properly prepared to defend. Such a scenario seems more than a little sketchy.

What is the difference between, on the one hand, the alleged antibodies that supposedly are generated in conjunction with an attenuated virus, and, on the other hand, the antibodies that supposedly are generated in conjunction with a non-attenuated virus? Why will the antibodies that allegedly are produced in relation to an attenuated virus be able to protect one, whereas the antibodies which, supposedly, are produced in relation to a non-attenuated virus will not be able to adequately protect an individual?

What is the antibody response mechanism allegedly responding to in each of the foregoing cases? What supposedly causes such a difference in immune response?

Some people are said to be able to develop a natural form of immunity through a process of being exposed to this or that virus irrespective of whether such viral entities are attenuated or not. What happens to that natural capacity when people are injected with a synthetic concoction of ingredients which, apparently, disrupts the natural, inborn capacity and renders the latter unable to deal with an alleged virus that is not attenuated?

There is also another line of questioning that an individual also might want to pursue in conjunction with the foregoing considerations. If viruses do not exist, then, what was in the concoction that was present in the vaccines being produced by Cutter Laboratories that caused illness, paralysis, and, all too frequently, death in some of those who received those injections?

If viruses do not exist, then, people who received the Cutter Laboratories vaccine did not die from a manufactured product in which viruses were improperly attenuated. They were ill, paralyzed, or dead because their biological terrains could have become poisoned by the toxins that might have been present in that vaccine.

If poisoned, then, why didn't everyone succumb to the toxins that might have been in the Cutter Laboratories vaccines? One possibility is that just as not everyone has the same sensitivity, or vulnerability, to an array of toxins that are present in everyday life, so too, not everyone who receives an injection with toxic potential will necessarily succumb in some immediate way to the presence of those toxins.

On the other hand, there might be a risk that the toxic load of those individuals who are not immediately affected will increase, nevertheless, as a result of whatever toxins might be present in a given vaccine. If so, then, such a toxic load could, in time, lead to the emergence of one, or another, mode of chronic disease that could be variably manifested in different individuals according to their circumstances.

Gaston Naessens, Enderlein, and Béchamp indicated that when the biological terrain of a given individual reaches a certain tipping point, then, it can be induced to transition away from a condition in which its symbiotic relationship with the microbiome that occupies it is dynamically stable. As a result, when such transitions away from symbiosis take place, various microorganisms within the microbiome might begin to enter into phases of their pleiomorphic life cycles that entail problems which require some form of detoxification that is directed toward helping the biological terrain to be able to re-acquire the symbiotic relationship that it previously enjoyed before it was destabilized by, for instance, some form of toxic load that had reached a tipping point and was induced to spill over into non-symbiotic relationships with one, or more, of the microorganisms that inhabit a microbiome that is present in different aspects of the biological terrain.

There is absolutely no way to prove that the reason why an individual who received a vaccine did not get sick in a certain fashion is due to that injection. To be sure, studies have been done in which the titer, or concentration, levels of certain elements – allegedly antibodies – are observed to increase over pre-vaccination concentrations, but no method presently exists which is capable of determining whether any of the molecular substances whose concentration levels are being measured are actually capable of helping to protect an individual against some given disease.

For instance, one might wish to reflect on the following considerations. Adjuvants – such as aluminum, usually in the form of aluminum hydroxide – are invariably added to the solutions that make up the contents of a vaccine, and the stated reason why those adjuvants are said to be necessary is because they have been shown to be able to help to increase the titer levels of the sorts of protein molecules – which, supposedly, are antibodies – that are believed to be able to protect an individual against this or that sort of infectious disease.

However, the presence of the foregoing sorts of adjuvants does nothing to protect the body against the potential toxicity of aluminum. For example, when, for whatever reason, the aluminum hydroxide from a vaccine becomes embedded in muscle tissue, it can lead to the onset of a disease known as Macrophagic Myofascitis.

In other words, here we have a case in which an antigen has been intentionally presented to the alleged immune system via a vaccine, and as a result of that presentation, antibodies are supposedly generated in response to the presence of that antigen/adjuvant. Yet, nonetheless, the antibodies which arise in conjunction with the presence of such an antigen are not able to defend against the toxicity that can be generated through the presence of aluminum.

In short, we appear to be confronted with a clear cut case in which the alleged antibodies that arise in response to the presence of an antigen (i.e., aluminum) cannot actually defend against the toxic potential of such an antigen. Consequently, irrespective of whether, or not, the concentrations of certain kinds of proteins – alleged to be antibodies – actually increase as a result of the presence of an adjuvant in the vaccine, nevertheless, a sort of 'proof of concept' has been demonstrated in which simply because certain kinds of proteins increase their concentrations in response to the presence of an adjuvant/antigen, one cannot conclude that those proteins necessarily have the capacity to effectively serve as protective antibodies.

One might have evidence that the concentration of something has increased following exposure to an adjuvant. However, there is no evidence which demonstrates that whatever it is that has increased in its concentration is capable of defending against certain kinds of allegedly infectious diseases.

After all, the increased concentrations of the alleged antibody which occurred in conjunction with being exposed to an adjuvant/antigen (say, aluminum hydroxide) cannot protect the body against the antigen that gave rise to it. Therefore, why should anyone suppose that such proteins – alleged to be antibodies – will be able to protect the body against any other kind of antigen?

On the other hand, if viruses do not exist but an individual receives a vaccine, and, then, becomes ill with the very disease that the vaccine is supposed to protect against – as was the case in the Cutter Laboratories affair – then, obviously, legitimate questions can be directed toward the possible toxicity of various components within the vaccine. For instance, could the contents of the vaccine have brought about the very illness that emerges following such a vaccination and against which the vaccine was supposed to protect a person?

Alternatively, one might ask, what is the actual nature of the disease that is manifesting itself? In other words, if a given disease is alleged to be caused by a certain kind of virus, yet such viruses cannot be proven to exist, then, what is the actual nature of the disease that previously was being attributed – falsely – to the virus, and, just as importantly, if a person who receives a vaccine comes down with the very disease against which that vaccine supposedly protects a person, yet, viruses do not actually exist, then, what is the contents of the vaccine – which are supposedly anti-viral in nature -- that would cause symptoms to appear which are similar to a naturally occurring form of pathology that cannot be attributed to a virus?

Suzanne Humphries and Roman Bystrianyk have put forth a great deal of evidence in their book *Dissolving Illusions* which indicate how programs of vaccination have had little, if anything to do, with the declines in incidence that have taken place with respect to various kinds of diseases such as measles, mumps, chicken pox, small pox, diphtheria, and poliomyelitis. All of those diseases were following a downward trend long before, and, therefore, quite independently of vaccine programs.

Moreover, proponents of vaccines cannot argue that the reason why the incidence of those diseases has continued to stay low, or ticked even slightly lower, is because of the intervention of vaccines. To make such an argument, one would have to be able to prove that all of the improvements in public health that have been made throughout the last half of the nineteenth century and during the first 50-60 years of the twentieth century were no longer continuing to impact the incidence of disease. In other words, one would have to be able to credibly argue that improvements in diet, quality of water, sanitation, personal hygiene, food security, as well as discontinuing the use of various kinds of pesticides – all of which, initially, led to the decline in the incidence of the aforementioned diseases quite independently of vaccine programs -- are no longer actively at work or continuing to exercise a downward pressure on the extent to which people might be vulnerable to this or that kind of disease.

Proponents of vaccination want vaccines to be able to take credit for the downward trend in certain kinds of diseases. However, those individuals have no scientific basis for doing so in a way that would be able to show indisputably that it is vaccines and only vaccines which are keeping the incidence of an array of disease in decline.

Moreover, in order to be able to advance the foregoing sorts of arguments, in a convincing manner, proponents of vaccines would have to be able to provide indisputable proof that viruses actually exist. Not only can't they do this, the so-called scientists on who they rely for their information refuse to even try to operate in accordance with the requirements of empirical science and, instead, just seem to want everyone to accept their biases, assumptions, and theories without examination or question.

In effect, such vaccine proponents want everyone to act like the individuals on the committee that had been put together by the Department of Health, Education, and Welfare for purposes of – supposedly – evaluating the efficacy and safety of the Salk vaccine. In other words, the proponents of vaccines want everyone to succumb to the pressures that are being exercised by said vaccine proponents to induce people to reach unnecessarily rapid, critically ill-considered, and evidentially impoverished conclusions concerning the alleged value of vaccinations.

In their book -- *Dissolving Illusions* -- Suzanne Humphries and Roman Bystrianyk note that during the Cutter Laboratories affair some of the adults also became ill with polio as a result of having had contact with individuals in their household who had been injected with the Salk vaccine. The authors indicate that the incidence rate of poliomyelitis among those who were vaccinated was somewhere in the range of between one in 100 to one in 600 injections, but no comparable rate of incidence is given for the aforementioned sorts of secondary, contact forms of poliomyelitis (people who were not vaccinated but had contact with people who were vaccinated).

The foregoing authors do state, however, that some of the secondary, contact forms of polio were quite serious. At least 13 people were sufficiently paralyzed that they needed to be placed in an iron lung, and five of those individuals died.

There also were reported cases in which babies that had been vaccinated were symptom-free but, apparently, live vaccines were found in their stool. As a result, apparently, a number of the mothers of those babies became ill, as did at least 39 neighbors of those same households in which vaccinated individuals lived.

Why did some babies remain symptom-free, while their mothers became seriously ill? Why did some babies remain symptom-free, but some of their neighbors become seriously ill?

Why did somewhere between 1 in 100 and 1 in 600 individuals become ill as a result of receiving the Salk vaccine, and why did somewhere between 99 in 100 or 599 in 600 remain free from the disease? How many of the neighbors of those who and had been injected and showed symptoms also become ill?

Some people have argued that the reason why so many people were unaffected by the "live" or non-attenuated virus that was alleged to be present in the Salk vaccine is because they already had developed a natural form of immunity. Not only is such a suggestion highly speculative, but one should add that if natural immunity was so widespread, then, why were so many people being vaccinated.

There are two broad ways the foregoing issues might be explored or investigated. One of those two processes would engage the foregoing questions from the point of view that viruses exist, while the other process would start from a perspective that discounted the existence of viruses and would want to know what it was in the vaccine's contents that was or were making some people ill as well as why only some people seemed susceptible or sensitive to the presence of such toxic materials.

Both of the foregoing approaches would likely acknowledge that shedding of some kind was taking place in those instances where secondary contact (via the individual who had been vaccinated) with the contents of the vaccine – whatever they might be – appeared to lead to the onset of polio symptoms. However, the more interesting questions tend to emerge in conjunction with those who are trying to determine what might be happening in cases where individuals are becoming sick – both through primary or secondary exposure – but no virus is present, because if no virus exists, then, what is causing the symptoms of those who become ill.

Urination, defecation, sweating, breathing, and nasal discharge are all ways in which the body seeks to detoxify and slough off toxins of one kind or another. Whether the toxins are a function of alleged viral infection or are a function of the materials that constitute the content of the vaccine, the body will try to find ways to slough them off, and, as a result, people, through secondary contact with such sloughed-off toxins – whatever their nature -- could become ill.

However, if there are no viruses present, then, why are some people getting sick through secondary contact with the vaccinated? Furthermore, if no viruses are present, then, what is causing the symptoms to be what they are? In addition, if there are no viruses present, then, what, if anything, is being detoxified – and, therefore, discharged – from the bodies of individuals who have been vaccinated (some of whom are symptom-free and some of whom are not), as well as from the bodies of individuals who are not symptom-free but have not been vaccinated, which might induce someone to become ill?

If there is no virus present, is the illness that arises through secondary contact (i.e., in people who were not vaccinated) necessarily a function of having been exposed to some sort of toxic discharge which was issuing from a person who has been vaccinated? Is it possible that illnesses arising in people who live in the same house as someone who has been vaccinated or who are neighbors of the latter sort of individual might not be due to exposure to a material toxin but, instead, could be due to some sort of resonance phenomenon?

Young female college students who live in the same dormitory often have their periods become relatively synchronized. In Couvade syndrome a man will mirror many of the same physical phenomena that are occurring in his pregnant partner including: A substantial gain in weight; alterations in hormonal patterns; morning sickness; insomnia, and so on.

Negative nocebo influences – just like their positive placebo counterparts – have been shown to have the potential to serve as powerful modulators that are capable of shaping the experiences and phenomenology of people that are exposed to such influences. Many people – as hypnosis, voodoo dynamics, and everyday advertising have demonstrated -- are suggestible to varying degrees.

Crowd contagion is a real phenomenon. Moreover, the energy levels, spirits, and sense of physical well-being of individuals can be pulled upward or pushed downward depending on the moods of those around them.

Experiments have been conducted which appear to indicate that being exposed to the frequencies of certain colors can have a debilitating effect on a person's sense of well-being. Moreover, as the frequency following research of Dr. Nick Begich or Veda Austin have indicated, as well as years of experience might suggest in which thoughts appear to have been sent to, or received from, my wife, we all are a lot more sensitive or vulnerable to the events that are going on around us than we often suppose is the case, and, therefore, to suppose that one can be influenced by another's physical condition – even to the point of becoming sick and mimicking whatever symptoms are associated with such an illness is not necessarily out of the question.

There is a lot more solid evidence in support of the idea that viruses do not exist than there is solid evidence in support of the idea that such entities do exist. People who are vaccinated and who might become ill as a result of toxins that are present in a given vaccine may display symptoms of the very disease against which the vaccine is supposed to protect, not because there is an unattenuated, live virus present in the vaccine but, instead, because the condition of dis-ease that has emerged in a biological terrain that has been destabilized by the toxins within a vaccine resonate with, or might follow the ideational and expectational frequencies that are associated with, such a disease. Such ideas, thoughts, and expectations have been talked about for years via families, among friends, within communities, in schools, during television programs, by doctors, and at medical facilities.

Toxic thoughts, ideas, emotions, anxieties, fears, expectations, beliefs, and frequencies can be shed into the environment just as easily as can various kinds of physical toxins. The effects of psychological forms of frequency following behavior can be every bit as powerful as the effects of frequency following behavior that are set in motion by material events.

The foregoing considerations are not trying to convey the idea that illness is all in one's head. Rather, what is being said is that we are being constantly inundated with all manner of frequencies.

Some of those frequencies which we follow in the form of our behaviors (which could include symptoms of one kind or another) are material in nature, while other frequencies that we follow in the form of our behaviors (which could include symptoms of one kind or another) are psychological, conceptual, emotional, and/or spiritual in nature. The condition of our biological terrains can be – either to our benefit or to our detriment -- as much a function of non-physical frequency following behavior as that condition can be a function of physical frequency following behavior.

Another set of controversies surrounding polio vaccines involved something called "Simian virus number 40" (SV40). Up until the 1980s (and some have argued that this continued on with some vaccines right up to the year 2000), many vaccines contained monkey kidney tissues as part of the culturing process that went into the manufacturing of vaccines.

Supposedly, there is evidence indicating that SV40 has been detected in different kinds of tumors, including various forms of brain tumors, lung mesotheliomas, as well as an assortment of tumors found in kidneys, bones, and breasts. In addition, when cultures believed to contain SV40 are injected into experimental animals or human volunteers, tumors have appeared, and, moreover, extensive genetic damage has been reported in conjunction with cell cultures that are believed to contain SV40.

Dr. Michael Carbone once likened SV40 to a first-rate military weapon. He made the foregoing reference because of his belief that SV40 is able to adversely impact at least four different cellular mechanism that play key roles in defending the body against the on-set of cancerous dynamics

Apparently, notwithstanding the foregoing sorts of evidence, there has been no smoking gun, so to speak, which definitively proves that SV40 actually causes a number of different kinds of cancer. Correlations have been established between the alleged presence of SV40 and the existence of cancer, but nothing, yet, has demonstrated how SV40 causes cancer.

Perhaps one of the reasons why no one has been able to show that SV40 causes cancer is because Simian virus 40 does not exist. Although cultures, tissues, and tumors are believed to contain SV40, nevertheless, believing that this is the case is not necessarily the same thing as this actually being the case.

If viruses do not exist, then, Simian virus 40 does not exist. To be sure, something might be present in certain cultures, tissues and tumors that is being identified as, or understood to be, or interpreted as SV40, but what is the nature of this 'something' and why is it being labeled SV40? In addition, individuals such as the aforementioned Dr. Carbone may have theories about how a putative virus such as SV40 might be able to interfere with, or undermine, different cellular processes, but what makes a theory a theory is that it lacks the proof which is needed to transform a conceptual idea into a concrete, existential fact.

As was in intimated in chapters 7 through 10 of the present book, no one has found an entity within the tissue of a human being or in a culture being grown in a Petri dish and, subsequently, has been able to properly and completely isolate that entity from all other materials other than itself, and, in addition, has been able to purify what has been isolated to ensure that only such an entity is present, and, which, then, has been opened up by investigators who, in turn, discover that the interior portion of that entity contains a coil of RNA or DNA which, when later sequenced through actual lab procedures and not through a set of arbitrary algorithms, gives expression to evidence, in the form of the dynamics that are set in motion by such genomic properties, which are capable of proving that such an entity is, indeed, a virus ... that is, it is a material 'something' capable of proving that such an entity is able to provide evidence which demonstrates that the genetic material contained within such an entity has the sort of information which would enable that entity to gain access to the interior of an organism, take over the cellular machinery responsible for replicating genes, and, after replicating its own genomic properties for an indeterminate number of times, would proceed to exit from such a cell, usually killing the host cell in the process of exiting from it, and, then, move on to gain entry into and replicate itself in other cells. Let it be said again – no one has succeeded in successfully performing the foregoing set of experimental procedures in a way that would constitute proof that the narratives being voiced by virologists, microbiologists, bacteriologists, immunologists, and medical doctors concerning the existence of viruses are, in fact, true.

To go from the general case to the particular case, no one has been able to show that whatever phenomenon or material that is being referred to as SV40 has been successfully taken through the foregoing set of experimental conditions and, thereby, revealed that its identity is actually that of a virus. "SV40" is a shorthand way of referring to an enormous set of assumptions, conjectures, and theories that purport to make hermeneutical sense of a given body of empirical data.

Cancerous conditions might have arisen in certain people who took the oral Sabin vaccine. Whether, or not, those conditions were due to some form of carcinogenic influence – labeled as "SV40" -- that might have been present in the vaccine is unknown. Whether, or not, such conditions were due to some form of frequency that was emanating from one, or more, substances or entities in the vaccine is not known.

A previously noted in chapter 5, Royal Rife actually was able to conduct a highly successful clinic at the University of Southern California – a clinic which was run with the assistance of a variety of competent medical doctors and microbiologists – in which he used frequencies to destroy four forms of microorganism that he had identified as being the cause of cancer as a result of extensive research and experimentation that had been carried out in conjunction with his extremely high-powered Universal microscope. Dr. Virginia Livingston-Wheeler had also identified a microorganism – Progenitor cryptocides – as being a cause of cancer.

Béchamp, Enderlein, Rife, and Naessens, along with others, had put forth considerable evidence to indicate that microorganisms were pleiomorphic/pleomorphic. That is, depending on circumstances, microorganisms could be induced to change their morphologies and functionality.

The four kinds of allegedly cancer-causing microorganisms identified by Rife, along with the allegedly cancer-causing microorganism identified by Dr. Livingston-Wheeler, as well as the multifaceted life cycles of pleiomorphic/pleomorphic microorganisms, including so-called phages to which Béchamp, Enderlein, and Naessens alluded, could all constitute candidates that give expression to the very entities that are believed to be present in a given cell, tissue, or tumor and which are being referred to as SV40 viruses but which are not, in fact, actually viruses.

Alternatively, what is being referred to as SV40 and what is being attributed to it (i.e., that it might be cancer causing) could actually be a function of ingredients which actually are known to be in the contents of vaccines and are not merely conjectured to be present in vaccines as is the case with SV40. Unfortunately, many of these other vaccine ingredients have never been properly tested for their carcinogenic potential either individually or in conjunction with some sort of negative synergistic dynamic that different vaccine ingredients might have with one another.

Moreover, every vaccine has its proprietary ingredients and processes which the public is not permitted to know because the original intention of the framers of the Constitution has been completely inverted and, as a result, corporations – an idea and set of legal dynamics that was antithetical to the values and beliefs of many American colonists/patriots -- have come to be able to enjoy more rights and protections than do actual people. Quite frankly, only individuals who have become corrupted in one way or another could believe that the financial and material health of corporations should be afforded more importance than the biological and mental health of actual human beings.

Consequently, there are proprietary dimensions of vaccines which could have short-term or chronic ramifications for the health of human beings which cannot be properly (i.e., independently, objectively, and thoroughly) explored or tested. As a result, what is being attributed to SV40 actually could be a function of one, or more, of the proprietary components that are present within a given vaccine.

In India, research has indicated that between 1996 and 2011 the number of cases of paralysis associated with alleged wild-type forms of polio virus have declined, while the numbers of cases diagnosed as AFP (i.e., Acute Flaccid Paralysis) have been trending upward by many tens of thousands of cases per year. Several questions concerning the foregoing research tend to bubble to the surface.

To begin with, previously, mention was made about how the CDC indicates that only 1% of individuals who test positive for polio (and testing entails its own set of problems) go on to develop some form of polio. In the light of such data, how can one be sure that the people who develop polio do so because of the presence of a wild-type of virus whose existence cannot be verified?

Secondly, Acute Flaccid Paralysis has been attributed to a bevy of possible causes. Among such possibilities are: Rabies, Guillain-Barré syndrome, transverse myelitus, Karwinskia tick bite paralysis, clostridium botulinum toxins, myasthenia gravis, and polio vaccines.

The one statistical trend of the Indian research that does stand out is the following one. Increases in the cases of AFP tends to correlate best with the cumulative number of doses of oral vaccine that have been given during the previous three years, and, therefore, the greater the number of doses that have been given, the higher is the increase in the number of cases of AFP that tends to be recorded.

Apparently, there seems to be something in the polio vaccine that might be causing an increase in cases of Acute Flaccid Paralysis. Or, alternatively, there is some other set of non-vaccine related factors that are going on in India which is causing an increase of AFP which, simultaneously for some reason, are also correlating highly with the number of doses of vaccine which are being given out over a three year period.

The strategy of the W.H.O. (World health Organization) and GAVI (Global Alliance for Vaccines and Immunizations) has been to double, triple, and quadruple down by imposing even more vaccines on individuals. Some children have received as many as 30 polio vaccines by the time they are five years old, and, yet, the so-called "experts" at W.H.O. and GAVI refuse to acknowledge the extent of their ignorance as well as the very real possibility that their vaccine programs are the reason why cases of Acute Flaccid Paralysis are reaching epidemic proportions in India and other localities.

There is at least one common denominator to the various kinds of tragedies discussed in the previous pages that have been engendered by various advocates of the allopathic system of medicine. The opioid crisis, the HIV-causes-AIDS fiasco, the chemical imbalance in the brain fiction, the polio travesty, the flatulence of the cancer industry, the arbitrary and misguided adventurism within virology, the ill-advised certainties of immunology, the oppressive phantasmagoria of vaccinology, along with so many other problems that have settled in like some toxic black mold beneath the sparkling veneer of alleged allopathic wizardry and technological knowhow – each of the foregoing issues seems to point in a similar direction.

More specifically, all too many of the practitioners and theoreticians of allopathic medicine appear to lack the humility, sensitivity, insight, and character that is needed to understand what is staring them in the face – namely, in far too many ways, they don't necessarily know what they are doing and, unfortunately, they don't seem to care that their ignorance is killing and harming people to the tune of hundreds of thousands of people per year. Any terrorist group one might care to mention would have been subject to wars and black ops that were dedicated to wiping out such terrorists for committing far few atrocities on a much more limited scale.

Moreover, one of the etiological starting points for the growth of such ignorance is the failure of many of the proponents of medicine to seriously engage the research and discoveries of people such as Béchamp, Enderlein, Rife, and Naessens who had a much better grasp of the life process – both in terms of wellbeing and pathology -- than many of the intellectually moribund descendents of a monomorphically limited Pasteur will ever be able achieve as long as such individuals continue to pay tribute to, and live in accordance with the values of, someone who was as corrupt, self-serving, ill-informed, self-aggrandizing, intuitively stunted, and intellectually challenged as their nineteenth century progenitor has proven himself to be.

None of what precedes this sentence is meant to be definitive. However, all of what precedes this sentence is intended as an introduction to possibilities which, hopefully, might induce readers to begin to critically reflect on what it means to be alive – physically, psychologically, scientifically, medically, philosophically, socially, politically, and spiritually.

What has been said in the current and previous chapters might not always be right. Nonetheless, I believe that everything which has been said, and is about to be said in the final chapter, is intended to point in a heuristically valuable direction.

.

Chapter 18: Rights, Medical Practice, and Public Health

In 1976, more than half a dozen military personnel were hospitalized at Fort Dix, New Jersey. One of those individuals died.

Samples were taken from the stricken individuals and analyzed by members of the New Jersey Department of Health. Those authorities claimed that while most of the sick military personnel seemed to be suffering from only a common strain of influenza, there were several anomalous strains that were forwarded to the Center for Disease Control and Prevention in Georgia for further examination.

Eventually, the CDC judged that those samples contained a form of H1N1 swine flu which seemed to have similarities to the allegedly lethal 1918 flu virus. As a result, on February 13, 1976, David Sencer, the Director of the CDC, released a memo calling for a program of mass immunization to be initiated.

A month later (and one wonders why it took so long for this to happen), President Gerald Ford was informed of the aforementioned CDC memo. Subsequently, a committee of experts -- including Albert Sabin and Jonas Salk -- was assembled with whom Ford might consult concerning the issue.

A Senate subcommittee was convened to explore the matter further. During those hearings, a representative from a drug company requested indemnity for whatever damages might arise out of such a mass immunization program, and another pharmaceutical company indicated that it would not sell vaccines to the government if the company was not indemnified in relation to those vaccines.

The House Appropriations Committee generated a bill which included 135 million dollars to underwrite the costs of the proposed mass immunization program. The bill was approved in early April, 1976.

Several insurance companies came forth. They indicated that they would not provide the pharmaceutical companies with any form of indemnification for product liability in conjunction with whatever flu vaccines might be manufactured for the mass immunization program.

The White House was informed that without product liability indemnification, the pharmaceutical companies were unwilling to move forward with the production of a vaccine. As a result, President

Ford put forth a proposal to Congress that would provide such product liability indemnity.

In July 1976 a conference was held and one of the attendees maintained that there was no similarity between what was transpiring at Fort Dix and what had happened in 1918. Later on during July, a researcher by the name of: J. Anthony Morris was dismissed from the FDA for insubordination but, subsequently, went public and announced that the vaccines being prepared were not safe.

Presumably, the topic of his announcement was, in some way, likely to have been connected to the charges of insubordination that had been levied against him by the FDA and for which he had been fired. In other words, based on his research, Morris, apparently, had been generating difficulties within the FDA over his concerns about vaccine safety, but the FDA didn't want to hear about those concerns and fired him because he persisted in airing them despite having been told to drop the matter.

A few days after Morris came out with his public warnings about vaccine safety, a number of vaccine manufacturers gave notice that they were going to discontinue producing vaccines that, supposedly, would protect people against the alleged flu outbreak. In other words, those companies were playing a game of "let's hold the American people hostage" as a way of trying to leverage the situation so that they could get the indemnity that they wanted.

In late July of 1976, President Ford urged Congress to pass a bill that would extend indemnity to the pharmaceutical companies with respect to the vaccine. In early August, President Ford held a press conference.

During the latter event, he again brought up the issue of indemnification. He urged Congress to pass an appropriate bill which would extend product liability to pharmaceutical companies that might manufacture a flu vaccine, and four days after the foregoing press conference took place, both houses of Congress passed a bill that extended product liability to companies which manufactured the flu vaccine.

In early September, the first vaccines were submitted to the FDA's Bureau of Biologics for safety testing. Approximately three weeks later, the first vaccines were released to the public.

Three weeks is not enough time to develop, let alone, test a vaccine. However, given that the vaccine manufacturers had been granted indemnity, concerns about safety might only get in the way of making money.

By early December of 1976, there had been a multiplicity of cases involving Guillain-Barré syndrome that were reported in at least eleven states. The CDC, itself, investigated those reports and indicated that there were four times as many cases of Guillain-Barré syndrome among vaccinated individuals as were occurring among non-vaccinated individuals.

The mass immunization program was suspended. Eventually, researchers determined that of the 45 million people who had received vaccinations during a six week period, there were more than 360 individuals who had been vaccinated that, subsequently, were diagnosed with Guillain-Barré syndrome during that period of time.

Whether, or not, other people who had been vaccinated might go on to develop long-term health issues as a result of being injected did not appear to be a research topic. The pharmaceutical industry only conducted "research" – if it can be called that -- concerning the issue of adverse effects that fell within a time frame that lasted just a few days or a few weeks, and, therefore, what might happen a few years down the line seemed to be irrelevant, and, yet, in the past various drugs and vaccines had to be recalled because adverse effects from those products didn't show up right away.

In effect, Phase IV of the FDA's four-step set of protocols is intended to see what might happen when a given product is authorized for commercial release and, thereby, let loose on the public. Phase IV is the permission that the FDA gives to the pharmaceutical industry to carry out experiments on the American public in order to see whether there might be problems which emerge over time within the general population that might not have been visible within the truncated nature of the testing process entailed by Phase III trials.

Following the suspension of the immunization program, discussions ensued about whether, or not, the outbreak of Guillain-Barré syndrome could really be causally traced to flu vaccines. In addition, some individuals asked whether it was better to err on the side of aggressive intervention or on the side of caution concerning these sorts of intervention programs.

The circumstances surrounding, and leading up to, the mass influenza immunization program of 1976 give expression to a great many of the issues that are entailed by the activity of vaccination. For example, there was the matter of the initial diagnosis.

On the basis of tests conducted at Fort Dix, most of the individuals who were hospitalized were showing, apparently, nothing more than what was considered to be a normal, run-of-the-mill form of influenza. However, there were several samples taken at Fort Dix that contained certain anomalies which were forwarded to the CDC for further analysis, and someone at the CDC indicated that those anomalies involved a form of flu that was similar to the strain of influenza which some people believed was the cause of the Great Influenza of 1918-1919.

There are a number of questions which surface in conjunction with the foregoing considerations. First, there is great deal of evidence – evidence that was available in 1976 – to indicate that claims concerning the existence of viruses (flu-like or otherwise) are not tenable.

If viruses do not exist, then, what credence should be given to tests which indicate that something is present which has never been properly isolated, purified, sequenced, and proven to be something that is capable of doing what a virus is supposed to be able to do? In 1976 – as is the case now – the notion of a virus was entirely entangled in unproven theoretical conjectures, suppositions, and assumptions which refused to acknowledge the existence of empirical evidence that contradicted those sorts of conjectures, suppositions, theories, and assumptions.

Once the people at Fort Dix separated out what they thought they understood, but did not actually know, from that which they were willing to acknowledge fell outside of what they believed – untenably - - they knew, they sent the latter materials to the CDC. People at the

CDC – who saw potential viral epidemics and pandemics practically everywhere they looked and who had conflicts of interest practically everywhere that other people looked – displayed the character of their expertise by declaring that what had not been identified by the researchers at Fort Dix was, in fact, a form of swine flu which was very similar to the virus that, supposedly, was responsible for so many deaths in 1918-1919.

In Chapter 7, a critical overview concerning the alleged piecing together of the 1918 influenza virus by Jeffrey Taubenberger and others was given. The upshot of that overview is there are many unanswered questions surrounding the Taubenberger flu project, and, when one adds such questions to the more general issue that no one has put forth convincing evidence that viruses of any kind actually exist – in the sense employed by virologists – then, one must treat the pronouncements of the CDC concerning the existence of this or that kind of virus with considerable caution.

In addition, the CDC's Advisory Committee on Immunization Practices (ACIP) recommends which vaccines should be added to the schedule of vaccines for children and teenagers. Many of the individuals who are members of that advisory committee hold patents for a variety of vaccines and also regularly receive grants from vaccine manufacturers to conduct related research, and, moreover, the CDC spends more than a third of its budget on buying and distributing vaccines.

Obviously, in light of the foregoing considerations, neither the CDC nor many of the members of the aforementioned Advisory Committee on Immunization Practices can be considered to be objective, independent researchers when it comes to the issue of the safety and efficacy of vaccines. Furthermore, given that most, if not all, members of the CDC have bought into the mythology of virology hook, line and sinker, then, those individuals cannot be assumed to be in a position to offer a unbiased, rigorously objective, fair, and independent assessment of the many claims of virologists concerning the existence of viruses or concerning the alleged need for anti-viral vaccines to counter such existentially-dubious entities.

As the testimony of CDC whistleblower Dr. William Thompson revealed, for 14 years a sizeable group of individuals at the CDC lied about the causal links between the thimerosal which was present in certain vaccines and the incidence of autism in black youths. The fact that such prevarication went on for such a long period of time and was covered up by the CDC indicates that there appears to be a culture of corruption that governs a great deal of what transpires within the CDC.

Among other things, there is often a revolving door policy which connects people working at the CDC with pharmaceutical companies for whom the former individuals later go to work, and this dynamic is part of the regulatory capture process that enables the pharmaceutical industry to control the CDC rather than to be properly regulated by that government agency. In other words, there are people who have worked for, are working for, and will work for the CDC who have been, are, or will be making decisions concerning pharmaceutical companies that could impact a given CDC employee's own future opportunities for lucrative jobs at such companies that offer compensation packages that are many times what can be offered to a government employee, and, therefore, one cannot trust that whatever decisions are forthcoming from those sorts of individuals necessarily will be made in the best interests of the American people rather than being made in accordance with the best interests of this or that pharmaceutical company.

Consequently, when someone like David Sencer, the Director of the CDC, issues a memo that there should be a program of mass immunization to thwart the alleged threat posed by the swine flu that, supposedly, has been detected in several individuals at Fort Dix, why should one treat such a memo with any degree of seriousness? What conflicts of interest might be compromising David Sencer's judgment on the matter?

Why should one accept pronouncements about the existence of viruses that are based on questionable science? Why should one comply with a government employee's theoretical – and, therefore, ideologically driven -- biases concerning virology and/or vaccines?

For reasons which usually have nothing to do with science, politicians are known to be a cautious lot who are not so much interested in what the truth of something might be as much as they try to be cognizant of the sorts of things for which they might be blamed later on. Consequently, President Ford -- or one, or more, of his advisors (none of whom necessarily understood anything about viruses or vaccines) – felt that notwithstanding the memo of the Director of the CDC calling for a mass program of immunization, there should be an "independent" committee of experts assembled to consider the matter.

The "optics" of the foregoing move is interesting. The federal government is already paying millions, if not billions, of dollars, to hundreds of "experts" at the CDC.

The CDC offers its judgment on the matter of the alleged swine flu threat. However, the President, perhaps at the behest of some of his political handlers, suggests that what is needed is some sort of 'blue ribbon' committee or panel that will be able to provide the President with a certain amount of cover that – before caving into the demands of pharmaceutical corporations – will offer the appearance of having consulted with "independent" counsel before moving ahead in whatever way they do that might, or might not, have anything to do with what such a committee recommends.

Thus, people such as Jonas Salk and Albert Sabin, are called upon to offer their expert opinion on the crisis that confronts the Ford administration. Salk and Sabin have both been portrayed as scientific and medical saints by the media, and, yet, the underbelly of that story is wrought with all manner of mistakes, errors, deaths, problematic science, and allegedly cancer-causing viruses.

Since few people know any of the back story involving the Salk and Sabin vaccines, President Ford – or one, or more, of his advisors – wish to leverage the public saint-like persona of those individuals, as well as the personae of "expertise" involving whatever other individuals might have been asked or induced to grace the advisory committee which is being formed, in order to be in a position to propagandistically convey the idea that the government is committed to making the right sort of decision when it comes to the issue of a program of mass immunization.

Whether President Ford or any of his advisors know anything about virology, microbiology, immunology, vaccinology, Salk, or Sabin is beside the point. They are in the image creating business and not the truth business.

The aforementioned committee of experts meets and discusses, among other things, the CDC recommendation for mass immunization. The Senate holds hearings on the issue, and during the latter sessions, the Senate is informed that vaccine manufacturers are reluctant to be willing to contribute their part (i.e., vaccines) to the idea of a mass immunization campaign unless they can be indemnified against product liability.

Here you have vaccine manufacturers who are so sure of their knowledge and understanding of virology and vaccinology that they are harboring reservations concerning the safety and efficacy of their products. Apparently, they do want to profit from what they do, but they don't want to be held accountable for what they do.

In other words, they want to be given indemnity for experimenting on the American public. The question is whether the federal government will be interested in authorizing the right of pharmaceutical corporations to be able to experiment on the American public.

A few days later, the answer to the foregoing question is made known. President Ford puts forth a proposal indicating that Congress should move ahead with some form of indemnity protection for those who might be manufacturing a flu vaccine.

In July of 1976, a conference is held in which some of the participants -- who, supposedly, are experts in their field -- indicate that there is absolutely no similarity between what allegedly had been discovered in conjunction with the Fort Dix illnesses and the alleged virus that supposedly ravaged populations in 1918-1919. Unfortunately, when it comes to governance, expertise is not about differentiating between reliable and problematic expertise but, rather, the issue of expertise tends to be decided in favor of those who, often for hidden reasons, have the ear of, or who are willing to subjugate themselves to, those who make the decisions.

Around roughly the same time as the aforementioned conference is taking place, J. Anthony Morris is fired by the FDA because he had the poor taste to question the safety of the vaccines that were being prepared for possible use in the mass immunization campaign being proposed by the CDC. The FDA is an agency of the government which has the legislatively granted power to authorize pharmaceutical companies to proceed with their experiments on the American public.

For whatever reason, President Ford – or, one, or more, of his advisors (none of whom necessarily know anything about issues of virology and vaccinology) – decides not to listen to, or might not even know about, the testimony of individuals such as J. Anthony Morris who are indicating that the flu vaccines are not safe. Once again, President Ford – either with knowledge that there might be safety concerns concerning the vaccine or in the absence of such understanding -- publically recommends that Congress needs to move forward with a bill that will indemnify vaccine manufacturers from being sued for product liability issues.

Whether the President or the people who are advising him have any understanding of the issues is not known. It is unknown whether the President or the people who are advising him are making the recommendation they are making because they fully understand the scientific and medical issues surrounding the swine flu claims, or because they have become beguiled by a medical and scientific paradigm that prevents them from seeing anything but what they are told to see and believe, or because while they might have little, or no, understanding of the medical and scientific issues with which they are confronted, nonetheless, they do have some insight into how politically and financially powerful vaccine manufacturers are, and, therefore, have an appreciation of the forces which help to shape their fate.

Thus, on the one hand, the CDC is recommending that the American people be experimented on with a program of mass immunization which is based on nothing more than its own biases, beliefs, conflicts of interests, and culture of corruption. On the other hand, the FDA is trying to silence one of its employees for having safety concerns with respect to the possibility that the American public might be exposed to a problematic product, and, by taking such actions, the FDA is clearly indicating that it is quite prepared to take whatever risks it deems necessary to carry out its program of vaccine experimentation on the American public.

Finally, on a number of occasions, the President of the United States has been pushing the idea that pharmaceutical companies should be freed from all concerns with indemnification. In other words, for whatever his ultimate reasons might be, he is advocating that pharmaceutical companies should be authorized by Congress to move forward with whatever experiments those companies care to conduct on the American people.

There are many members of Congress who are ideologically and/or financially committed to promoting the protection and enhancement of the rights of corporations over the rights of the people. There are many doctors and lawyers in Congress who are ideologically committed to, and biased toward, the mythology of virology and vaccinology, and despite provisions in the first amendment that "Congress shall make no law respecting an establishment of religion ..." – and what is an ideological commitment to various kinds of assumptions, conjectures, theories, mythologies, and biases but a form of religion – Congress proceeds to heed the words of the White House and grants pharmaceutical companies the indemnity which they have sought and, thereby, has authorized such companies to conduct experiments on the American people.

Make no mistake. If one (whether this is the CDC, the FDA, the President, Congress, or the pharmaceutical companies) cannot ensure that a product will not adversely affect the physical well-being of someone who consumes or uses that product, then, those who are authorizing or manufacturing such products are engaged in an experimental process. How is it that American governmental officials prosecuted Nazis for experimenting on human beings without the informed consent of the latter, but, 30, or so, years later, many of those same government officials are falling all over themselves to find ways of authorizing pharmaceutical companies to do precisely the same sort of thing in conjunction with the American people as was done during the second world war by the Nazis?

People who were vaccinated with the Swine flu vaccine for which the manufacturers were granted indemnity protections against product liability were four times more likely to be diagnosed with Guillain-Barré syndrome than were people who did not receive that vaccine. Proponents of those vaccines sought to argue that the causal links between the vaccine and Guillain-Barré syndrome were questionable, and, yet, without embarrassment, those same people argued on the basis of mere conjecture, assumptions, biases, theories, and problematic experimental evidence that vaccines which could not be shown to be safe and effective (and, therefore, for which pharmaceutical companies needed to be granted indemnity) should be permitted to be experimentally administered to the American public in order, allegedly, to protect the latter against an entity – namely, the flu virus – that has not, yet, been proven to exist.

Everything that is wrong with public health policy in America is a subtext of the 1976 Swine Flu fiasco. However, insult was added to injury when ten years later, during the Reagan administration, something known as the 'National Childhood Vaccine Injury Act of 1986' was approved by both houses of Congress and signed into law by President Reagan.

Despite signing the foregoing Act into law, President Reagan had mixed feelings concerning its authorization. More specifically, he was concerned that the American people were being empowered to be able to extract money from the federal government as compensation for injuries attributed to vaccines without having to prove that manufacturers were actually liable for those injuries.

In other words, apparently, President Reagan didn't trust the American people. Despite the fact that it has been pharmaceutical companies that, for years, had been prosecuted by the federal government, again and again, for criminally and civilly defrauding the American public, and despite the fact that President Reagan had little, or no, proof that the American people were about to embark on a campaign to fleece the federal government of unjustly gained forms of compensation for alleged vaccine injuries, President Reagan was questioning the wisdom of a program that might offer children (and their parents) some form of financial protection should injuries arise in conjunction with the taking of certain vaccines.

Prior to signing the Omnibus Health Bill – of which the National Childhood Vaccine Injury Act was a part – President Regan had threatened to veto the whole Omnibus Health Bill precisely because of his concerns about the possible ramifications of the part of that Bill which dealt with the National Childhood Vaccine Injury Act. He was talked in off the ledge by his Vice-President, George H.W. Bush, and James Baker, who, at the time, was Secretary of the Treasury.

Bush had ties with the pharmaceutical industry. He had served on the Board of Directors for one of its members.

Apparently, Bush also knew what President Reagan didn't seem to understand. The National Childhood Vaccine Injury Act was not about providing a means of extracting money from vaccine manufacturers because the Act actually indemnified those manufacturers against product liability.

The foregoing Act made the federal government the protectors and guardians of corporate reputations. Any person who pursued compensation for vaccine injuries would be going up against the federal government and not vaccine manufacturers.

The Department of Justice was being used to not only protect the reputation of vaccine manufactures, but, as well, it was also being used to protect the way that the CDC, the FDA, the NIH, and the U.S. Congress were collaborating with one another to serve the interests of the pharmaceutical industry and a system of allopathic medicine. Consequently, the National Childhood Vaccine Injury Act was not intended to help protect children by providing compensation for possible vaccine injuries, but, rather that Act was intended to protect the allopathic medical system against those whom such a system was injuring on a regular basis.

The National Childhood Vaccine Injury Act was part of the managed care system that was at the heart of allopathic medicine. In other words, the Department of Justice would be used to manage compensation claims so that, superficially, the government would be seen to be serving the interests of the American people by ensuring that those who deserved compensation received it, but in reality, the Department of Justice was being used to protect the allopathic medical system against any kind of legal discovery that would be able to demonstrate that there were serious problems with the whole notion of the vaccine schedule for children and teenagers. It was all part of a managed health care system that would enable the government to be able to continue authorizing the pharmaceutical industry to continue experimenting on the American people by managing the sorts of injury complaints that could be levied against the vaccine process and, thereby, be able to help hide from the public the actual extent of the damage that was being perpetrated upon the American people – especially its children and youth.

The U.S. District Court was empowered to determine who, according to the provisions of the National Childhood Vaccine Injury Act, should and should not receive compensation. One wonders why a decision was made – and by whom -- to engage such issues through an adversarial process in which the parents of children who might have been vaccine injured were required to hire lawyers to undertake a lengthy, expensive, process of gathering research, procuring expert witnesses, and pursuing litigation before an arbitrarily established Vaccine Court in which those parents would have to face-off against lawyers who were being fully financed by the government as well as be required to have to deal with the appointed "Masters" of the Court who not only were being paid by the government but either didn't necessarily know all that much concerning the medical and scientific issues about which they were supposed to be making "fair" judgments, or were so brainwashed by an allopathic approach to medicine that they had virtually no capacity to reach independent conclusions concerning the sort of mendacity and delusional behavior that governs much of virology and vaccinology.

Processes of mediation might have been better suited to deal with a multiplicity of issues that likely were to be entailed by claims of vaccine injury. Moreover, such a program could have been organized in a manner that would have made issues involving fairness, money, time, expertise, research and resources accessible to everyone.

Unfortunately, the program set in motion by the National Childhood Vaccine Injury Act enabled the Department of Health and Human Services as well as the Department of Justice to be solely responsible for making up the rules by which the Vaccine Court was to operate. For instance, only certain kinds of injuries were recognized by the government as medical problems that might be accepted -- with the right kind of evidence, expert witnesses, and so on – as, possibly, being due to vaccines, and this list of "approved" injury possibilities was known as the Vaccine Injury Table.

The Secretary of Health and Human Services has sole discretion with respect to what might be recognized as a possible vaccine-related injury and, therefore, be able to qualify as an item that would appear in the aforementioned Table. There is no Congressional oversight concerning those decisions.

Persuasive cases might be able to be assembled that sought compensation for what were considered to be off-table vaccine related injuries. However, many off-table vaccine-related injuries were kept off-table precisely because defensible cases could be made that certain vaccines might have led to modalities of injury that were not included in the Vaccine Table, and as long as such gate-keeping practices were in place, parents had no way of redressing the situation because vaccine manufacturers had been indemnified with respect to product liability in those matters.

Over the years, HHS has aggressively restricted the kinds of complaints that could be addressed through the Vaccine Injury Table. Yet, the original intent of the Act had been to provide Health and Human Services with the authority to be able to expand, not restrict, what kinds of problems would appear in the Vaccine Injury Table, and, therefore, one can't help but wonder what forces have been acting on various Secretaries, and other members, of HHS to induce them to act in a way that was contrary to what had been discussed and agreed upon before the National Childhood Vaccine Injury Act was passed.

The Department of Health and Human Services also has responsibility for ensuring that the American people know about the existence of the Childhood Vaccine Injury program so that members of the public would be aware that such a possibility existed and, if necessary, would be familiar with the basic steps and conditions that were entailed by the process of filing claims. Unfortunately – and, very likely, intentionally so -- the HHS did very little to make sure that the public knew about the program.

Furthermore, the Department of Justice had complete authority to shape the rules of the Court as it deemed fit. Thus, without any form of Congressional interference or oversight, the Department of Justice could: Interpret, revise, or change the way the Vaccine Court operated, as well as be able to determine who could or would be appointed to serve as a "Special Master" in those courts.

Unfortunately, across a number of different Presidential administrations, personnel in the Department of Justice abused the foregoing license and often acted against the interests of justice. For example, the original intent of the National Childhood Vaccine Injury Act was to operate in a way that, on average, would bring about the settlement of claims in a year or less.

However, not too long after the inception of the foregoing Act, the average length of cases began to increase to two or three years and more. In the 1990s the average length of many cases took five, or more, years to settle (and not necessarily in favor of the families filing the claims).

One of the primary reasons underlying the substantial increases in the average length of settlement times for various cases had to do with the manner in which different Secretaries of HHS have been arbitrarily changing the definitions of terms to be found within the Vaccine Injury Table. For instance, the notion of encephalopathy – brain injury – was interpreted in such a way that made the term almost impossible to be considered applicable to any claim because the meaning of the term was based on a report by the Institute of Medicine that professed neutrality on the issue of whether, or not, vaccines could be linked to certain kinds of brain injuries.

The Institute of Medicine was a supposedly independent, non-governmental body. Yet, its research and opinions were thoroughly influenced and shaped by the principles of allopathic medicine, and, therefore, the idea that vaccines might – on a regular basis -- cause injuries was, in most respects, not part of its lexicon.

Another example of the foregoing sort of problem arises in connection with a "severity clause" which was established as a requirement for even being able to file a claim for compensation (claims which might be denied despite being able to meet the conditions for filing them). For example, in order to be able to satisfy the severity clause requirement, petitioners had to be able to show that a child had been suffering from some injury for more than six months and, moreover, that at least $1,000 dollars in unreimbursed medical expenses had accrued with respect to that injury. Furthermore, if the claim for compensation was being made on behalf of a dead child, then, the petitioners had to provide proof that the death was caused by a given vaccine.

Setting a time period of six months during which some sort of injury has to have been proven to exist is completely arbitrary.

Oftentimes, for instance, neurological issues are difficult to identify or quantify and various doctors might arrive at totally different conclusions as to whether, or not, something is amiss. If symptoms come and go, then how does one demonstrate that a condition has been on-going for at least six months, or if one's family has no health insurance or can't afford to see a doctor, then, how does one go about proving that a given condition has lasted for at least six months?

Furthermore, setting a minimum of $1,000 in unreimbursed medical expenses concerning a given injury is completely arbitrary. The fact that an insurance company might have reimbursed medical expenses concerning some sort of injury has nothing to do with whether, or not, such an injury is vaccine-related, nor does it have anything to do the following issue -- namely, if an injury has been caused by a vaccine, then, that injury should be provided with compensation quite independently of whether, or not, some sort of reimbursement for on-going medical expenses has been taking place.

In addition, roving that a death was due to a vaccine injury is often an arbitrary exercise because many of the people who sign death certificates are ideologically committed to – and not evidentially persuaded by -- the notion that vaccines cannot cause someone's death.

The foregoing severity clause also often makes it difficult to comply with another arbitrary feature of the petition process – namely, the statute of limitations for either death due to possible vaccine injury (which is two years) or non-lethal forms of possible vaccine-related injuries (which is three years). Given that HHS has done a very poor job in publicizing the existence of the Childhood Vaccine Injury compensation program, if one has to wait for more than six months to file a compensation petition, then, by the time one finds out about the program – assuming one does – and begins to explore one's options, one is almost out of time to file a petition.

The foregoing problem comes into even sharper focus when one realizes that petitioners must be able to find experts who will be willing to testify on their behalf. This is a very difficult task to accomplish because the manner in which the medical system is set up often entails the possibility that those who testify against such a system could run the risk of losing their medical licenses or be threatened in some other way (such as through the loss of business or impediments to career advancement).

For a variety of reasons, trying to find an expert who will be willing to testify on one's behalf can be a time-consuming process for petitioners. By the time they are able to satisfy the requirements entailed by the aforementioned severity clause, and, then, subsequently, they come to learn about the National Childhood Vaccine Injury Act, and, then, they go in search of legal and expert witnesses, such would-be petitioners often are pushing up against the statute of limitations that arbitrarily have been set by the Department of Justice.

In the meantime, the would-be petitioners need to be able to work, and, as a result, they don't have all kinds of time to: Undertake research, make appointments, or attend meetings, and so on. Moreover, during this same period of time, potential petitioners are trying to deal with all of the financial, medical, social, emotional, marital, and family difficulties that are associated with a child who, for whatever reason, has suffered some sort of severe, possibly vaccine-related injury.

Any statute of limitations policy that fails to take into account the foregoing issues is not just arbitrary. It also is completely devoid of even a hint of compassion and lacks – perhaps intentionally so – the slightest bit of common sense concerning how difficult life can be, and how emotionally exhausting and physically draining life can be, for people who are trying to grapple with on-going tragedy.

One might also note that in contradistinction to the way in which most state and federal court systems are operated, there is no period of discovery which is permitted to those who petition the Vaccine Court. The alleged purpose of such a limitation on rights was intended to serve Congress's original intent that petitions involving the National Childhood Vaccine Injury Act should be decided quickly.

However, as noted previously, the average length of vaccine court cases have increased substantially over the years. Therefore, quick decisions are not the norm, and, as a result, losing the right for discovery becomes just one more obstacle that has been placed in the way of petitioners concerning their opportunity for fair and just treatment.

While Court Masters do have some discretion to extend to themselves a certain period of time in order to reach a decision, nonetheless, petitioners are not afforded the same degrees of freedom. Therefore, irrespective of whatever evidence individuals might try to uncover in order to determine whether, or not, they even have a case for which a petition can be filed, such efforts merely are eating up the time which has been allotted to them under the statute of limitations.

Although Congress was supposed to exercise continued oversight responsibilities in conjunction with the implementation of the National Childhood Vaccine Injury Act, it failed to do so. 13 years passed before the General Accounting Office – which is required by law to regularly review government programs like the National Childhood Vaccine Injury Act that involve trust funds of one kind or another – issued a report indicating, among other things, that claims were not being settled in a timely manner.

The trust fund which provides the money that is used to cover the legal fees, administrative costs, and compensation awards entailed by the Vaccine Court's operations is derived from an excise tax that is exacted on every dose of a vaccine which is sold. The amount of the tax is approximately $0.75, but by the time certain branches of the government take a cut of the proceeds, the amount has been estimated to have become whittled down to $0.56.

Irrespective of the amount of money that ends up in the trust fund, that sum is increasing. The Department of Health and Human Services, in conjunction with the Department of Justice, have established a Maginot-like line of defenses and obstacles which make it very, very difficult for families with children who might have been injured as a result of being vaccinated to be able to receive some sort of compensation, and, therefore, the trust fund has been going up, not down.

According to Wayne Rohde (*The Vaccine Court: The Dark Truth of America's Vaccine Injury Compensation Program*), the Department of Justice has refused to respond to Freedom of Information requests concerning how much of the trust fund – which is taking in more than it is paying out – is directed toward paying the salaries of the lawyers the government uses to prosecute vaccine injury claims, and the ridiculous excuse that is cited for refusing to disclose such information is that such information is a matter of legal privilege because divulging it could tip off one's adversaries about various strategies that are being used to prosecute cases. There is also controversy about whether, or not, the accumulated funds are being used to bankroll various kinds of research projects or are being used, surreptitiously, to balance the books for this or that department.

In addition, vaccine manufacturers complained that since more money is coming in to the trust fund than is being paid out, then, perhaps, the amount of the excise tax that is being charged per vaccine injection is too high and, therefore, should be reduced. Apparently, being given indemnity is not enough, and such corporations would like more profits as well.

Aside from all of the foregoing sorts of structural problems that have been summarized over the last five, or so pages, and which arbitrarily – and, therefore, adversely – affect petitions for compensation with respect to possible vaccine-related injuries, there are also elements of corruption that surface from time to time with respect to the manner in which the Department of Justice engages the National Childhood Vaccine Injury Act. For instance, consider the 'Autism General Order #1' that -- with the best of intentions -- was issued in July of 2002 by Chief Special Master Gary Golkiewicz but which, subsequently, became entangled within some corrupt machinations that were perpetrated by various individuals within the federal government.

More specifically the Autism General Order #1 was intended to set up the Omnibus Autism Proceedings (which didn't take place until 2007 and 2008) that would investigate the possibility that certain vaccines on the childhood schedule were believed to be responsible -- directly or indirectly -- for increases in cases of autism that were being diagnosed. The Order was intended to serve as a way of dealing with a large number of petitions (at least 5,500) that had been filed in conjunction with the Childhood Vaccine Injury Act and which sought compensation for autistic conditions that the petitioners were causally attributing to certain vaccines which were claimed to have been laced with thimerosal (mercury).

Essentially, the purpose of Autism General Order #1 was to establish a process (the Omnibus Autism Proceedings) for conducting hearings concerning three test cases – representing most of the 5,500 petitioners – that would be investigated in order to determine if a clear-cut decision could be reached concerning whether, or not, certain vaccines which contained thimerosal could be considered to have caused vaccine-related injuries according to the provisions of the Childhood Vaccine Injury Act. Whatever decision was reached in conjunction with those test cases would be used as a template for making decisions concerning compensation involving those kinds of cases moving forward.

There was a somewhat parallel dynamic taking place in Congress around the same time as Autism General Order #1 was being issued. More specifically, Dr. William Frist, a senator from Tennessee, was said to have surreptitiously placed a section into the 2002 Homeland Security Act which, on the one hand, prevented anyone from suing manufactures who used thimerosal in their vaccines, and, on the other hand, required all complaints seeking financial compensation to be filed in the form of a petition under the provisions of the National Childhood Vaccine Injury Act.

Dr. Frist is a member of a family that owns Hospital Corporation of America, the largest hospital oriented corporation in the United States. Moreover, as will be noted shortly, William Frist also seemed to have been implicated in another surreptitious Congressional action in conjunction with a second piece of legislation known at the PREP Act of 2005-2006.

Whatever the activities of Dr. Frist might have been in 2002 or 2005, one of the investigatory proceedings set in motion by the aforementioned Autism General Order #1 was scheduled to take place in 2007. To make a much longer story more manageable, the 2007 Omnibus Autism Proceedings revolved around several key issues. First, the lawyers for the Department of Justice wanted to introduce a report by a Dr. Bustin which had been used by the British government to discredit a finding of the O'Leary labs that contained data indicating that autism and vaccines might be linked.

The petitioners wanted time to study the material which was to be introduced into evidence by the American federal government so that the former individuals would be in a position to put forth evidence that might rebut the Bustin report. Although the Special Master had the discretionary authority to allow the petitioners the time they requested for studying the Bustin document, but, for reasons that seem rather elusive, the Special Master refused the petitioners the time they needed to be able to study and critically reflect on a report which was to be placed into evidence.

Toward the latter stages of this particular Vaccine Court hearing, Dr. Bustin was called to testify in support of the report that he had written for the British government which critiqued evidence that had been presented by the O'Leary labs concerning another case involving Dr. Andy Wakefield's research indicating that there might be some sort of tie between a particular vaccine and the emergence of certain kinds of medical conditions. Because the plaintiffs had not been granted the time by the Special Masters that the former individuals needed to be able to properly study the Bustin report, they could not effectively counter what was in the report or Dr. Bustin's testimony concerning his own report.

Many observers believe that the Bustin report along with the doctor's testimony concerning his own report, together with the Court-forced inability of the plaintiffs to be able to counter such evidence effectively was a key turning point of the hearings. Although the Vaccine Court would not announce its decision for another year and a half, the fate of the plaintiffs had been sealed as a result of what transpired in conjunction with the report and testimony of Dr. Bustin – especially as a result of the decision of the Special Masters to not grant time to the plaintiffs to be able to mount a defense against the report so that the witness could be properly cross-examined.

Subsequently, the lawyers for the government also wanted to introduce into evidence the opinion of a Dr. Andrew Zimmerman who was a pediatric neurologist from Baltimore. Six weeks before the legal proceedings Of 2007 had begun Dr. Zimmerman had written a letter to government lawyers stating his opinion that he had found no connection between the vaccine that had been received by a young girl and the emergence of autism later on, and, in addition, Dr. Zimmerman felt that the autism that did emerge was due to genetic factors and not due to a vaccine.

Although Dr. Zimmerman's letter was introduced into evidence during the legal proceedings, Dr. Zimmerman was not called by the government lawyers to give testimony in support of that document.

Generally speaking, if the written opinion of an individual is entered into evidence, then, the person who wrote that opinion is called on to offer testimony to confirm and verify what has been written. If such an individual is not called on to testify, then, the written words can be considered to be a form of hearsay because it lacks the sorts of procedural foundations that are needed to show that the contents of the document are substantive and, therefore, are capable of being defended.

However, the special masters conducting the hearing permitted the letter to stand as evidence without requiring the person who had written that letter to give testimony. The Zimmerman document was subsequently used to discredit every claim seeking compensation for the occurrence of autism as a result of thimerosal having been present in a vaccine taken by the individual who became autistic.

Later on, after the Court proceedings were over, evidence was uncovered indicating that Dr. Zimmerman actually had reversed his earlier opinion in another petition case – which had been sealed – and in that sealed testimony he stated that he did believe there was a link between autism and the presence of thimerosal in a vaccine. Although the lawyers for the federal government knew about the second, reversed medical position, they kept that information from the Court even while they were using Dr. Zimmerman's first opinion to win their case.

The most likely reason why government lawyers didn't call Dr. Zimmerman to testify in their case is because he might have mentioned – and, perhaps, at some point, probably would have mentioned – how he actually did believe that autism could be caused by the presence of thimerosal in a vaccine. In other words, the government lawyers were willing to concede the loss of one case (Poling v. HHS) involving the reversed testimony of Dr. Zimmerman in order to ensure that such testimony would be sealed and, then, those same lawyers proceeded to use testimony which had been recanted during the sealed testimony in order to prosecute a case that would not be sealed but would be used as a template for making decisions through the Vaccine Court which would deny all future cases involving claims concerning a link between the presence of thimerosal in vaccines and autism.

However, as despicable as the actions of the government lawyers were in the foregoing matter, what is less apparent – but, perhaps, equally concerning – are the actions of the special masters with respect to that same case. Why did they permit a letter that was not backed up by in-person testimony to stand as evidence in the Hazlehurst v HHS trial -- especially given that the letter in question was later used as the evidential basis for denying thousands of petitions made in conjunction with the National Childhood Vaccine Injury Act?

Following the end of the Hazlehurst v. HHS hearing in 2007 but before the Special Masters reached their 2009 decisions concerning the three test cases involved in the Omnibus Autism Proceedings (which the Hazlehurst case was part of), the parents of Hannah Poling decided in early 2008 to file a motion which sought to unseal their case so that it could be discussed with the media because, among other things, evidence presented in their case demonstrated that there was a link between thimerosal in vaccines and the incidence of autism. The respondents and their overlords in the Department of Justice opposed the foregoing motion because whatever their rationalized legal arguments might have been, they didn't want the public to know how they had maneuvered to keep information from the public which indicated that there was link between thimerosal and autism.

A status conference -- involving a special master, the respondent (i.e., the federal government) and the plaintiff (the Poling family) – was convened to discuss the motion. On the basis of what transpired during that status conference, the motion which the Poling family had filed with the Vaccine Court was eventually denied, and, as a result, evidence put forth in the Poling case indicating that there was, indeed, a link between thimerosal and autisms continued to be officially buried ... although, obviously, the information did get leaked unofficially.

In early 2009, the special masters who had been assigned to oversee the three test cases involved in the Omnibus Autism Proceedings came down with their decisions. All of the decisions went against the plaintiffs who had been claiming that there was a causal link between thimerosal and autism.

In the Cedillo v. HHS decision, Special Master George Hastings stipulated that he had studied the evidence for many months and was convinced that while the family itself had acted in good faith, nonetheless, the Special Master believed that the doctors who had advised the Cedillo family concerning the possibility of a connection between the vaccination and a subsequent medical condition which emerged in Michelle Cedillo were not only in error but, in some way, those physicians had perpetrated acts of "gross medical misjudgment." Given that the Poling case – to which the Special Master did not have access -- entailed evidence that there was a link between vaccines and certain kinds of injuries, and given that the CDC had been covering up evidence for, by that time, seven years – to which the Special Master likely did not have access – that indicated how there was a link between vaccines and the emergence of certain medical conditions, one wonders what the nature of the evidence was that convinced the Special Master that not only had the physicians advising the Cedillo family been in error but they had been guilty of "gross medical misjudgment?"

While one cannot expect a Special Master to be able to come to a decision based on evidence to which he does not have access (e.g., the Poling case and the CDC cover-up concerning the link between vaccinations and autism), nonetheless, if an individual is going to tar the reputations of a number of physicians with the charge that they were guilty of "gross medical misjudgment), then, one might presume that such charges are going to be backed up by a detailed account concerning the nature of such misjudgment. Stating that one has studied the evidence for months and that one has become convinced that such is the case is not really an adequate response.

Isn't it possible that the physicians who were advising the Cedillo family had, in good faith, arrived at a conclusion that merely differed with the conclusion which had been reached by the Special Master? What was it about the perspective of the physicians who were advising the Cedillo family that, in the opinion of the Special Master, rendered the judgment on which the former perspective had been based to be something which involved "gross medical misjudgment?"

Why would the Special Master give more credence to, and consider to be more persuasive, one set of arguments rather than another? Would such judgments have anything to do with the philosophical lenses through which he was framing the evidence being given in the Cedillo case?

What does the Special Master actually know about pleiomorphism/pleomorphism, monomorphism, Pasteur, Béchamp, Enderlein, Rife, the Universal Microscope, Naessens, the Somatoscope, virology, microzymas, endobionts, somatids, microbiological life cycles, the microbiome, the biological terrain, immunology, junk DNA, evolution, epigenetics, resonance, frequency following behavior, structured water, field theory, quantum mechanics, entanglement, non-local dynamics, energy, or any of the other topics that might have a material relevance to the sorts of judgments he is making? Furthermore, if a given individual did know a lot about such issues and had learned to develop a truly independent opinion concerning those matters, I doubt very much that he or she would ever have been permitted to become a Special Master.

The Vaccine Court reminds me of the "legal" proceedings that were established in the story by Stephen Vincent Benét entitled "The Devil and Daniel Webster" in which a fictionalized version of Daniel Webster is induced to represent a farmer who has sold his (the farmer's) soul to the Devil in order to change the fortunes of his (the farmer's) community for a set period of time. Without in any way wishing to refer to various Secretaries for the Department of Health and Human Services, or to the members of the Department of Justice, or to the lawyers representing the DOJ before the Vaccine Court, as giving expression to the Devil, and without in any wishing to refer to the individuals who are appointed to be Special Masters as being like the ghostly denizens who are brought in to make up the jury in "The Devil and Daniel Webster" story, nonetheless, there is a distinct resonance between the way in which the HHS, the DOJ, and the Special Masters go about their business in the Vaccine Court and the way in which the Devil and his henchmen go about their business in the Stephen Vincent Benét story – namely, the game in both cases is rigged in favor of the biases, assumptions, theories, ideas, beliefs, values, and vested interests of the individuals who are overseeing what transpires in those two respective courts.

Just as the National Childhood Vaccine Injury Act added insult to injury when President Ford and Congress officially decided to grant indemnity to those who manufacture vaccines for children, even more monstrous forms of injury and insult were imposed on the American people when several pieces of legislation were introduced following 9/11. For example, the oxymoronically titled Patriot Act of 2001 could be considered a candidate for such monstrous legislation because it actually provides governmental tools through which patriots can be oppressed rather than be protected but, officially is known as: 'Uniting and Strengthening America By Providing Appropriate Tools Required to Intercept and Obstruct Terrorism Act of 2001' – although one should note in passing, the Act is devoid of tools for intercepting and obstructing acts of terrorism by the American government against its own people or against innocent people in other countries.

The 342-page Patriot Act was, supposedly: Written, introduced into Congress, debated, subjected to several votes, re-issued in 'compromised' form, helped along by a number of anthrax attacks containing weaponized materials known as the Ames strain because the origins of those materials had been traced to a government experimental lab in Iowa, and finally passed in to law approximately six weeks following the events of 9/11. The Act was minimally debated as it wormed its way through the catacombs of Congress, and, moreover, there is evidence to indicate that not only had most members of Congress read little, or anything at all, of the bill that became an Act which would adversely affect the lives of millions of American citizens, but, as well, there is evidence to indicate that a different version of the Act came into play in the early morning hours before members of Congress had assembled to take a final vote on something that, apparently, was other than they believed it to be.

In 2004, the Project Bioshield Act was signed into law by President George W. Bush. Among other things, the Act served as a method through which a lot of tax-payer money could be transferred to the pharmaceutical industry whenever there was a declared public emergency involving bioterrorism or bioterrorism-like events, and one of the ways in which pharmaceutical companies stood to reap a financial windfall was because the Act indicated that if no one purchased the materials produced by the pharmaceutical companies during such emergencies, then, the U.S. government would guarantee that it would become the buyer of last resort and purchase all of the unsold products that had been manufactured in response to some declared emergency concerning an alleged bioterrorism pronouncement.

Most unexpectedly – but not really – the pharmaceutical industry indicated that it was dissatisfied with the limited extent of the provisions that were present in the Project Bioshield Act. They not only wanted whatever money could be generated via that Act, but, as well, they wanted indemnity concerning product liability not just in conjunction with the sorts of protection that were afforded by the National Childhood Vaccine Injury Act in relation to babies, children, and teenagers, but they also wanted indemnity with respect to all pharmaceutical products that might be sold to adults, as well, during declared emergencies.

Several years were to pass before the foregoing idea was translated into governmental action. This took place at 11:20 P.M. on December 17, 2005 when Dr. William Frist -- whose family owned the largest hospital-related business in America and who was a Senator from Tennessee (who, as previously noted, had been said to have been involved in surreptitiously altering the 2002 Homeland Security Act so that it would include provisions that would prevent people from suing vaccine makers for product liability independently of the jurisdiction of the aforementioned Vaccine Court), walked over to the chambers for the U.S. House of Representatives where pretty nearly everyone had left for the day after authorizing the 2006 Defense Appropriations bill, and handed the Speaker of the House a 40-plus page addendum to the Defense Appropriation bill that was to be referred to as "Division E" but which had not been read by, or voted on, by members of the House.

The PREP Act – or, Division E -- is short-hand for the "Pubic Readiness and Emergency Preparedness' Act. This Act indicates that the Secretary of Health and Human Services has the authority to declare emergencies concerning whatever the Secretary deems to be a threat to public health, and, as well, the Act specifies that anyone who produces or supplies what are considered to be covered countermeasures (involving pharmaceuticals, vaccines, technological mechanisms, and software) in response to such declared emergencies cannot be held liable for whatever part they might play in "the development, manufacture, testing, distribution, or administration" of the foregoing sorts of products (except in cases of willful misconduct that have been acknowledged to be such by the Attorney General of the United States). Under the provisions of the foregoing Act, no matter how experimental and untested a given product might be and irrespective of whether, or not, people died or were severely injured or became seriously ill as a result of using, or being given, such covered countermeasures, then, as long as there was no action involved in products which the U.S. Attorney General was willing to officially acknowledge as giving expression to an act of willful misconduct with respect to such covered countermeasures, then, there was – and is -- complete indemnity concerning product liability.

On December 22, 2005, David Obey -- a 36-year member of Congress from Wisconsin who was the ranking member of the House Appropriations Committee -- made a statement on the floor of the House attesting to the fact that Senator William Frist had made arrangements with the Speaker of the House (Dennis Hastert) to attach a 40 page addendum (which no one in the House had read or voted on) to the Defense Appropriations Bill for 2006, and the addendum was to be referred to as "Section E". Representative Obey indicated that the aforementioned 40 page addendum – which he held in his hand and referred to as he gave his statement -- was entirely directed toward providing an across-the-board sort of product liability for an array of pharmaceutical goods.

When Congress re-convened after the Christmas break, the foregoing issue went dark. In other words, no one followed up on Obey's December 22, 2005 statement from the floor of the House, and this included the individual who made the official statement.

One can only wonder why someone might go to the trouble of making sure that a statement alleging Congressional misconduct – which named names – would be given from the floor of the House so that, among other things, it might be included in the Congressional Record and, then, that individual would do nothing more to further his original effort. Of course, under such mysterious circumstances, one might be willing to entertain the possibility that either he and/or his family might have been threatened in some way if he were to have pursued the matter any further.

Almost one hundred years prior (1905) to the PREP Act (2005), the Supreme Court of the United States upheld a decision of the Supreme Court of Massachusetts which, previously, had ruled that a Board of Health located in Cambridge Massachusetts had the right to fine any person within its jurisdiction who did not comply with the directive of that Board to be vaccinated for smallpox. The foregoing judgment was rendered in Jacobson v. Massachusetts.

Some of the details leading up to the foregoing legal case are as follows. In 1902, there had been an outbreak of smallpox in Cambridge, and based on a Massachusetts state statute that empowered local boards of health to take measures that, when necessary, would enhance public safety, the board of health in Cambridge issued an edict which indicated that anyone who failed to be vaccinated against smallpox would – per the provisions of the state statute – have to pay a fine of $5.00, a not inconsiderable amount of money at the time.

The state statute governing the issue did not indicate that such vaccinations were mandatory, but, apparently, it indicated only that failure to comply with the statute would result in a fine being levied against the individual who refused to comply with state law. There is also some ambiguity surrounding the foregoing state statute about what would happen if a given individual continued to resist being vaccinated after paying the initial fine ... in other words, could they be fined again.

Henning Jacobson, who was the father of a boy, had refused to comply with the Cambridge board of health's edict concerning the issue of vaccination. Mr. Jacobson told local authorities that both he and his son had experienced some adverse reactions during previous encounters with the vaccination process.

The Massachusetts Supreme Court was of the opinion that the issue before it was not really a matter of whether, or not, someone became vaccinated. The Court indicated that the existing statute did not authorize mandatory vaccinations but, rather, only authorized the imposing of a fine for non-compliance, and, therefore, the fact that Mr. Jacobson and his son had experienced adverse effects in conjunction with previous instances of vaccination was irrelevant to the issue.

However, if the original state statute indicated that only a fine could be levied for non-compliance with an official edict concerning vaccination, then, one wonders why such a statute would specify that boards of health were authorized to require vaccinations "when necessary for public health and safety." How does a fine promote health and safety if a vaccination is considered to be "necessary" for enhancing – presumably -- public health and safety?

If one could substitute a fine for a vaccination, then, one might wish to question how 'necessary' a given vaccination actually might be with respect to the issue of public health and safety. Moreover, if public health and safety are the primary focus of a given statute, then, why aren't the adverse reactions of recipients of vaccinations also a relevant issue since such reactions are threats to public health and safety as well?

Jacobson appealed the decision of the Massachusetts Supreme Court to the Supreme Court. As noted earlier, the latter Court upheld the decision of the Massachusetts Supreme Court.

Apparently, many people were, and are, of the opinion (perhaps including the members of the 1905 U.S. Supreme Court) that, supposedly, the Constitution clearly indicates (presumably, via the 10th Amendment) that whatever has not been delegated to the federal government by that document, nor prohibited to the state governments by that same document falls within the purview of the sovereign authority of states. Maybe such issues are not as cut and dried as some seem to want to suppose is the case.

Rather curiously, many people read through the Bill of Rights and, somehow, come to the conclusion that the issue of sovereignty is an either-or sort of issue between states and the federal government. More specifically, such people seem to believe that whatever powers are itemized in the Constitution as belonging to the federal government fall outside of the authority of state governments, while everything else – as long as the Constitution does not prohibit such considerations to the states – falls within the power and authority of state governments.

How anyone can read through the first nine amendments – which are entirely directed toward the rights of individuals and which place limits on what governments can do with respect to those rights – and, then, conclude that the tenth amendment is all about state's rights has not only been failing to pay attention to what has been taking place in the first nine amendments of the Bill of Rights, but, as well, apparently such individuals can't read. The tenth amendment does not divvy up powers between the federal government and the states, but, rather, divvies up the power among the federal government, the state governments, and the people.

Roger Sherman added the words "or to the people" to the Tenth Amendment. Those words were accepted without comment or debate.

If the federal government and the state governments were the only two realms of sovereignty that were of Constitutional importance, then, there would have been no need for Roger Sherman to add the foregoing words that he did to the Tenth Amendment. The issue of individual rights – and not necessarily state's rights -- came up again and again during many of the Ratification conventions that had been convened to discuss, debate, and vote on whether, or not, to accept the 1787 Philadelphia constitutional document, and the people who were bringing up the issue of rights were representing their local communities and not the states in which those communities were located.

Furthermore, to add weight to the foregoing considerations, the Ninth Amendment specified that "the enumeration in the Constitution, of certain rights, shall not be construed to deny or disparage others retained by the people" … not retained by the states, but "retained by the people." Since powers concerning public health and safety had not been specifically assigned to the federal government by the Constitution, nor forbidden to the states, then, such powers belong to the states and the people.

Consequently, if a state seeks to exercise power over individuals with respect to, say, issues of health and safety, then, according to the Ninth Amendment, such a state must avoid denying and disparaging the unenumerated rights of the people which include issues of health and safety since those kinds of rights have not been delegated specifically to the federal government nor prohibited to the states, and, therefore, also have not been prohibited to the people.

Does a state have the authority to indicate what the boards of health in local communities can and can't do? Not necessarily, because the issue has not, yet, been settled as to what might constitute the unenumerated rights of the people which the state could be denying or disparaging through its statutes.

Similarly, does a local board of health have the authority to determine what individuals can and can't do? Not necessarily, because the issue has not, yet, been settled as to what might constitute the unenumerated rights of the people which a given board of health might be denying or disparaging through its edicts.

Does the United States Supreme Court have the authority to indicate what states can and cannot do with respect to the unenumerated rights of individuals? No, it doesn't, because to claim that it does have such authority would, potentially, constitute a form of denying and disparaging the unenumerated rights that are assigned to individuals within those states under the provisions of the Ninth and Tenth amendments.

In fact, the United States Supreme Court should not even have legal standing in those sorts of matters. More specifically, anything that it seeks to establish in such cases would constitute, potentially, a form of denying and disparaging the unenumerated rights of individuals, and, therefore, the most appropriate action the Supreme Court might take in those cases would be to recuse itself or recommend that the matter be delegated to some independent mediating agent (a lesser court of some kind) in which the federal government would help individuals and states to come to workable ways of resolving certain kinds of conflicts involving the sovereignty of individuals and the sovereignty of states.

The sovereignty of the federal government, the states, and individuals are all limited in nature. None of their modalities of sovereignty are absolute and all encompassing, and both the devil and Divinity are in the details of how one goes about getting those different kinds of sovereignty to constructively – and not destructively -- work with one another.

Justice John Marshall used the term "police powers" to refer to the alleged right of states to pass laws that, supposedly, were intended to establish conditions which were believed to be conducive to the realization of such things as peace, education, health, morals, and so-called good order. However, when Justice Marshall refers to police powers in the manner that he does, he actually seems to be violating the provisions of the Constitution.

By claiming that states had the sort of authority known as "police powers" which could impose on its citizens various kinds policies and programs, he was engaged in a process that appears to be denying and disparaging various, possible, unenumerated rights of the people. "We the People" are sovereign individuals and, therefore, individuals who should not be treated merely as forms of state-owned chattel that the state could do with as it wished.

Issues of 'peace, education, health, morals, and so-called good order' all cut across issues that, on the one hand, constitute forms of unenumerated rights which neither the federal nor state governments can automatically deny or decry, and, simultaneously, on the other hand, such issues also touch upon, if not imply or entail, an array of principles that tend to be woven into religious frameworks about which the federal Congress can make no laws respecting or establishing those principles nor prohibiting the free exercise thereof. Moreover, both the Ninth and Tenth amendments indicate that the absence of federal authority in such matters does not automatically give states the right to jump into the breach and dictate what individuals can and cannot do with respect to giving expression to processes of peace, education, health, morals, and/or good order.

There is a need for some organized form of 'give and take' concerning boundary disputes in which the sovereignty of states clashes with the sovereignty of individuals (more on this a little later). Historically, states have often tended to deny the legitimacy of such boundary disputes concerning conflicting issues of sovereignty involving individuals and the states, and, historically, the federal government has often let the states get away with denying and decrying the unenumerated rights and reserved powers of the people, but whenever the federal government has permitted this to take place, the federal government has failed to live up to the Constitutional guarantee of providing the states with a republican form of government that protects the provisions of, among other things, the Ninth and Tenth amendments.

The Bill of Rights – including the Tenth Amendment -- is about the rights of individuals, not just the rights of states. Under the provisions of the Constitution, the sovereign authority to establish programs concerning peace, education, health, morals, and good order belongs to the people and not just to the states, and, therefore, responsibility for working out co-operative ways of addressing those kinds of issues in a manner that protects and enhances the health and safety of individuals, as well as the collective, will be incumbent on individuals as well as both state and federal forms of governance.

As indicated earlier, historically, states usually have sought to usurp the sovereignty that has been afforded to the people via the Bill of Rights and, as a result, states have sought to claim authority for determining how to pursue peace, education, health, morals, and good order. However, contrary to the opinion of many individuals, the 1787 Philadelphia constitution was never about giving priority to the idea that the majority should rule.

In fact, one of the primary driving forces of people, such as Madison, for wanting to formulate a new modality of governance had to do with their revulsion concerning the sort of mob rule that often seemed to be dominating the dynamics of governance not only on the state level but on the national level as well, and, in the process, mob rule was threatening what individuals such as Madison believed were their personal, sovereign rights. Democracy wouldn't let Madison and the other "framers" of the constitution do what they wanted to do, and, consequently, they sought to establish a republican form of government in which certain principles would place limits on how the majority might intervene in the lives of individuals and in the dynamics of governance.

Returning to the Jacobson case, neither the Massachusetts state government nor the Cambridge Board of Health knew: What smallpox was; what caused it; what would prevent it, or what might cure it. They knew that people who exhibited the symptoms associated with smallpox often became very ill and often died.

When Justice Harland provided an overview in his judicial opinion concerning what he believed was true with respect to the issue of smallpox, he was wrong in almost every detail. More specifically, if one did not cherry pick the data as Justice Harland had in his decision, the evidence available at the beginning of the twentieth century concerning the smallpox vaccination did not actually indicate that the vaccination was either safe or effective.

For example, there were many people who had not been vaccinated but, nevertheless, did not get sick and die. In addition, considerable data existed indicating that there were many people who had been vaccinated but, nonetheless, they did become sick and died, and, as well, there also was a certain amount of evidence to indicate that people who had received the vaccination actually brought smallpox into communities which, previously, had not experienced those kinds of outbreaks.

Finally, there was the experience of places such as Leicester, England. For decades, the people in that city had discontinued all forms of vaccination in conjunction with smallpox and, yet, the incidence of both outbreaks and deaths had dropped precipitously.

In 1902 – as well as later on -- the Massachusetts state government could not put forth a credible case which demonstrated that the best way to protect the health and safety of the public would be by way of a program of vaccination. Moreover, even if the state authorities could have put forth such an argument, there was still the issue of whether fining Mr. Jacobson for not complying with the vaccination program was, on the one hand, a form of denying and decrying his unenumerated rights under the Ninth Amendment as well as, on the other hand, a form of undermining powers of sovereignty that had been reserved to him – as one of the individuals to whom Roger Sherman's added words "or the people" alluded – under the Tenth Amendment.

When someone wishes to make foxes the guardians of a hen house, then, the hens will be confronted with possibilities that are both problematic and, often, deadly. When certain individuals who have vested interests wish to make the federal and state governments guardians of what constitutes a process of denying and decrying the rights of individuals under the Ninth Amendment, or, alternatively, such individuals wish to make federal and state governments guardians of what the natures of the sovereign powers are that have been reserved for the people under the Tenth Amendment, then the people – both individually and collectively -- are likely to become entangled in a network of deadly and debilitating possibilities such as happened in the 1976 swine flu vaccination fiasco, or the 1986 National Childhood Vaccine Injury Act, or the Bio Act of 2002 or the PREP Act of 2005-2006.

None of the foregoing considerations is intended to soft-pedal the very real problem which remains. That is, on the one hand, how can the rights and powers that constitute the sovereignty which has been reserved for the people as individuals, and, therefore, which cannot be denied or decried, be reconciled with, on the other hand, the rights and powers that constitute the sovereignty of state forms of governance which are acknowledged by the Constitution because such rights and powers have not been assigned to the federal government nor prohibited to the states (or the people)?

Those individuals that like to speak in terms of "liberty" and "freedom" as being the primary principles of a republic do not appear to have been able to successfully resolve the conundrum which arises when one's person modality of freedom and liberty chafes against the manner in which another person pursues a different conception of freedom and liberty. If one person is a socialist and another person is a capitalist, do those individuals not realize that there are likely to be conflicts and tensions – possibly irreconcilable ones – that are generated through the manner in which their respective notions of freedoms and liberties engage one another?

Not all libertarians, socialists, capitalists, liberals, conservatives, independents, atheists, or religious proponents will define or seek to realize the notions of "liberty" and "freedom" in the same way. So, what does one do when one kind of a seemingly immovable object meets another kind of apparently immovable object?

The traditional way, for better or worse, has been to have some source of authority (king, governor, ruler, sovereign, judge, priest, imam, rabbi, guru,) resolve the issue for us. However, if we – the people – are the ones who are sovereign, then, how do we go about interacting with one another in ways that will only minimally (a very slippery term) deny or decry our respective rights or interfere with the respective powers that have been reserved for people -- as individuals as well as collectively?

The Supreme Court of the United States does not appear to have any constitutional standing in the foregoing issues because almost any decision it makes in such a context is likely to result in denying or decrying someone's unenumerated rights or is likely to result in undermining the powers that have not have assigned to the federal government or prohibited to the states but, instead have been reserved for the states or the people. On the other hand, the federal government does appear to have a moral and constitutional responsibility under Article IV, section 4 to ensure that the states are provided with a republican form of government, and part of carrying out such a responsibility is to ensure that the states are not denying or decrying the unenumerated rights and reserved powers of the people ... rights and powers which exist quite independently of whatever powers have been reserved for the states after one removes those powers which have been specifically assigned to the federal government or which have been forbidden to the states.

Moreover, state governments do not have preeminent authority over the issue of individual sovereignty. If states were to try to claim the foregoing kind of authority, then, the exercise of that authority would almost invariably involve denying or decrying the unenumerated rights of the people as individuals, as well as interfere with the sovereign powers that have been reserved for the people and not just the states ... and, in a sense, such authority has been forbidden to the states (in a, yet-to-be-determined way) under the Ninth and Tenth amendments

Various justices of the Supreme Court have confirmed that while the Constitution protects individual liberties, nonetheless, liberties are not an absolute right. Consequently, according to those jurists, there are times that a duty of care exists for which people – as individuals and as part of a collective – have a responsibility to go about establishing reasonable forms of constraint and restraint on the actions of people – both as individuals and as a collective – in order to promote or protect the health and safety of the people, both as individuals and as part of a collective.

The problem is that, over the last several hundred years, various justices have had different ideas about the notion of what constitutes reasonable forms of constraint and restraint that can be placed on the people, whether considered as individuals or as part of a collective. Law books are filled with decisions and precedents which give expression to the opinions of jurists who – in voicing such decisions -- frequently seem to be actively engaged in the process of denying and decrying the unenumerated rights of the people, as well as interfering with the powers that have been reserved for the people, both individually and collectively.

In the 1905 Jacobson decision, the Supreme Court of the United States indicated that the local board of health was qualified to make decisions concerning public health and safety. In what sense was the local board of health qualified to make such a decision?

To be sure, in order to be elected to, or appointed to, such a board, individuals are likely to have gone through some set of a vetting dynamic that, at least in the eyes of some individuals (often with vested interests), supposedly will render the people who are elected or appointed as being qualified to make certain kinds of decisions. To what extent, and in what ways, will the decisions of such allegedly qualified people deny and decry the unenumerated rights of people who have gone about life and become qualified in ways that are at odds with the modes of qualification through which board of health members might have gone?

Isn't it arbitrary – and, perhaps, even unreasonable, if not oppressive -- to automatically suppose that the qualifications of the members of a board of health are necessarily better and, in some way, superior to the qualifications of someone who is not a member of such a board of health? What is the metric that is to be used to decide between the two kinds of qualification, and irrespective of which metric one selects for deciding those issues, how does one reconcile the use of such a metric with the potential for denying or decrying the unenumerated rights of the people, considered both as individuals and as part of a collective?

In the Jacobson case, the Supreme Court stipulated that state legislatures had the prerogative to decide how to deal with issues such as epidemics as long as the manner in which they did so was not oppressive, arbitrary, or unreasonable. However, reasonable questions can be raised about the extent to which the statutes that are passed by state legislative bodies might be arbitrary, oppressive, or unreasonable in various ways, and, therefore, one had a reasonable right to be concerned about the implications which the foregoing sorts of questions pose with respect to the potential of state legislatures to actively be engaged in denying and decrying the unenumerated rights of the people to determine their (the people's) own way for engaging the challenges associated with the outbreak of smallpox?

The Supreme Court of the United States indicated that the Massachusetts state legislature had proceeded on the basis of a theory which considered vaccination to be the best, and most effective, way to counter the potential threat of a smallpox outbreak that imperiled an entire population. However, the theory on which the Massachusetts based its legislation not only could not necessarily be shown to constitute the best and most effective way to counter a possible epidemic, but, as well, such a theory directly contravenes – and, therefore, denies and decries -- the unenumerated right of Mr. Jacobson to engage the smallpox situation in a different way. Consequently, given that however deadly a smallpox outbreak might be, no population has ever been wiped out, then, one cannot necessarily say that the presence of smallpox imperils an entire population, and, as a result, the Supreme Court of the United States has offered no metric which would identify the state's theory of smallpox to be superior to Mr. Jacobson's theory of smallpox, and, consequently, the Court – contrary to the principles which it cited as being central to how governments need to conduct themselves -- was being unreasonable, arbitrary, and oppressive in the Jacobson decision.

In the opening sentences of the Supreme Court's decision in the Jacobson case, references are made to the idea that one cannot cite the Preamble to the Constitution as constituting a credible counter to the authority of states to issue statutes which oppose the inclination of individuals – taken singly or collectively -- to attempt to realize some generalized form of justice, tranquility, welfare, defense, or liberty. Justice Harlan, who wrote the majority decision, indicates that the Preamble does not confer any substantive power upon government, and in order for government to be able to act, the powers on which it draws must be specified within the Constitution or be implied by such specific powers.

By giving expression to the foregoing sort of perspective, Justice Harlan, as well as those who concurred with him, seem to have forgotten that the Ninth and Tenth amendments actually authorize the people – considered both individually and collectively – to bring the Preamble to life. Justice, tranquility, welfare, defense and liberty all are implied by the unenumerated rights of, and powers that have been reserved for, the people under, respectively, the Ninth and Tenth amendments.

The Preamble does not begin with: "We the government" but, instead, begins with "We the people." According to the Preamble, the Constitution exists to enable the people, and not government, to "form a more perfect union.

While the federal and state governments have their roles to play in bringing about such a more perfect union, that task does not belong to just government. Ultimately, the challenge to form a more perfect union belongs to us all, and what Justice Harlan is seeking to do appears to be a form of "bait and switch" in which people – right from the very beginning -- are induced to believe that the Constitution is about certain possibilities – namely, justice, tranquility, defense, welfare, and liberty (goals and purposes to which everyone aspires) – but, then, he does an about face and proceeds to stipulate that such words are ghostly, and not substantive, and, therefore, can be ignored, just as so many jurists (including Justice Harlan) attempt to deny and disparage the unenumerated rights of the Ninth amendment and the reserved powers to which the Tenth Amendment alludes.

Justice Harlan, then, goes on to refer to an observation of Chief Justice Marshall that the spirit of an instrument – such as the Constitution – needs to be respected as much as the letter of that instrument. However, he proceeds to abrogate the aforementioned observation of Chief Justice Marshall by claiming that in the Jacobson case there is no need to look at anything except the "plain, obvious meanings of the Constitution" which he claims "must control" the Court's decision.

The author of the majority opinion in the Jacobson case does not say what the spirit of the Constitution is, and he does not put forth arguments which explain why certain words should relegate such a spirit to irrelevance, and he does not explain why certain words in the Constitution "must control" the decision. In fact, he does not actually identify the precise words in the Constitution which he believes "must control" what is decided or why all of the other words of the Constitution might not have certain kinds of modulating or controlling influences as well.

Justice Harlan talks about "experts" and he talks about "common knowledge" during his decision in the Jacobson case. Furthermore, without going into any detail, he dismisses the arguments that were put forth by those who were representing Mr. Jacobson because, in effect, those sorts of ideas clash with, and differ from, the opinion of those individuals who Justice Harland considers to be experts and who operate out of the sort of "knowledge" that Justice Harland is prepared to recognize as being knowledge.

References are made by Justice Harlan concerning what he believes to have been established medical knowledge for nearly a century concerning the issue of vaccination. All one can do is cringe at the epistemological shallowness that is being displayed by Justice Harlan in his comments concerning so-called "experts" and what constitutes "common knowledge " because, clearly, he doesn't know as much as he, apparently, thinks he does.

He indicates that because courts, legislatures, and the medical profession have, for quite some time, operated out of a consensus concerning such matters as vaccination, then, even if Mr. Jacobson had brought in his own expert witnesses on the matter, nonetheless, that kind of testimony would not have mattered. In other words, the understandings of those who wield power already were formed on the issue of vaccination, and, therefore, legislatures are within their rights to pass statutes that are based on understandings which might not be correct but must be accepted because such understanding is consonant with the people who are recognized by the system as being experts and who are responsible for determining what constitutes knowledge – common or otherwise -- and, this amounts to being nothing more than a circular argument which has not been independently corroborated.

In his legal opinion, Justice Harlan mentions that States do not give up their police powers simply because they have become members of a constitutional union. Yet, unfortunately, Justice Harland does not appear to take into consideration the idea that people – as individuals - - should not be expected to give up their sovereignty merely because they become members within a constitutional union.

He goes on to stipulate that while the Court has made no attempt to define the limits of the police powers of the state, nevertheless, he indicates that the court does acknowledge the right of the State to pass statutes involving health provisions of every kind, including those that pertain to the issue of quarantine. At this point, he qualifies his remarks by indicating that the State must go about the business of protecting public safety and health through reasonable means, and, as well, he maintains that however a given State decides to proceed in the formulating and enforcement of its police powers, it cannot do so in a way that will interfere with what transpires in other states, nor can it do so in a way that would cause such legislation to come into conflict with the operations to which the General Government is entitled under the provisions of the Constitution.

Justice Harlan talks about the rights of States and he talks about the rights of the federal government. However, he does not talk about the unenumerated rights of the people that cannot be denied or decried under the Ninth Amendment, nor does he explore the powers that are reserved to the people – and not just the states -- under the Tenth Amendment.

Instead, Justice Harlan dismisses the perspective of Mr. Jacobson out of hand because it is not consonant with what the State and the Court have accepted as constituting expertise and knowledge. As a result, the most important issues before the Court – namely, what constitutes 'expertise', 'knowledge', and how does one reconcile matters of expertise and knowledge with the unenumerated rights and reserved powers which, constitutionally, have been delegated to the people – are never critically examined.

The author of the majority opinion in the Jacobson case maintains that governments have been instituted to seek and secure the prosperity, protection, happiness, safety, and common good of the people rather than to promote the interests of any one human being.

Furthermore, he claims that the legislature has the authority to determine what might be entailed by the foregoing notions of prosperity, protection, happiness, safety, and common good.

Nowhere in the Constitution are governments authorized to seek and secure the prosperity, protection, happiness, safety, and common good of the people. Nowhere in the Constitution are legislatures identified as bodies that have the sole right to determine what is entailed by those ideas.

The Constitution gives expression to a set of provisions that is intended to assist "We the People" to form a more perfect union through the establishment of justice, tranquility, defense, welfare, and liberty. The method set forth in the unamended Constitution that, supposedly, was intended to assist people to realize their respective aspirations comes in the form of a guarantee – namely, Article IV, section 4 which states: "The United States shall guarantee to every state in this union a republican form of government ...."

Republicanism is not just a matter of having a tri-partite form of government in which each of the branches has been provided with certain rights and powers that are different from one another, but, in some mysterious fashion, are considered to be equal to each other. Republicanism is a moral philosophy that became popular during the Enlightenment period – a period that overlaps with the American Revolution as well as with the writing, discussing, and ratifying of an amended Constitution.

Republicanism requires the members of the three branches of government to adhere to a set of moral principles. Those principles require them to be: Objective, non-partisan, honest, independent, dis-interested in seeking personal gain, noble, unbiased, self-sacrificing, courageous, honorable, sincere, compassionate, critically reflective, virtuous, and opposed to serving as judges in their own causes.

In other words, the Constitution does not tell people what to do. It does tell them how they are to go about doing whatever they do.

The opinion that Justice Harlan is issuing in the Jacobson case is not: Objective, non-partisan, independent, unbiased, courageous, honorable, or critically reflective, and, therefore, it stands in violation of the requirements of the guarantee clause concerning the responsibility of individuals in government to provide a republican form of government to the states. Furthermore, one might note in passing that Article IV, section 4 does not indicate that a republican form of government is guaranteed to the governments of different states, but, rather, the guarantee is to states as bodies of "We the People."

Justice Harlan adds insult to injury with respect to the way in which he violates the constitutional guarantee of republicanism because he is seeking to serve as a judge in his own cause – something that is antithetical to the idea of republicanism. He is serving as a judge in his own cause by putting forth a decision that gives expression to his beliefs about what constitutes: Expertise, knowledge, medical opinion, common understanding, the nature of the Preamble, vaccinations, the pre-eminence of the letter of the law over the spirit of the law, and the right of legislatures to decided what constitutes the nature of public health, public safety, and the common good.

As an individual, Justice Harlan is entitled to believe in whatever he likes. However, as a member of the federal government, he is not entitled to seek to impose his beliefs on to other people – such as Mr. Jacobson and his child – because by doing so he is serving as a judge in his own cause.

If someone should object to the foregoing point and say words to the effect of: 'how would judges ever be able to decide matters if they are not permitted to act on what they believe,' one might respond by indicating that, perhaps, judges should seek some other way of going about their business because their current way of doing things not only enables them to serve as judges in their own causes by imposing their beliefs onto other people, but, as well, often induces them to take part in activities that deny and decry the unenumerated rights of the people as well as ignores the powers that have been reserved to "we the people" quite independently of the federal government and the state governments.

In addition, judging matters after the fact – as the Supreme Court system tends to do – seems to be an ill-advised kind of idea. Why not try to resolve problems of governance before they are dumped onto the people rather than only after the dogs of legislative wars have been released into the public to perpetrate whatever rabid forms of financial, environmental, political, legal, technological, social, martial, scientific, medical, educational, or spiritual damage such legislation often tends to inflict on the public?

Congress has been forbidden to make any law that either establishes religion or prohibits the free exercise thereof. Yet, pretty much everything that Congress does is an exercise in establishing or prohibiting religious activities of some kind.

After all, religion does not have to be about submitting to God or a Supreme Deity, but, rather, religion also can be about how an individual goes about submitting to one's understanding of the relationship one has with whatever one considers reality to be. A person's sense of the sacred comes out of such an understanding. An individual's sense of duty is a function of that kind of an understanding. The metrics one uses to evaluate experience reflects such an understanding.

Therefore, in light of the foregoing considerations, what are members of Congress engaged in doing when they pass most instruments of legislation? Are they going to pass legislation that doesn't speak to their values and beliefs or which doesn't reflect their sense of the sacred or which fails to acknowledge their ideas about the sorts of duties of care that give expression to what they believe constitutes a framework of legality?

However, there is a difference between, on the one hand, a group of people reaching a common conclusion based on investigatory research that is: Unbiased, non-partisan, objective, fair, honest, sincere, noble, honorable, and self-sacrificing, and, on the other hand, a group of people who democratically vote for a given conclusion without having gone through a rigorous process that is: Unbiased, non-partisan, objective, fair, honest, sincere, noble, honorable and self-sacrificing. Consequently, the duty of care that must govern those who govern is to provide a form of government which is based on principles of republican morality that are independent of one's likes and dislikes or religious beliefs.

Maybe, the job of Supreme Court jurists should not be a matter of making judgments about whether some given action of government is consonant with someone's arbitrary notion concerning the alleged meaning of the Constitution. Perhaps, such jurists should be the guardians of Article IV, section 4 and, thereby, ensure that everybody in government is operating in accordance with the moral principles of republican government ... indeed, ensuring that members of Congress are complying with the principles of republican morality prior to making legislation official rather than waiting until after such legislation has been passed and already let loose upon society with potentially damaging consequences.

Perhaps, the test of the constitutionality of a law is whether, or not, that law conforms to principles of republican morality. Maybe, constitutionality is not a function of all the hermeneutical dancing and posturing that takes place in the current legal system and which tends to lead to whatever arbitrary, conflicting, inconsistent precedents that might issue forth from those sorts of dynamics.

When what is considered legal is required to give expression to conditions of republican morality such as being: Objective, honest, honorable, unbiased, non-partisan, sincere, self-sacrificing, noble, compassionate, and independent, then differentiating between what is legal and what is illegal tends to become fairly clear and relatively transparent. When what is considered legal requires one to trace a lot of theoretical ideas through an arbitrary network of precedents and decisions that are often devoid of qualities of republican character, then, what is meant by the idea of law becomes a lot more convoluted, murky, and likely to serve vested interests or the way of power.

The way of power loves to entangle people in webs of case law because such laws lend themselves to endless rounds of disputation, uncertainty, confusion, hermeneutical cleverness, manipulative tactics, and ambiguous decisions. The way of sovereignty encourages people to find and use constructive methods for pushing back the horizons of ignorance concerning one's quest to discover the truth about the nature of one's relationship with reality.

Sovereignty has to do with uncovering one's essential nature. The way of power does everything it can to undermine such a quest.

Sovereignty has nothing to do with trying to impose one's ideas on other people. The way of power cannot survive unless it seeks to impose its ideas on other people.

Sovereignty is about establishing a dynamic balance between the principles of: "neither control, nor be controlled" in order to establish the degrees of freedom that are needed to work toward realizing one's essential potential. The way of power is about seeking to maximize the ways in which one can effectively circumscribe the lives of others, while minimizing the ways that the "other" can problematically affect one's attempt to circumscribe the lives of others.

Maybe constitutionality is simply a matter of whether, or not, the legislative branch, the executive branch, and the judicial branch are attempting to carry out their duties of office in an: Honorable, unbiased, non-partisan, compassionate, disinterested, virtuous, noble, and objective manner. Maybe constitutionality is simply a matter of whether, or not, government officials refrain from serving as judges in their own causes and, in the process, enacting a form of governance which will assist "We the People" to establish justice, tranquility, defense, the common good, and liberty by enabling the people to develop their unenumerated rights and reserved powers in a manner that will help the latter individuals to realize the aspirations that are set forth in the Preamble and the amended Constitution.

It is not up to Justice Harlan – or those who concurred with his opinion -- to figure out what was, or should have been, meant by the 1780 provision of the Massachusetts constitution in which "the whole people covenants with each citizen, and each citizen with the whole people" for the common good. Moreover, notwithstanding the possibility that a government might have been instituted for purposes of establishing: Protection, happiness, safety, prosperity and the common good, nevertheless, governments often fail with respect to such intentions of institution government, and, therefore, perhaps Mr. Jacobson and his child should not be held hostage to a situation in which good intentions might have turned problematic ... a possibility that Justice Harlan does not ever seriously investigate or critically reflect upon.

According to Justice Harland – quoting approvingly from a recently decided case known as 'Viemeister v. White, President &c' –

"A common belief, like common knowledge, does not require evidence to establish its existence, but may be acted upon without proof by the legislature and courts .... The fact the belief is not universal is not controlling, for there is scarcely any belief that is accepted by everyone. The possibility that the belief may be wrong and that science may yet show it to be wrong, is not conclusive, for the legislature has the right to pass laws which, according to the common belief of the people, are adapted to prevent the spread of contagious diseases ... for what the people believe is for the common welfare must be accepted as tending to promote the common welfare, whether it does in fact or not. Any other basis would conflict with the spirit of the Constitution, and would sanction measures opposed to a republican form of government."

The foregoing quotation is filled with a series of claims. Absolutely no evidence has been cited, or arguments developed, within the context of such claims, or introduced separately by Justice Harland, to indicate that any of those claims actually are consonant with the 'spirit of the Constitution' (which has been left unspecified) or are consonant with a 'republican form of government' (which also has been left unspecified).

The foregoing words which are cited by Justice Harland do nothing to "prevent the spread of contagious diseases" that are even more devastating and lethal than smallpox. More specifically, those quoted words do nothing to stop the contagious spread of willful blindness, ignorance, and arrogance to which they give expression.

Republican government is not about the notion that the majority rules. To speak about a democratic form of republican government is oxymoronic.

Justice Harland does not seem to be interested in helping "We the people" to discover truths that will enable them – both individually and collectively -- to seek real forms of well-being though which, for example, the biological terrain of a human being can be maintained in, or be shown ways to recover, a condition of symbiotic stability with the microbiome that occupies it. Apparently, Justice Harland could have cared less whether the people who are in charge of a state or community are delusional, as long as, in good faith (whatever that might mean) they are prepared to operate in accordance with narratives that are not tenable.

Instead, he seems to be more interested in identifying the sources of control that can be used to place untenable, and, therefore, oppressive, 'police power' limits on how people can go about seeking and trying to live in accordance with principles that are capable of constructively serving their well-being rather than problematically serving the interests of someone's arbitrary notion of the public good. If Justice Harland were correct about the way that governance ought to work, the American Revolution would never have taken place because everyone would have agreed that as long as someone is in power, what such people believe or do doesn't matter as long as it is considered to give expression to "common knowledge" and done in good faith.

Republican government is rooted in principles of republican morality. If one jettisons the latter, the former cannot exist.

A member of a republican form of government – which is what a U.S. Supreme Court Justice is – cannot endorse a majority-rules-democratically-oriented-approach to state government without denying and decrying the unenumerated rights and reserved powers of the people who live in such a state. Since the guarantee of a republican form of government is specifically directed to states and not to the governments of those states, then, to side with the police powers of a given state government over against the unenumerated rights and reserved powers of the people of that state to which they are entitled under the Constitution is to contravene the principles of republican morality that are embedded in Article IV, Section 4 of the Constitution.

The U.S. Supreme Court has no standing in issues that pertain to specifying the nature of the unenumerated rights and reserved powers that belong to the states or the people. That Court only has standing in issues that pertain to whether, or not, the specific powers and rights that have been assigned by the Constitution to the federal government are being undermined, or impinged upon, in some fashion, and even here representatives of the federal government must tread very carefully less they go about the business of governance in a manner in which they become judges in their own cause ... a cardinal sin in republican morality.

A process, or dynamic, or system, or framework is needed to mediate such issues. Unfortunately, such a process, dynamic, system, or framework has never been established in over 236 years of Constitutional history.

In Tolkien's story concerning the Hobbits and the ensuing trilogy of tales, a ring that was fashioned through occult mans grants the wearer, a superficial and peripheral capacity for invisibility. More importantly, one of the ring's essential power was the capacity to not only control all other rings of power, but, as well, to be able to dominate the wills of the users of those other rings.

The ring could, on occasion, expand in size and, thereby, escape from the individual wearing it. The ring's capacity to be able to accomplish such escapes was, perhaps, an indication that the way of power is dedicated to itself and is beholden to no living being, whether that living being is a Hobbit, wizard, or otherwise.

According to the historical narrative which is created by Tolkien, Déagol, a Stoor hobbit, finds the occult ring during a fishing trip. Sméagol, a friend and relative who had accompanied Déagol on the trip, is drawn to the ring's power and desires it, and as such, the first sign of corruption is that the individual is drawn to the ring in a manner that suggests the sort of frequency following behavior that was discussed during an earlier chapter of the present book.

Sméagol asks Déagol to give the ring as a birthday gift, but this "request" is denied. Evidence that the request was not a request soon surfaces when Sméagol strangles his alleged friend in order to possess the ring.

Sméagol stares into the abyss of his monstrous, ring-inspired deed, and becomes transformed. The ring quickly corrupts his body, mind, and spirit, and in the process turns Sméagol into the monstrous Gollum who comes to see power as being "precious."

Executive, judicial, and legislative office are like Tolkien's ring of power. It is a potentially corrupting set of influences that induce people to become monstrous because their only desire is to hold on to the ring because of the power they acquire via the ring to control others and whatever lesser rings of power those individuals might wear.

The ring's grip on the Gollum – his Precious -- is such that he is never prepared to give it up willingly. Such tends to be the way of public office as well in which people are reluctant to let go of the ring of power which seduces those who forget the principles of republican morality which are supposed to govern how elected and appointed offices are to be used.

In Tolkien's tale, the occult ring of power can only be destroyed by being thrown into the volcanic fires of Mount Doom (where it originally had been forged), and, this is the task which Frodo Baggins sets out to accomplish. Similarly, the occult potential of power associated with public office can only be destroyed by throwing that potential back into the volcanic cauldron in which it was forged – namely, the Constitutional process – so that the ring of power's seductive, occult nature can be melted away by the fiery, rigorous dynamics inherent in the moral principles of republicanism.

Most jurists – whether working at the federal level or the state level – are not prepared to relinquish their hold on the ring of power which has lured them into appointed or elected office. They believe that they have the right – by virtue of the ring of power they wear – to consistently deny and decry the unenumerated rights and reserved powers of "We the people," and because of the corrupting influence of the ring of power which they wear, they believe they have the right to ignore the guarantee of republican government which has been given in Article IV, section 4 of the Constitution, and an important dimension of such a guarantee is to ensure that no one – on either the federal or state level – denies and decries the unenumerated rights and reserved powers that have been assigned to the people under the Ninth and Tenth amendments.

Under the provisions of the Constitution, the Judicial Branch of the federal government has the authority to set up inferior courts, and it has the capacity to establish grand juries that have the authority to subpoena witnesses, investigate issues, and render decisions concerning how the government should move forward in certain matters. However, since the federal government has no actual constitutional standing with respect to the determination of any of the specifics entailed by the unenumerated rights and reserved powers of the people under the Ninth and Tenth amendments because to do so would be a potential form of denying and decrying those very unenumerated rights and reserved powers, the inferior court that needs to be set up to handle disputes between the states and the people with respect to such rights and powers should be a process of mediation involving a grand-jury like capacity to: Subpoena witnesses, investigate, and provide directives to the federal land state governments as to how to proceed in any given conflict, but the members of the grand jury-like body in such an inferior court of mediation would be made up of members of the public who – as with any jury selection process – would be vetted to ensure that they will be able to abide by the moral principles of republicanism that are to govern such deliberations.

The members of such a meditational form of grand jury would not be permanent but, rather, as is the case with any grand jury, would only be appointed for a limited period of time. Moreover, the vetting process through which the foregoing grand jury-like members are chosen would permit the federal government, the state, and the people so many opportunities – both with and without cause – to reject potential jury members in order to assemble a group of people who might best be able to give expression to the principles of republicanism during their tenure as members of such a grand –jury like mediation group.

The decisions of any given mediation group need not be tied to previous precedents that were generated by previous groups. Moreover, each group gets to set their own set of operating procedures for tackling whatever conflicts they are seeking to mediate.

There should be one such group for every state in the union. Thus, this grand jury-like mediation process should be decentralized, not centralized, which means that the decisions reached by one grand jury-like mediation group need not reflect the decisions that are arrived at by such groups in other states.

The commonality which binds all the foregoing grand jury-like mediation groups is that they operate in accordance with the moral principles of republicanism. The specific decisions reached by such groups are not reviewable by the Supreme Court – because to do so would risk being a form of denying or decrying unenumerated rights and reserved powers -- but the process through which such decisions were reached are reviewable under Article IV, section 4, and if found wanting, can be rejected by the Supreme Court.

However, such judgments of the Supreme Court would, themselves, be reviewable by an oversight committee to ensure that the members of the Supreme Court had conducted themselves in accordance with the requirements of the moral principles of republicanism. The members of the oversight committee would be selected through the same kind of vetting process that governed the selection of the grand jury-like mediation groups, and like the grand jury-like mediation groups, its members would be drawn from the federal government, state governments, and the people in such a way that the people had majority control of the process.

The foregoing sort of arrangement is not about instituting democratic principles of majority rules. Rather, the intent is to ensure that the people have a major say in how their unenumerated rights and reserved powers are delineated, and, as such, is intended as a procedural rule which serves the moral principles inherent in a republican form of governance rather than succumbing to the arbitrariness that tends to bedevil democratic processes of voting.

While the majority of the members of the foregoing grand jury-like mediation groups should be drawn from the people, there also should be representatives from both the federal government and the state government who are members of such groups, and just as members of the public need to be vetted to ensure that they are willing to abide by the moral principles of republicanism, so too, the representatives from the federal and state governments need to be vetted and, therefore, representatives of the federal government, state government, and the people should have a set number of opportunities – both for cause and without cause – to reject any given candidate for the group.

Whatever decisions are reached by such groups which are not rejected by the Supreme Court under Article IV, section 4, will stand throughout the period of time for which the grand jury-like mediation group has been convened. Those decisions will continue to stand until such time as some subsequent grand jury-like mediation group changes direction in conjunction with whatever sort of conflict is being mediated by a subsequent group of mediators.

The foregoing groups are not intended to operate through an adversarial process. They are intended to be co-operative, investigatory, problem solving or resolving bodies that cannot be controlled by the states, the federal government, or individuals with vested interests who are incapable of operating within a context that is governed by moral principles of republicanism.

There is no continuity-of-government issue entailed by any of the foregoing. There is only a continuity-of-constitution issue in which moral principles of republicanism are to be preserved which are guaranteed by Article IV, section 4 of the Constitution.

Executive orders can only be issued for the purpose of improving the administration of the executive branch so that it operates in greater conformity to the requirements of republican government. Consequently, any other kind of executive order that is intended to serve as a form of legislation that is to be imposed on the general populace not only inappropriately usurps the role of the legislature but, as well, interferes with, undermines, and, therefore, inherently denies and decries the unenumerated rights and reserved powers of the people.

There can be no institution of martial law that abrogates the provisions of the Constitution because to do so nullifies the guarantee of a republican form of government that has been made to the states. There can never be a form of martial law which is established or led by the police, the military, the National Guard, FEMA, or any other agency of either the federal or state governments because to do so would be to undermine the unenumerated rights and reserved powers of the people under the Ninth and Tenth amendments.

There is no Constitutional provision for suspending the Constitution. Martial law – to whatever extent it can be said to exist in any given instance -- is entirely directed toward preserving the continuity of the constitution rather than being directed toward the continuity of any given form of governance by means of policing, military operations, the deployment of the National Guard, or the policies of FEMA, or emergency declarations of Health and Human Services.

Based on what has been said up to this point, the continuity of the Constitution is most likely to be best served when the federal government operates in accordance with the moral principles of republicanism that are guaranteed in Article IV, section 4 and, in addition, when those operations are supported by means of the sort of decentralized forums of republican (in the moral sense) grand jury-like mediation group dynamics that have been outlined during the foregoing discussion.

The FDA, the CDC, the National Institute of Health and its subsidiary agencies, the Department of Defense, as well as the Department of Health and Human Services (along with other departments of the Executive Branch), the nineteen intelligence agencies which exist within the federal government, the NSA, the FBI, the Judicial Branch (especially in the guise of the Supreme Court) and the Legislative Branch have all been responsible, on numerous occasions, for contravening the guarantee clause of Article IV, Section 4 of the Constitution, as well as running rough shot over the unenumerated rights and reserved powers that have been delegated to "We the people" under the Ninth and Tenth amendments respectively. Evidence in support of the foregoing claim has been put forward in the present chapter, along with other chapters of this book, as well in a number of other books that are listed in the bibliography.

In a number of his books, Chalmers Johnson refers to, and critically explores, the SOFA contracts that the United States military forces on countries where it seeks to establish bases ... some 700-800 of them in the vast majority of countries in the world. SOFA is the acronym for the Status of Forces Agreement that governs the "relationship" between the U.S. Military and the countries with whom such contracts are negotiated.

The SOFA contracts ensure that the U.S. military has final say in virtually every aspect of those so-called "relationships." They are not agreements of reciprocity and co-operation, but, rather, they are occupational directives in which, for all intense purposes, the military considers itself to be above whatever local laws exist.

Irrespective of any environmental, social, political, legal, personal, or institutional crimes that might be committed by the U.S. military during the tenure of a given SOFA contract, the U.S. military is virtually untouchable or uncontrollable according to the provisions of those contracts. Consequently, SOFA contracts take away the sovereignty of the people upon whom they are imposed.

From the very beginning of America – going back to the Articles of Confederation, if not before – the national government has instituted an array of SOFA contracts with the people of the United States. As was, and continues to be, the case with respect to all of the SOFA contracts – sometimes known as treaties – that were established in conjunction with the indigenous peoples of America, the federal government has continually reneged on the guarantee clause of Article IV, section 4 of the Constitution, and, as well, continually denied and decried the unenumerated rights and reserved powers of the people of the United States (which includes all people of color – including whites), and in the process, the federal government has prevented many, if not most, Americans from being able to realize the purposes for which the union, supposedly, was formed – that is, to enable "We the people" to form a more perfect union through being enabled to establish specific ways of resolving problems involving justice, tranquility, defense, welfare, and liberty by means of the Ninth and Tenth amendments.

T.S. Eliot once wrote:

> "We shall not cease from exploration
> And the end of all our exploring
> Will be to arrive where we started
> And know the place for the first time.
> Through the unknown, remembered gate
> When the last of earth left to discover
> Is that which was the beginning;
> At the source of the longest river
> The voice of the hidden waterfall
> And the children in the apple-tree
> Not known, because not looked for
> But heard, half-heard, in the stillness
> Between two waves of the sea."

Life is, from beginning to end, a process of exploration. Where does one arrive at the end of that exploratory dynamic? ... an end to which I am very much closer than I ever was before?

One arrives at the realization of how much one does not know, and, for the very first time, one begins to understand the nature of the ignorance that characterizes so much of the existential point from which we began our quest.

Gates of knowledge to which individuals such as: Béchamp, Enderlein, Rife, Naessens, Pollack, Goffman, Begich, Emoto, Austin, Breggin, Lanka, Kaufman, Cowan, Carey, Firstenberg, Hillman, Mullis McMakin, Humphries, Bystrianyk, Tennant, Arp, Mullins, Popp, Shelldrake, Wood, and many others give expression. Yet, though such individuals might be remembered, they often are still unknown.

Their efforts – both individually and collectively -- allude to a mysterious source from which the long, winding river of life flows and which remains to be discovered by the remnants of lowly earth. Hidden realities of beauty that are engaged through the creative play of young, inquiring minds which are unknown due to a lack of curiosity on the part of so many concerning those journeys.

Yet, nonetheless, their voices resonate with frequencies both heard and unheard within two waves involving Being and manifestation. Between those two, we will know the nature of our ignorance for the very first time.

Bibliography

Addeo, Edmond G – The Woman Who Cured Cancer: The Story of Cancer Pioneer Virginia Livingston-Wheeler, MD. and the Discovery of the Cancer-Causing Microbe, Basic Health Publications, 2014.

Angell, Marcia Dr. – The Truth About the Drug Companies, Random House, 2004.

Arp, Halton – Seeing Red: Red Shifts, Cosmology, and Academic Science, Apeiron, 1997.

Austin, Veda -- The Secret Intelligence of Water, Lifestyle Entrepreneurs Press, 2020.

Ball, Philip – Beyond Weird: Why Everything You Thought You Knew About Quantum Mechanics is Different, Vintage, 2018.

Banks, Nancy Turner Dr.– Aids, Opium, Diamonds, and Empire: The Deadly Virus of International Greed, iUniverse, 2010.

Barry, John M. – The Great Influenza, Penguin Books, 2018.

Béchamp, Antoine – The Blood and Its Third Element, A Distant Mirror, 2017.

Becker, Robert O. and Marino, Andrew A. – Electromagnetism and Life, Cassandra Publishing, 2010.

Begich, Nick Dr. – Controlling The Human Mind, Earthpulse Press, 2006.

Bird, Christopher, The Persecution and Trial of Gaston Naessens, H.J. Kramer, Inc., 1991.

Blakeway, Jill – Energy Medicine: The Science and Mystery of Healing, Harper Wave, 2019.

Breggin, Peter R. Dr. -- Toxic Psychiatry, St. Martin's Press, 1991.

Breggin, Peter R. Dr. and Breggin, Ginger Ross – Talking Back to Prozac, Open Road Media, 1994.

Breggin, Peter R. Dr. – Medication Madness, St. Martin's Press, 2008.

Breggin, Peter R. Dr. and Breggin, Ginger Ross – COVID-19 and the Predators: We Are The Prey, Lake Edge Press, 2021.

Broadwater, Jeff – George Mason: The Forgotten Founder, The University of North Carolina Press, 2006.

Cancer Tutor – "How the Flexner Report Hijacked Natural Medicine", 2020

Carey, Nessa – The Epigenetics Revolution, Columbia University Press, 2012.

Carey, Nessa – Junk DNA, Columbia University Press, 2015

Carter, James P. Dr. – Racketeering in Medicine: The Suppression of Alternatives, Hampton Roads Publishing Company, 1992.

Close, Frank – The Infinity Puzzle: Quantum Field Theory and the Hunt for an Orderly Universe, Perseus Book Group, 2011.

Coleman, Vernon Dr. – Anyone Who Tells You Vaccines are Safe and Effective is Lying. Here's The Proof, 2014.

Cowan, Thomas Dr. – Human Heart Cosmic Heart, Chelsea Green Publishing, 2016.

Cowan, Thomas Dr. – Vaccines, Autoimmunity, and the Changing Nature of Childhood Illnesses, Chelsea Green Publishing, 2018.

Cowan, Thomas Dr. – Cancer and the New Biology of Water, Chelsea Green Publishing, 2019.

Cowan, Thomas Dr. and Morell, Sally Fallon – The Truth About Cotagion: Exploring Theories of How Disease Spread, Skyhorse, 2021.

Debaun, Daniel T. and Debaun, Ryan P. – Radiation Nation: The Fallout of Modern Technology, Archangel Ink, 2017.

Dettmer, Phillip – Immune: A Journey Into the Mysterious System That Keeps You Alive, Random House, 2021.

Emoto, Masaru (translated by David A. Thayne) – The Hidden Messages in Water, Simon and Schuster, 2001.

Engelbrecht, Torsten; Köhnlein, Claus; Bailey, Samantha; and Scoglio, Stefano – Virus Mania: How the Medical Industry Continually Invents Epidemics Making Billion-Dollar Profits at Our Expense, Books On Demand, 2021.

Firstenberg, Arthur – The Invisible Rainbow: A History of Electricity and Life, Chelsea Green Publishing, 2020.

Flexner, Abraham – Medical Education In The United States and Canada: A Report To The Carnegie Foundation For The Advancement of Teaching, The Carnegie Foundation, 1910 (Reproduced in 1972).

Gilder, Louisa – The Age of Entanglement: When Quantum Physics Was Reborn, Alfred A. Knopf, 2008.

Habakus, Louise Kuo and Holland, Mary (Editors) – Vaccine Epidemic, Skyhorse Publishing, 2012.

Hawthorne, Fran – Inside the FDA, John Wiley & Sons, 2005.

Hickey, Steve and Roberts, Hilary – Tarnished Gold: The Sickness of Evidence-based Medicine, 2011.

Hillman, Harold – 'New Considerations about the Structure of the Membrane of the Living Animal Cell,' Pub Med, 1994.

Hossenfelder, Sabine Dr. – Physicist Despairs Over Vacuum Energy, YouTube, 2022.

Hume, Ethel Douglas and Pearson, R.B. – Béchamp or Pasteur? A Lost Chapter in the History of Biology, Pasteur: Plagiarist, Imposter, A Distant Mirror, 2017.

Humphries, Suzanne Dr. -- Rising From the Dead, Independently Published, 2016.

Humphries, Suzanne Dr. and Bystrianyk, Roman – Dissolving Illusions: Disease, Vaccines, and the Forgotten History, Create Space, 2012.

Jacobson v. Massachusetts, 197 U.S. 11, Supreme Court of the United States, 1905.

Johnson, Chalmers – Nemesis: The Last Days of the American Republic, Henry Holt and Company, 2006.

Jureidini, Jon and McHenry, Leemon -- The Illusion of Evidence-Based Medicine, Wakefield Press, 2020.

Kennedy, Jr., Robert – The Real Anthony Fauci: Bill Gates, Big Pharma, and the Global War on Democracy and Public Health, Skyhorse Publishing, 2021.

Kiernan, Denise and D'Agnese, Joseph -- Signing Their Rights Away, Quirk Books, 2019.

Kolodny, Andrew Dr. – "How FDA Failures Contributed to the Opioid Crisis," AMA Journal of Ethics, August 2020.

Lanka, Stefan – "The Misconception Called Virus: Measles As an Example", WissenschaffPlus Magazine, 2020.

Lanka, Stefan – "Misinterpretation: Virus II", WissenschaffPlus Magazine, 2020.

Lester, Dawn and Parker, David – What Really Makes You Ill: Why Everything You Thought You Knew About Disease is Wrong, Independently Published, 2019.

Leung, Brent – House of Numbers, Knowledge Matters Productions, 2009.

Lipton, Bruce – The Biology of Belief, Hay House Inc, 2015.

Lynes, Barry – The Cancer Cure That Worked!, BioMed Publishing Group, 1987.

Macy, Beth – Dopesick: Dealers, Doctors, and the Drug Company that Addicted America, Back Bay Books, 2018.

Maier, Pauline – From Resistance to Revolution, Alfred Knopf, 1972.

Maier, Pauline – Ratification: The People Debate the Constitution, Simon and Schuster, 2010.

Kumar, Manjit – Quantum: Einstein, Bohr, and the Great Debate About the Nature of Reality, W.W. Norton, 2008.

Maready, Forest – Unvaccinated, Feels Like Fire, 2018.

Mariner, Wendy K., Annas, George J. and Glantz, Leonard H. – Jacobson v Massachusetts: It's Not Your Great-Great-Grandfather's Public Health Law, American Journal of Public Health, April 2005, Volume 95, No.4.

McBean Eleanor – The Poisoned Needle, 1957.

McMakin, Carolyn – The Resonance Effect, North Atlantic Books, 2017.

McTaggart, Lynne – The Field: The Quest for the Secret Force of the Universe, Harper Collins E-books, 2001.

Merola, Eric – Burzynski: Cancer Is Serious Business – Extended Edition, 2011.

Milham, Samuel – Dirty Electricity: Electrification and the Diseases of Civilization, Second Edition, iUniverse, 2012.

Moskowitz, Richard – Vaccines: A Reappraisal, Skyhorse Publishing, 2017.

Moss, Ralph – Doctored Results: The Suppression of Laetrile at Sloan-Kettering Institute for Cancer Research, Equinox Press, 2014.

Mullins, Eustace – Murder by Injection, The National Council for Medical Research, 1988.

Obey, David – Statement on Defense Appropriations Correction Bill: A Shameful End to a Shameful Congress, December 22, 2005.

Obukhanych, Tetana – Vaccine Illusion, 2012.

Pannier, Samantha T., African Americans, Women and the 1910 Flexner Report: Progressive Medical Reform and Professional Exclusion, Honors Thesis, University of Utah, 2016.

Penston, James -- Fiction and Fantasy in Medical Research, The London Press, 2003.

Pollack, Gerald – The Fourth Phase of Water, E-book Architects, 2013.

Ponesse, Julie – My Choice: The Ethical Case Against COVID-19 Vaccine Mandates, The Democracy Fund, 2021.

Poyet, Marie Ange and Lambert, Didier – Injecting Aluminum – Cinema Libre Studio, 2017.

Rohde, Wayne – The Vaccine Court, Skyhorse Publishing, 2014.

Shelldrake, Rupert – The Presence of the Past: Morphic Resonance and the Habits of Nature, Vintage Books, 1989.

Sjursen, Daniel – A True History of the United States, Steerforth Press, 2021.

Smolin, Lee – Three Roads to Quantum Gravity, Basic Books, 2011.

St. Fleur, Nicholas – "How One 1910 Report Curtailed Black Medical Education for Over a Century", Listen, 2023

Stone, Mike – Viroliegy: Exposing the Lies of Germ Theory and Virology Using Their Own Sources, Viroliegy.com, 2020-2023.

Taleb, Nassim Nicholas – Fooled by Randomness: The Hidden Role of Chance in Life and in the Markets, 2nd Edition, Random House, 2004.

Taleb, Nassim Nicholas, The Black Swan: The Impact of the Highly Improbable, Random House, 2010.

Tennant, Jerry – "Healing is Voltage: The Physics of Emotion" EU2017, YouTube.

Trebing, William Dr., Good-by Germ Theory, 6th Edition, Xlibris Corporation, 2006.

Weigel, Günter, A Comprehensive Guide to Sanum Therapy According to Prof. Enderlein, Semmelweis-Verlag, 2001.

Whitehouse, Anab – Beyond Democracy, Bilquees Press, 2018.

Whitehouse, Anab – Cosmological Frontiers, Bilquees Pr. 2018.

Whitehouse, Anab – Educational Horizons, Bilquees Press, 2018.

Whitehouse, Anab – Evolution Unredacted, Bilquees Press, 2018.

Whitehouse, Anab -- Framing 9/11, 3rd Ed., Bilquees Press, 2018.

Whitehouse, Anab – Observations Concerning My Encounter with COVID-19 (?), Bilquees Press, 2021.

Whitehouse, Anab – Quantum Queries, Bilquees Press, 2018.

Whitehouse, Anab – Quest for Sovereignty, Bilquees Press, 2018.

Whitehouse, Anab – Searching for Sovereignty, Bilquees Press, 2018.

Whitehouse, Anab – Sovereignty and the Constitution: An Unexpurgated Guided Tour, Bilquees Press, 2021.

Whitehouse, Anab – Sovereignty: A Play In Three Acts, Bilquees Press, 2018.

Whitehouse, Anab -- The People Amendments, Bilquees Press, 2018

Whitehouse, Anab – The Spirit of Religion, Bilquees Press, 2018.

Whitehouse, Anab – Tolstoy: A Very Human Journey, Bilquees Press, 2019.

Wilcox, Brett -- Jabbed, Skyhorse Publishing, 2018.

Wolf, Naomi – The Bodies of Others, All Seasons Press, 2022.

Wood, Gordon – The Radicalism of the American Revolution, Vintage Books, 1993.

Wood, Patrick – Technocracy: The Hard Road to World Order, Coherent Publishing, 2018.